Controversies in Diseases of the Aorta

Guest Editor

JOHN A. ELEFTERIADES, MD

CARDIOLOGY CLINICS

www.cardiology.theclinics.com

Consulting Editor

MICHAEL H. CRAWFORD, MD

May 2010 • Volume 28 • Number 2

SAUNDERS an imprint of ELSEVIER, Inc.

W.B. SAUNDERS COMPANY
A Division of Elsevier Inc.

1600 John F. Kennedy Blvd. • Suite 1800 • Philadelphia, PA 19103-2899

http://www.theclinics.com

CARDIOLOGY CLINICS Volume 28, Number 2
May 2010 ISSN 0733-8651, ISBN-13: 978-1-4377-1801-0

Editor: Barbara Cohen-Kligerman

Cardiology Clinics (ISSN 0733-8651) is published quarterly by Elsevier Inc., 360 Park Avenue South, New York, NY 10010-1710. Months of issue are February, May, August, and November. Business and Editorial Offices: 1600 John F. Kennedy Blvd., Ste. 1800, Philadelphia, PA 19103-2899. Customer Service Office: 3251 Riverport Lane, Maryland Heights, MO 63043. Periodicals postage paid at New York, NY and additional mailing offices. Subscription prices are $264.00 per year for US individuals, $416.00 per year for US institutions, $132.00 per year for US students and residents, $322.00 per year for Canadian individuals, $517.00 per year for Canadian institutions, $374.00 per year for international individuals, $517.00 per year for international institutions and $187.00 per year for Canadian and international students/residents. To receive student/resident rate, orders must be accompanied by name of affiliated institution, data of term, and the *signature* of program/residency coordinator on institution letterhead. Orders will be billed at individual rate until proof of status is received. Foreign air speed delivery is included in all *Clinics* subscription prices. All prices are subject to change without notice. **POSTMASTER:** Send address changes to *Cardiology Clinics*, Elsevier Health Sciences Division, Subscription Customer Service, 3251 Riverport Lane, Maryland Heights, MO 63043. **Customer Service: 1-800-654-2452 (U.S. and Canada); 314-447-8871 (outside U.S. and Canada). Fax: 314-447-8029. E-mail: journalscustomerservice-usa@elsevier.com (for print support); journalsonlinesupport-usa@elsevier.com (for online support).**

Reprints. For copies of 100 or more, of articles in this publication, please contact the Commercial Reprints Department, Elsevier Inc., 360 Park Avenue South, New York, NY 10010-1710. Tel.: 212-633-3812; Fax: 212-462-1935; E-mail: reprints@elsevier.com.

Cardiology Clinics is also published in Spanish by McGraw-Hill Interamericana Editores S. A., P.O. Box 5-237, 06500, Mexico D. F., Mexico; in Portuguese by Reichmann and Alfonso Editores Rio de Janeiro, Brazil; and in Greek by Dimitrios P. Lagos, 8 Pondon Street, GR115-28 Ilissia, Greece.

Cardiology Clinics is covered in *MEDLINE/PubMed (Index Medicus)*, *Excerpta Medica*, *The Cumulative Index to Nursing and Allied Health Literature* (CINAHL).

Printed and bound in the United Kingdom

Transferred to Digital Print 2011

Contributors

CONSULTING EDITOR

MICHAEL H. CRAWFORD, MD
Professor of Medicine, University of California,
San Francisco; Lucie Stern Chair in Cardiology
and Chief of Clinical Cardiology, University
of California, San Francisco Medical Center,
San Francisco, California

GUEST EDITOR

JOHN A. ELEFTERIADES, MD
William W.L. Glenn Professor and Chief,
Section of Cardiac Surgery, Department of
Surgery, Yale University School of Medicine,
Yale-New Haven Hospital, New Haven,
Connecticut

AUTHORS

MICHAEL ARCARESE, MD
Section of Cardiology, Yale University School
of Medicine, New Haven, Connecticut

JEAN BACHET, MD, FEBTCS
Senior Cardiovascular Consultant,
Department of Cardiovascular Surgery,
Zayed Military Hospital, Abu Dhabi,
United Arab Emirates

DONALD M. BOTTA JR, MD
Cardiac Surgery, Yale School of Medicine,
New Haven, Connecticut

ALICIA A. CARLSON, MS
Department of Internal Medicine,
University of Texas Health Science
Center at Houston, Houston, Texas

MICHAEL A. COADY, MD, MPH
Division of Cardiothoracic Surgery,
Alpert School of Medicine at Brown University,
Rhode Island Hospital, Providence,
Rhode Island

MICHAEL J. COLLINS, MD
Division of Cardiothoracic Surgery,
Department of Surgery, Yale-New Haven
Hospital, Yale University School of Medicine,
New Haven, Connecticut

JOSEPH S. COSELLI, MD
Professor and Cullen Foundation Endowed
Chair, Division of Cardiothoracic Surgery,
Michael E. DeBakey Department of Surgery,
Baylor College of Medicine; Chief, Section
of Adult Cardiac Surgery, The Texas Heart
Institute at St Luke's Episcopal Hospital,
Houston, Texas

PETER DANYI, MD, MPH, MBA
Cardiology Fellow, Virginia Commonwealth
University, Richmond, Virginia

ANNO DIEGELER, MD, PhD
Professor of Medicine and Director,
Department of Cardiovascular Surgery,
Cardiovascular Clinic, Herz- und
Gefaess-Klinik, Bad Neustadt, Germany

JOHN A. ELEFTERIADES, MD
William W.L. Glenn Professor and
Chief, Section of Cardiac Surgery,
Department of Surgery, Yale University
School of Medicine, Yale-New Haven
Hospital, New Haven, Connecticut

SAMMY ELMARIAH, MD
Fellow in Cardiovascular Disease,
The Marie-Josee and Henry R. Kravis
Center for Cardiovascular Health,
The Zena and Michael A. Wiener
Cardiovascular Institute, The Mount
Sinai School of Medicine, New York,
New York

ANTHONY L. ESTRERA, MD
Associate Professor, Department of
Cardiothoracic and Vascular Surgery,
University of Texas Medical School,
Memorial Hermann Heart and Vascular
Institute, Houston, Texas

EMILY A. FARKAS, MD
Assistant Professor of Surgery,
Cardiothoracic Surgery, Saint Louis
University School of Medicine, St Louis,
Missouri

ROSSELLA FATTORI, MD
Cardiovascular Radiology Unit, Cardiovascular
Department, University Hospital S. Orsola,
Bologna, Italy

MARINA FELDMAN, MD
Section of Cardiac Surgery, Yale University
School of Medicine, New Haven,
Connecticut

VALENTIN FUSTER, MD, PhD
Richard Gorlin, MD/Heart Research
Foundation, Professor of Medicine/Cardiology,
The Marie-Josee and Henry R. Kravis Center
for Cardiovascular Health, The Zena and
Michael A. Wiener Cardiovascular Institute,
The Mount Sinai School of Medicine, New
York, New York; President of Science,
Centro Nacional de Investigaciones
Cardiovasculares, Madrid, Spain

ARNAR GEIRSSON, MD
Assistant Professor of Surgery, Section of
Cardiac Surgery, Yale University School of
Medicine, New Haven, Connecticut

JAIME GERBER, MD, FACC
Section of Cardiology, Yale University School
of Medicine, New Haven, Cardiology
Associates of New Haven, Guilford,
Connecticut

M.J. JACOBS, MD, PhD
Professor of Surgery, Department of
Vascular Surgery, European Vascular Center
Aachen-Maastricht, University Hospital of the
Rheinisch-Westfälische Technische
Hochschule-University Aachen, Aachen,
Germany; Department of Surgery, University
Hospital Maastricht, Maastricht,
The Netherlands

ION S. JOVIN, MD, ScD
Assistant Professor of Medicine, Department
of Medicine, Virginia Commonwealth
University; Director, Cardiac Catheterization
Laboratories, McGuire VAMC, Richmond,
Virginia

T.A. KOEPPEL, MD
Associate Professor of Surgery, Department
of Vascular Surgery, European Vascular Center
Aachen-Maastricht, University Hospital of the
Rheinisch-Westfälische Technische Hochschule-
University Aachen, Aachen, Germany

AMIT KORACH, MD
Lecturer and Attending Surgeon, Department
of Cardiothoracic Surgery, Hadassah Medical
Center, Hebrew University, Ein-Kerem,
Jerusalem, Israel

MOSES LEBOVITS, BA, JD
Daniels, Fine, Israel, Schonbuch and Lebovits,
LLP, Los Angeles, California

ARISTIDIS LENOS, MD
Consultant, Department of Cardiovascular
Surgery, Cardiovascular Clinic, Herz- und
Gefaess-Klinik, Bad Neustadt, Germany

STEVE L. LIAO, MD
Instructor of Medicine, James J. Peters
Veteran Affairs Medical Center, Cardiovascular
Division, Department of Medicine, Bronx;
The Marie-Josee and Henry R. Kravis Center
for Cardiovascular Health, The Zena and
Michael A. Wiener Cardiovascular Institute,
The Mount Sinai School of Medicine,
New York, New York

W.H. MESS, MD, PhD
Professor of Neurophysiology, Department
of Clinical Neurophysiology, European
Vascular Center Aachen-Maastricht, University
Hospital Maastricht, Maastricht,
The Netherlands

DIANNA M. MILEWICZ, MD, PhD
Department of Internal Medicine,
University of Texas Health Science
Center at Houston, Houston, Texas

ATHENA POPPAS, MD
Division of Cardiology, Alpert School of
Medicine at Brown University, Rhode Island
Hospital, Providence, Rhode Island

ELLEN S. REGALADO, MS
Department of Internal Medicine,
University of Texas Health Science
Center at Houston, Houston, Texas

MICHAEL P. ROBICH, MD
Division of Cardiothoracic Surgery, Alpert
School of Medicine at Brown University, Rhode
Island Hospital, Providence, Rhode Island

HAZIM J. SAFI, MD
Professor and Chairman, Department of
Cardiothoracic and Vascular Surgery,
University of Texas Medical School, Memorial
Hermann Heart and Vascular Institute,
Houston, Texas

RAINER SCHMITT, MD, PhD
Professor of Medicine and Director,
Department of Radiology, Cardiovascular
Clinic, Herz- und Gefaess-Klinik, Bad
Neustadt, Germany

BRETT A. SEALOVE, MD
Fellow in Cardiovascular Disease,
The Marie-Josee and Henry R. Kravis
Center for Cardiovascular Health,
The Zena and Michael A. Wiener
Cardiovascular Institute, The Mount
Sinai School of Medicine, New York,
New York

FRANK W. SELLKE, MD
Division of Cardiothoracic Surgery, Alpert
School of Medicine at Brown University,
Rhode Island Hospital, Providence, Rhode
Island

OZ M. SHAPIRA, MD
Professor and Chief, Department of
Cardiothoracic Surgery, Hadassah Medical
Center, Hebrew University, Ein-Kerem,
Jerusalem, Israel

PHILIP H. STOCKWELL, MD
Division of Cardiology, Alpert School of
Medicine at Brown University, Rhode
Island Hospital, Providence, Rhode Island

PETER I. TSAI, MD
Assistant Professor, Division of Cardiothoracic
Surgery, Michael E. DeBakey Department of
Surgery, Baylor College of Medicine,
Houston, Texas

YUICHI UEDA, MD
Professor and Chairman, Division of Cardiac
Surgery, Department of Surgery, Nagoya
University Graduate School of Medicine,
Nagoya, Japan

PAUL P. URBANSKI, MD, PhD
Professor of Medicine, Senior Consultant,
Department of Cardiovascular Surgery,
Cardiovascular Clinic, Herz- und
Gefaess-Klinik, Bad Neustadt, Germany

SARINA VAN DER ZEE, MD
Fellow in Cardiovascular Disease,
The Marie-Josee and Henry R. Kravis
Center for Cardiovascular Health,
The Zena and Michael A. Wiener
Cardiovascular Institute, The Mount
Sinai School of Medicine, New York,
New York

ORI WALD, MD, PhD
Resident, Department of Cardiothoracic
Surgery, Hadassah Medical Center,
Hebrew University, Ein-Kerem, Jerusalem,
Israel

Contents

the prevention of catastrophic aortic complications. Aortic aneurysm is a worthy opponent on all fronts, and clinicians should continue actively to evaluate all potential diagnostic and therapeutic adjuncts with high levels of scientific scrutiny and rigor, so that the understanding and management of this disease process evolves in a complementary, rather than duplicative, manner. In the meantime, proteomics, genomics, and metabolomics continue to represent a muse of sorts in scientific circles, but clinicians are responsible for verifying the relevance and meaningful application of its postulates as they apply to individual patients within the context of efficient and effective global health care delivery.

Young athletes with unknown moderate enlargement of the ascending aorta are prone to aortic dissection during exertion. This dissection is linked to transient, severe hypertension during intense athletic effort. Promising young athletes are dying from this phenomenon. For this reason, the author suggests routine echocardiographic examination of young athletes.

The death of a young athlete is a particularly devastating moment in any society because these individuals represent our strengths and physical prowess as human beings. For this reason, the concept of preparticipation screening has captured attention. A routine screening program applied nonselectively to a particular population in the hopes of reducing morbidity and mortality from a disease must meet certain criteria to be useful. This article examines the scope of the problem from the perspective of acute aortic syndrome and aortic death; and reviews ways, if any, to systematically screen the population to help eradicate this wanton killer of gifted young athletes.

Discussion of the potential legal exposure of a health care provider for the failure to diagnose and treat a medical condition is premised on multiple considerations. The questions asked before taking legal action are if the case has merit, if the harm was caused by the act of omission or commission, if the damages were suffered as a result of that conduct, and the chances of success and the economic reality of pursuing the claim. The highly lethal nature of an acute aortic dissection makes it essential for the physician to recognize patients who are more likely to present atypically, and to aggressively pursue the diagnosis of acute aortic dissection. Whether the physician is ultimately liable for the poor outcome will depend not just on the breach of the standard of care, but whether it was a legal cause of the poor outcome. A poor outcome in and of itself does not create legal liability.

advanced aneurysmal disease, new insights into the pathogenesis of aortic aneurysm have resulted in an interest in targeting these pathways and reducing the rate of aneurysm expansion. The renin-angiotensin system is known to play a role in inflammation and aneurysm formation through nuclear factor-κB and expression of matrix degrading enzymes. Recent work also suggests that angiotensin receptor blockade may also disrupt transforming growth factor β1 signaling, resulting in a reduced rate of aneurysm expansion. These animal data, combined with recent retrospective trials showing markedly reduced rates of aortic root dilation in patients with Marfan syndrome treated with angiotensin receptor blockers, suggest a powerful role for angiotensin receptor blockers in the treatment of aortic aneurysms.

Thoracic aortic aneurysm is a major health problem with multiple causes and potentially devastating consequences. At present, no large randomized trial has shown that medical therapy can significantly slow or halt the progressive dilatation that eventually leads to dissection and rupture. Surgical therapy, on the other hand, is very effective at preventing these feared complications. A recent study suggested that angiotensin-receptor blocking agents slow the development of aneurysm dilatation in Marfan syndrome. The authors argue that because of the multiple possible causes of aneurysm formation and the potential downsides of therapy, the available evidence is not strong enough to suggest that all patients with thoracic aortic aneurysm should be treated with angiotensin-receptor blocking agents.

Bicuspid aortic valve (BAV) is the most frequently occurring congenital cardiac anomaly, affecting 1% to 2% of the population. BAV disease is increasingly recognized as a disease of the entire proximal aorta up to the level of the ligamentum arteriosum. The recent unfolding of the genetic and biologic background of the disease and the accumulating data regarding the natural history of BAV-associated aortic dilatation have accrued multiple levels of evidence strongly supporting early surgical intervention.

Bicuspid aortic valve (BAV)-associated aortopathy is a complex phenomenon, and the current lack of univocal interpretation of its causes and treatment can be ascribed to the multiform nature of its clinical presentation. Although there is strong bias in the literature favoring more aggressive treatment of ascending aortic dilatation in patients with BAV, evidence supporting this opinion is lacking. This review discusses some of the relevant issues relating to causation to facilitate a better analysis of the current recommendations used to guide surgical management, and concludes that treatment should be tailored by individual valvular pathology, clinical phenotype, and relevant comorbidities, using well-documented evidence-based clinical size criteria.

Acute aortic dissection remains the most common of all aortic catastrophes and is associated with significant morbidity and mortality. Urgent surgical intervention should be considered in all patients with acute type A aortic dissection. Immediate repair is performed for those who are hypotensive due to rupture and tamponade and who exhibit malperfusion of the coronary, cerebrovascular, visceral, or peripheral arterial systems. Selective delayed management with eventual repair may be assumed in patients with type A intramural hematoma and in those with coma (potential neurologic devastation), assuming that neurologic status improves. Urgent repair should not be precluded in patients presenting with active stroke, older age, and previous cardiac surgery. Ultimately, each patient should be individualized and the decision to intervene left to the surgeon.

This article considers the role for interval or permanent medical therapy for specific groups of acute type A aortic dissection patients. These include patients with extremely advanced age or prohibitive comorbidities, realized stroke, prior aortic valve replacement, and those who have already survived several days after onset of symptoms. This consideration represents a "back to the future" paradigm shift reminiscent of the earliest recommendations before surgical therapy was feasible or safe.

The number of supporters of complete arch replacement in the surgery of acute type A aortic dissection has been steadily increasing as a result of cerebral perfusion techniques that enable the extension of safe circulatory arrest time. However, there is no agreement in the surgical community on an optimal surgical approach, especially the distal extension of aortic repair. For a meta-analysis, dividing the patients into various subgroups according to the extent of dissection would be necessary. Until now, such classifications have not taken hold, although they are recommended. This article presents the authors' experiences during their uniform procedures in diagnostics and surgical strategy.

Acute type A dissection is one of the most lethal conditions that surgeons encounter. Advances in surgical techniques and perioperative management have resulted in acceptable short- and long-term outcomes. Traditionally, the surgical approach involves a conservative extent of aortic arch resection. Recently, some groups have advocated a more aggressive approach wherein the entire aortic arch is re-placed or an adjuvant descending aortic stent graft placed. This article reviews the literature pertaining to extent of distal aortic replacement in acute type A aortic dissection, arguing that a conservative approach is associated with more favorable outcome.

Paraplegia is one of the most severe complications of the repair of open descending thoracic aortic aneurysms and thoracoabdominal aortic aneurysms. To reduce these complications, a comprehensive strategy for spinal cord protection is manda-tory. Motor evoked potentials provide the surgeon with important information about spinal cord integrity throughout the operation. Neuroprotective measures include extracorporeal circulation, cerebrospinal fluid drainage, hypothermia, and selective segmental artery revascularization.

Thoracoabdominal aortic aneurysms (TAAAs) have a dismal natural history that fre-quently necessitates surgical repair, but such repairs sometimes result in paraplegia and paraparesis. To reduce the risk of these complications, intraoperative monitor-ing of spinal cord motor evoked potentials (MEPs) can be used to guide TAAA repair procedures and may potentially minimize spinal cord ischemia. However, the use of MEP monitoring techniques requires important changes to anesthetic management, entails certain risks, and has important contraindications.

The technical simplicity of retrograde cerebral perfusion (RCP) together with a highly favorable effect upon stroke rates and survival after aortic arch surgery justifies con-tinued clinical use of RCP in patients requiring hypothermic circulatory arrest (HCA), in particular patients with dissecting or atheromatous arch branches. In clinical prac-tice, using RCP can provide effective brain protection in HCA for about 40 to 60 min-utes, although there is a time limitation.

Straight deep hypothermic circulatory arrest (DHCA) is a technique available for brain preservation during deep hypothermic arrest in aortic arch replacement. In this article, the author discusses the practice of straight DHCA in his institute and the advantage of this technique over other brain preservation techniques.

Cardiology Clinics

Foreword

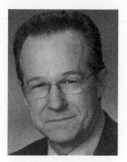

Michael H. Crawford, MD
Consulting Editor

In the 10 years since Dr Elefteriades guest edited a 1999 issue of *Cardiology Clinics* on diseases of the aorta, many new developments have occurred. Like all new diagnostics or treatments, many are controversial. Dr Elefteriades and the outstanding expert authors he has recruited to write this issue approached these new developments with debate-style articles: pro-con, for-against. This format makes for lively reading and helps clarify the issues with these new developments. For example, the genetics of certain aortic diseases are known: Should we do genetic testing? Are biomarkers for aortic disease useful? Type A (proximal ascending aorta tear) dissection management generates 2 debates: traditional surgery versus endovascular repair and extended arch resection or not. Should we intervene earlier in ascending aortic dilation associated with bicuspid valve? Does medical therapy work in aortic dissection, especially β-blockers and angiotensin receptor blockers? Does monitoring of motor evoked potentials make thoracoabdominal aneurysm resection safer? Should doctors be held liable for missing the diagnosis of aortic dissection? Should all athletes be screened for aortic disease? How do we protect the brain during aortic arch procedures?

Dr Elefteriades leads one of the best investigative units in the world for diseases of the aorta at Yale University. I was delighted that he agreed to guest edit again. It is a testament to his commitment to teaching others about this orphan organ. The debate format is an innovative way to present new information, and I am sure it will make the subject matter easier to remember. Aortic disease is a frequent source of physician litigation, so learning about aortic diseases and their recognition and management is especially important today.

Michael H. Crawford, MD
Division of Cardiology
Department of Medicine
University of California
San Francisco Medical Center
505 Parnassus Avenue, Box 0124
San Francisco, CA 94143-0124, USA

E-mail address:
crawfordm@medicine.ucsf.edu

doi:10.1016/j.ccl.2010.03.001

Preface

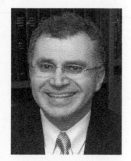

John A. Elefteriades, MD
Guest Editor

In the preface to an issue of *Cardiology Clinics* entitled *Diseases of the Aorta* published just over 10 years ago, I made two assertions:

1. That the aorta is "much more than a tube," with a complex physiology of its own and even an active participation with the heart in the symphony of mechanically propelling the blood, and
2. That the aorta is an "orphan" organ, with no nonsurgical specialty dedicated specifically to its study and treatment.

Now, a decade later, the first assertion is truer than ever. The complexity of the aorta, physiologically and hemodynamically, is becoming ever more impressive. The aorta certainly *is* much more than a tube for connecting the heart to the vital organs.

However, the aorta is no longer an orphan. In fact, with the advent of endovascular therapies, multiple specialties now claim the aorta as their own, including not only cardiac and vascular surgery (the traditional aortic specialists) but also interventional radiology and cardiology (General cardiologists have always had interest and expertise in the proximal aorta, which is visible on echocardiography, but less involvement with the more distal aorta.).

It is becoming increasingly more important to organize and disseminate accurate and up-to-date information on the pathology and treatment of the aorta.

In this issue, we take a written debate format. We identify several fundamental issues of controversy in aortic disease. We assign essayists to both PRO and CON points of view on each issue. These recognized authorities make their best arguments (Please keep in mind that we have specifically asked the authors to take a polarized point of view; this polarization on complex issues is an inherent feature of the debate format. In actual fact, the chosen topics are invariably complex issues, with shades of gray; the expressed viewpoints are taken in a polarized fashion, specifically for the debate format.).

By choosing a debate format, we aim to make this issue the written equivalent of lively oral debates, with the added benefit of readers having all the information and figures and references permanently available and organized in one written volume.

At the conclusion of each PRO and CON topic, the Guest Editor summarizes the key points presented by each author in bulleted sidebars to facilitate study and subsequent review. At the end of the bulleted summaries, a scale indicates where the weight of evidence appears to fall. This last feature is not intended as a critique of the essays themselves, which were polarized specifically at the Guest Editor's request, but rather as an assessment of how the well-presented data balance out.

We hope that both novice and expert aortic physicians, students, and paraprofessionals will find some information in this issue that is new and important in their work.

John A. Elefteriades, MD
Section of Cardiac Surgery
Department of Surgery
Yale University School of Medicine
Yale-New Haven Hospital
PO Box 208039
New Haven, CT 06520-8039, USA

E-mail address:
john.elefteriades@yale.edu

Cardiol Clin 28 (2010) xvii
doi:10.1016/j.ccl.2010.02.006

Genetic Testing in Aortic Aneurysm Disease: PRO

Dianna M. Milewicz, MD, PhD*, Alicia A. Carlson, MS,
Ellen S. Regalado, MS

KEYWORDS

- Familial thoracic aortic aneurysm and dissection
- Marfan syndrome • Loeys Dietz syndrome
- *FBN1* • *TGFBR1* • *TGFBR2* • *MYH11* • *ACTA2*

Aortic aneurysms and dissections are the major diseases affecting the aorta in the thoracic cavity. Thoracic aortic aneurysms tend to be asymptomatic and may not be diagnosed until a catastrophic event occurs, typically an acute aortic dissection. An aortic dissection occurs when the blood in the aortic lumen enters the wall through an intimal tear and dissects along the plane of the aortic wall, leading to the creation of a false lumen. Aortic dissections originate primarily in the ascending aorta just above the aortic valve (ascending or type A dissections), but can also occur in the descending thoracic aorta just distal to the origin of the left subclavian artery (descending or type B). Rupture and dissection of an aneurysm is associated with a high degree of morbidity, mortality, and medical expenditure despite continued improvements in surgical techniques. In contrast, prophylactic repair of an ascending aortic aneurysm before rupture or dissection is associated with very low morbidity and mortality, leading to the current recommendation to repair the ascending aorta when a stable aortic aneurysm enlarges to a diameter of 5.0 to 5.5 cm.[1] Therefore, prevention of untimely death from aortic dissections depends on the early identification of individuals predisposed to thoracic aortic disease, careful monitoring of the diameter of the ascending aorta, and timely surgical repair of diseased segments.[2,3] Monitoring of the ascending aorta involves imaging of the entire ascending aorta and obtaining standard measurements at the level of the annulus, sinuses of Valsalva, supraaortic ridge or sinotubular junction, and the proximal ascending aorta. If the ascending aorta is not well visualized by echocardiogram, further imaging by CT or MRI scan is recommended.

It has been recognized for many years that there are genetic syndromes that predispose individuals to thoracic aortic aneurysms leading to type A dissections (referred to as TAAD). Most prominent among these syndromes is Marfan syndrome (MFS), where virtually every affected patient will have ascending aortic disease during their lifetime. More recently, Loeys-Dietz syndrome (LDS) has been described, with a similar high risk for thoracic aortic disease. The majority of patients with TAAD do not have a characterized genetic syndrome. Despite the lack of syndromic features, many of these patients do have an inherited predisposition for TAAD, and current data indicate that there are many genes that predispose individuals to nonsyndromic inherited TAAD. Four genes have been identified for familial TAAD, and these genes account for approximately 20% of familial inheritance of TAAD.

Supported by grants from the NIH, (P50HL083794-01 and RO1 HL62594), and the Vivian Smith Foundation. D.M.M. is a Doris Duke Distinguished Clinical Scientist.
Department of Internal Medicine, University of Texas Health Science Center at Houston, 6431 Fannin Street MSB 6.100, Houston, TX 77030, USA
* Corresponding author.
E-mail address: Dianna.m.milewicz@uth.tmc.edu

Cardiol Clin 28 (2010) 191–197
doi:10.1016/j.ccl.2010.01.017

MARFAN SYNDROME AND LOEYS-DIETZ SYNDROME

Marfan syndrome is an autosomal dominant syndrome with pleiotropic manifestations that involve the skeletal (pectus deformities, kyphoscoliosis, dolichostenomelia, arachnodactyly, and other features), ocular (ectopia lentis), pulmonary (apical lung blebs and pneumothoraxes), integumentary (striae), and cardiovascular system (TAAD and valvular insufficiencies). Progressive dilation of the aortic root, culminating in aortic dissection, is the major cause of morbidity and mortality in MFS patients.[2,4,5] The management of aortic disease in MFS patients is well established.[1]

MFS is the result of heterozygous mutations in the fibrillin-1 gene (FBN1) on chromosome 15. Fibrillin-1 is a large 35-kDa cysteine-rich glycoprotein that is a major component of extracellular matrix structures called microfibrils, which are found at the periphery of elastic fibers. Over 600 FBN1 mutations have been identified in patients with MFS (http://www.umd.be:2030/), and the majority of the mutations are missense mutations predicted to disrupt just one amino acid out of the 2871 amino acids that comprise fibrillin-1. In addition to MFS, FBN1 mutations may also result in a range of isolated clinical manifestations, including isolated ectopia lentis, skeletal features of MFS, and familial TAAD.[6–10]

The current diagnostic criteria, termed the Ghent criteria, rely primarily on the cardiovascular, ocular, and skeletal features for the diagnosis of MFS. Genetic testing, involving direct sequencing of FBN1 and the identification of a mutation in the gene, is problematic for a number of reasons: (1) FBN1 is a large gene and sequencing of all 65 exons is an expensive undertaking; (2) not all rare genetic variants cause MFS but may instead cause isolated ectopia lentis, skeletal features of MFS, familial TAAD, or no phenotype; (3) sequencing is not required to make a diagnosis when major features are present in the cardiac, ocular, and skeletal systems, such as the case of classic MFS; and (4) FBN1 sequencing only identifies mutations in 72%–91% of patients with classic MFS, suggesting that some mutations in the gene are "cryptic."[11,12] Therefore, direct sequencing of FBN1 is currently not extensively used to confirm the diagnosis of MFS in an individual with classic features of MFS. However, identifying the causative FBN1 mutation leading to MFS in an individual can be useful to determine if other relatives are affected and for prenatal diagnosis.

More than a decade ago, genetic heterogeneity for MFS was proposed and a second locus for MFS, termed the MFS2 locus, was mapped to chromosome 3p24-25.[13,14] This locus was identified using a single large family, and whether or not the affected family members met the diagnostic criteria for MFS was controversial.[15] A heterozygous mutation in the gene encoding the transforming growth factor-β type 2 receptor (TGFBR2) was identified as the cause of disease in this family. TGFBR2 missense mutations in the intracellular domain of the receptor were identified in three additional families with MFS.

Mutations in both TGFBR2 and the transforming growth factor-β type 1 receptor gene (TGFBR1) have also been reported in a syndrome characterized by TAAD, arterial aneurysms and tortuosity, craniosynostosis, hypertelorism, cleft palate, bifid uvula, congenital heart disease, thin and translucent skin, and skeletal features of MFS, termed Loeys-Dietz aortic aneurysm syndrome or LDS. LDS patients experience rupture or dissection of the aorta at young ages, and dissections have occurred with aortic diameters less than 4.5 cm.[16] In addition, people with LDS have diffuse vascular disease, characterized by aneurysms and dissections of other arteries, including the cerebrovascular arteries and arteries branching off of the aorta. Almost all mutations identified are heterozygous missense mutations disrupting the intracellular kinase domain of these receptors, a domain critical for receptor cellular signaling with ligand binding.

In patients with TAAD and syndromic features of LDS, identification of a TGFBR1 or TGFBR2 mutation confirms the diagnosis of LDS. Therefore, sequencing of these genes plays a role in the diagnosis of LDS, and genetic testing should be considered in any patient with thoracic aortic disease and features of LDS. Currently, it is not known how often patients with aortic disease and features of LDS test negative for mutations in these genes.

Most current data support the conclusion that MFS patients with lens dislocation have underlying FBN1 mutation. In patients who meet the diagnostic criteria for MFS but have features of LDS, genetic testing for a TGFBR1 or TGFBR2 mutation should be considered. Any MFS patient with a TGFBR1 or TGFBR2 mutation needs to be examined for features of LDS and clinically managed based on the underlying TGFBR1 or TGFBR2 mutation.

Confirmation of a TGFBR1 or TGFBR2 mutation changes the clinical management of the patient. Individuals harboring mutations in these genes have a propensity for rupture and dissection of the aorta at a younger age and smaller aortic diameters, and therefore aggressive management of ascending aortic aneurysms is currently recommended.[16–18] In addition, these patients should be monitored for aneurysms and dissections of other arteries. LDS patients do well with vascular surgical repair and do not have the friable and thin tissues observed in vascular Ehlers-Danlos syndrome (EDS) patients. In addition, there are other management recommendations for complications involving systems other than the vascular system in LDS patients.[16,19]

FAMILIAL THORACIC AORTIC ANEURYSMS AND DISSECTIONS

Although it has been clearly established for the past 40 years that patients with MFS are predisposed to TAAD, the genetic contribution to nonsyndromic TAAD was only defined in the past 10 years. The first family with multiple members with TAAD in whom MFS and vascular EDS was excluded was reported in 1989.[20] The contribution of genetic factors to the cause of nonsyndromic TAAD was more recently established with familial aggregation studies demonstrating that up to 19% of TAAD patients had a first degree relative with TAAD.[21,22] These studies also showed that individuals with a family history presented with disease at a significantly younger age than those with sporadic aneurysms.[22,23]

Characterization of families with multiple members with TAAD indicated that the majority demonstrated an autosomal dominant mode of inheritance with decreased penetrance and variable expression with respect to the age of onset of the aortic disease, the location of the aneurysm, and the degree of aortic dilatation before dissection.[23,24] Imaging of the aorta of at risk family members to identify asymptomatic aneurysms proved to be a critical aspect to identifying the mode of inheritance of TAAD. An age-related onset of aortic disease was evident in almost all families, with more individuals presenting with aortic disease as they age. In addition, there is a marked variability in the age of onset of the aortic disease within families that is more pronounced than the variability observed in families with MFS. Another factor, complicating identification of the mode of inheritance, is that family members can inherit the disease gene but not have aortic manifestations even at advanced ages. This incomplete penetrance of the phenotype in family members inheriting the genetic defect occurs primarily in women.

There is variability in the clinical features in families with multiple members with TAAD. In a small subset of TAAD families, family members experience aortic dissection with no aortic dilatation.

There is also variability of the cardiovascular diseases segregating in the families with the TAAD. The association of bicuspid aortic valve (BAV) and TAAD as a familial condition has been frequently reported in the literature, leading to the suggestion that BAV and TAAD are manifestations of a single gene defect.[25–28] Family members can have BAV, TAAD, or both cardiovascular conditions. Similar to other TAAD families, the inheritance of the predisposition is autosomal dominant with incomplete penetrance.[28] In addition, patent ductus arteriosus can segregate with TAAD in families.[29,30]

The region of the initial ascending aortic enlargement is another variable observed in TAAD families. Whereas some families manifest ascending aneurysms involving the sinuses of Valsalva, similar to patients with MFS and LDS, other families present with aneurysms that spare the sinuses of Valsalva and, instead, occur in the ascending aorta and often extend into the arch of the aorta. Aneurysms involving the ascending aorta are typically associated with long-standing hypertension. The ascending aorta represents the most common location for thoracic aortic aneurysms.

Therefore, TAAD is frequently inherited in families. In addition to the TAAD segregating in these families, family members can have aneurysms and dissection of other arteries, including the abdominal aorta, cerebrovascular, or peripheral arteries. Relatives of patients with a family history of TAAD should undergo screening for aortic disease and any associated vascular disease, and referral to a geneticist should be considered for all families with multiple members with TAAD.

The clinical heterogeneity observed in the TAAD families predicted an underlying genetic heterogeneity for the disease. Four causative genes have been identified for familial TAAD. *TGFBR1* and *TGFBR2* mutations cause familial TAAD in the absence of features of LDS. In addition, the genes encoding smooth muscle-specific myosin heavy chain (*MYH11*) and smooth muscle-specific α-actin (*ACTA2*) also cause familial TAAD.[31–33]

TGFBR1 and *TGFBR2* Mutations in Familial Thoracic Aortic Aneurysms and Dissections

TGFBR2 mutations are responsible for less than 5% of familial TAAD.[31] Strikingly, *TGFBR2* mutations that alter arginine 460 (R460) in the intracellular domain of the receptor are common in these families, indicating a strong genotype-phenotype correlation.[31,34] On physical examination, these families do not have features of LDS (ie, hypertelorism, bifid uvula or cleft palate, or craniosynostosis). Arterial tortuosity and translucent skin are absent in the subset of family members that have been evaluated for these features. Although the vast majority of affected individuals in these families present with TAAD, some have subsequently developed descending aortic disease and aneurysms of other arteries, including cerebral, carotid, and popliteal aneurysms. Three individuals with the TGFBR2 R460 mutation have had dissections before reaching an aortic diameter of 5.0 cm. The smallest documented aortic diameter was 4.2 cm. Dissection of the thoracic aorta with minimal dilatation therefore supports the recommendation to prophylactically repair the aorta when an individual who carries the mutation reaches an aortic diameter of 4.2 cm.[31]

Multigenerational TAAD families with TGFBR1 mutations have also been described, and some affected members of these families do not have any features of LDS.[35] In fact, the first family reported with familial TAAD, in which MFS and vascular EDS were excluded, has a TGFBR1 mutation as the cause of the disease.[20] Therefore, TGFBR1 mutations can also lead to familial TAAD, but are a rare cause of the disease.

Therefore, TGFBR1 and TGFBR2 mutations lead to a spectrum of disease severity with LDS and early onset aortic disease (as young as 6 months of age) anchoring the spectrum at one end. At the other end of the severity spectrum are multigenerational families with TGFBR1 or TGFBR2 mutations who do not have features of LDS on physical examination. Some of these patients will have arterial tortuosity of the aorta or cerebrovascular arteries or minimal physical findings such as thin skin and bluish sclera. This fact raises the issue of whether patients at the mild end of the spectrum should be classified as having LDS or familial TAAD or just classified as having a TGFBR1 or TGFBR2 mutation.

The initial published descriptions of patients with LDS did not distinguish the features in patients with TGFBR1 mutations from features in patients with TGFBR2 mutations. Although these initial studies suggested the vascular disease management is the same whether the underlying mutation is in TGFBR1 or TGFBR2, recent studies have indicated that the vascular disease may differ based on the underlying gene mutated. There are numerous reports of aortic dissections at small aortic diameters in patients with TGFBR2 mutations and no reports of individuals with stable aneurysms greater than 5.0 cm in diameter. In contrast, there are TGFBR1 patients reported with stable aneurysms over 5.0 cm in diameter or who dissected at aortic diameters greater than

5.5 cm.[35] Further studies are needed to define the ideal clinical management of familial TAAD patients with TGFBR1 mutations.

Clearly, patients with TAAD and features of LDS, including minor features such as thin, translucent skin and atrophic scars, should be tested for a TGFBR1 or TGFBR2 mutation. The authors also recommend that TAAD families in which affected members go on to have aneurysms or dissections of other arteries, or have family members who present with dissections or aneurysms of other arteries, be tested for mutations in these genes. Even though these genes are responsible for only 1% to 4% of familial TAAD, the potentially lifesaving and powerful information provided when the underlying mutation is identified raises the possibility that all familial TAAD patients should be tested.

MUTATIONS IN GENES FOR THE SMOOTH MUSCLE-SPECIFIC ISOFORMS OF α-ACTIN (ACTA2) AND β-MYOSIN (MYH11)

The defective gene causing TAAD associated with patent ductus arteriosus (PDA) in a large French family was identified as MYH11, which encodes the smooth muscle cell (SMC)-specific myosin heavy chain, a major component of the contractile unit in SMCs.[36] Sequencing DNA from three unrelated families with TAAD associated with PDA identified MYH11 mutations in two of these families[37]; the remaining family had a TGFBR2 mutation as the cause of the TAAD and PDA. Subsequent analysis of 93 unrelated families with TAAD without PDA failed to identify any MYH11 mutations. The spectrum of MYH11 mutations identified for the familial TAAD-PDA phenotype is currently limited to four mutations: a small deletion, a splice site mutation, and two missense mutations. Therefore, MYH11 mutations are responsible for disease in the rare family with TAAD associated with PDA and are not a common cause of familial TAAD.

The authors identified that mutations in another SMC-specific contractile protein, α-actin (ACTA2), also cause familial TAAD.[33,38] Sequencing of 98 unrelated TAAD families revealed mutations in 14 families, indicating that ACTA2 mutations were responsible for approximately 14% of familial TAAD and the most common genetic defect identified for this condition to date.[33] Missense mutations are found throughout the protein, including recurrent mutations found in unrelated families, and predicted to produce a defective protein. Surprisingly, in the large family that was used to map the ACTA2 gene, the R149C mutation segregated completely with the skin rash livedo reticularis, indicating this clinical feature is a marker of the mutant gene. In contrast to TAAD characterized by enlargement of the ascending aorta, livedo reticularis is a vascular rash due to occlusion of the dermal vessels. Other features identified as associated in a subset of families with ACTA2 mutations included iris flocculi, PDA, and BAV. The penetrance of TAAD in family members heterozygous for ACTA2 mutations is low, with only half of ACTA2 mutation carriers presenting with aortic disease, a finding that differs from other identified loci and genes for familial TAAD. The majority of affected individuals presented with acute type A dissections or type B dissections, with 16 of 24 deaths in ACTA2 carriers occurring due to type A dissections. Only 2 of 13 individuals experienced type A dissections with a documented ascending aortic diameter less than 5.0 cm. Therefore, the risk for dissection at smaller aortic diameters differs from TGFBR2 mutations. In addition, aortic dissections occurred in three individuals under 20 years of age and two women died of dissections post partum. Finally, three boys had type B dissections complicated by rupture or aneurysm formation at the ages of 13, 16, and 21 years.

Further linkage analysis and association studies from 20 families with ACTA2 mutations uncovered a concurrent predisposition among mutation carriers for occlusive vascular diseases, including early-onset ischemic stroke and coronary artery disease (CAD).[39] Included in the premature strokes were cases of primary moyamoya disease, an early stroke syndrome characterized by bilateral occlusion of the distal internal carotid artery and collateral vessel formation, thereby establishing the first causal link between a genetic mutation and idiopathic moyamoya disease.[39] These occlusive lesions occur in young and middle-aged adults despite minimal or absent risk factors for vascular disease, such as hyperlipidemia, smoking, or diabetes. Thus, for ACTA2 mutations, affected patients are not only predisposed to thoracic aortic disease, but also premature CAD and stroke. Genotype–phenotype correlations have emerged from these initial family studies. Interestingly, the arginine 258 ACTA2 mutation is seen in families with TAAD and premature stroke, whereas other mutations predisposed to TAAD and CAD (alterations in arginine 149 or arginine 118).

The frequency of ACTA2 mutations in familial TAAD suggests that diagnostic sequencing of this gene should be considered in all familial TAAD patients. Genetic testing for MYH11 mutations should be considered in families with members with TAAD and PDA. It is not established which variants in MYH11 predispose to aortic disease and further studies may be necessary to determine if a MYH11 genetic variant is causative. If MYH11 is negative, testing for ACTA2 and TGFBR1 or TGFBR2 should also be considered in TAAD-PDA families.

Although the screening and management of thoracic aortic disease can follow the management for all familial TAAD, the extent and frequency of screening for CAD or cerebrovascular disease is not as clearly delineated. Screening for CAD is recommended in ACTA2 mutation carriers but data on which to base guidelines, such as the age at which screening should be initiated and how frequently this screening should happen, is still lacking. Screening for cerebrovascular disease is also recommended with the same unanswered questions. Carriers of ACTA2 mutations known to predispose to moyamoya disease should be considered for cerebrovascular imaging at a young age since this condition responds favorably to neurosurgical treatments. Further clinical studies are needed to determine the most effective management of the diffuse and diverse vascular diseases in patients with ACTA2 mutations.

SUMMARY

The authors have summarized the known genes causing a genetic predisposition to thoracic aortic disease and have provided information on the gene-specific phenotypes and gene-based recommendations for clinical management. Referral of patients with features of genetic syndromes or familial TAAD to a geneticist should be considered. In addition, a subset of patients with thoracic aortic disease need genetic testing. As the costs for diagnostic sequencing decreases and insurance companies more readily cover the costs, sequencing of the known genes should be done in all familial TAAD patients, which is already the approach at many centers. Identification of the causative gene is powerful information for the patient and family members, allowing for early identification of additional family members at risk for aortic disease and gene-based specific management. The GeneTests Web site (http://www.genetests.org) provides a directory of genetics specialists and a list of laboratories offering genetic testing for the genes that cause MFS, LDS, and familial TAAD. The four genes identified only account for 20% of familial TAAD, and therefore, there are further genes to be identified and general management guidelines are applied to these patients. At the same time, the genes identified to date have indicated that in the future, gene-specific management of the vascular diseases associated with specific mutations will provide the best care, a so-called personalized medicine approach to thoracic disease management based on the underlying mutation.

REFERENCES

1. Milewicz DM, Dietz HC, Miller DC. Treatment of aortic disease in patients with Marfan syndrome. Circulation 2005;111:e150–7.
2. Finkbohner R, Johnston D, Crawford ES, et al. Marfan syndrome. Long-term survival and complications after aortic aneurysm repair. Circulation 1995;91:728–33.
3. Silverman DI, Gray J, Roman MJ, et al. Family history of severe cardiovascular disease in Marfan syndrome is associated with increased aortic diameter and decreased survival. J Am Coll Cardiol 1995;26:1062–7.
4. Silverman DI, Burton KJ, Gray J, et al. Life expectancy in the Marfan syndrome. Am J Cardiol 1995;75:157–60.
5. van Karnebeek CD, Naeff MS, Mulder BJ, et al. Natural history of cardiovascular manifestations in Marfan syndrome. Arch Dis Child 2001;84:129–37.
6. Milewicz DM, Grossfield J, Cao SN, et al. A mutation in FBN1 disrupts profibrillin processing and results in isolated skeletal features of the Marfan syndrome. J Clin Invest 1995;95:2373–8.
7. Milewicz DM, Michael K, Fisher N, et al. Fibrillin-1 FBN1 mutations in patients with thoracic aortic aneurysms. Circulation 1996;94:2708–11.
8. Francke U, Berg MA, Tynan K, et al. A Gly1127Ser mutation in an EGF-like domain of the fibrillin-1 gene is a risk factor for ascending aortic-aneurysm and dissection. Am J Hum Genet 1995;56:1287–96.
9. Ades LC, Sreetharan D, Onikul E, et al. Segregation of a novel FBN1 gene mutation, G1796E, with kyphoscoliosis and radiographic evidence of vertebral dysplasia in three generations. Am J Med Genet 2002;109:261–70.
10. Katzke S, Booms P, Tiecke F, et al. TGGE screening of the entire FBN1 coding sequence in 126 individuals with marfan syndrome and related fibrillinopathies. Hum Mutat 2002;20:197–208.
11. Stheneur C, Collod-Beroud G, Faivre L, et al. Identification of the minimal combination of clinical features in probands for efficient mutation detection in the FBN1 gene. Eur J Hum Genet 2009;17:1121–8.
12. Loeys B, De Backer J, Van Acker P, et al. Comprehensive molecular screening of the FBN1 gene favors locus homogeneity of classical Marfan syndrome. Hum Mutat 2004;24:140–6.
13. Boileau C, Jondeau G, Babron MC, et al. Autosomal dominant Marfan-like connective-tissue disorder with aortic dilation and skeletal anomalies not linked to the fibrillin genes. Am J Hum Genet 1993;53:46–54 [see comments].
14. Collod G, Babron MC, Jondeau G, et al. A second locus for Marfan syndrome maps to chromosome 3p24.2-p25. Nat Genet 1994;8:264–8 [see comments].
15. Dietz H, Francke U, Furthmayr H, et al. The question of heterogeneity in Marfan syndrome. Nat Genet 1995;9:228–31.
16. Loeys BL, Schwarze U, Holm T, et al. Aneurysm syndromes caused by mutations in the TGF-beta receptor. N Engl J Med 2006;355:788–98.
17. LeMaire SA, Pannu H, Tran-Fadulu V, et al. Severe aortic and arterial aneurysms associated with a TGFBR2 mutation. Nat Clin Pract Cardiovasc Med 2007;4:167–71.
18. Williams JA, Loeys BL, Nwakanma LU, et al. Early surgical experience with Loeys-Dietz: a new syndrome of aggressive thoracic aortic aneurysm disease. Ann Thorac Surg 2007;83:S757–63.
19. Loeys BL, Chen J, Neptune ER, et al. A syndrome of altered cardiovascular, craniofacial, neurocognitive and skeletal development caused by mutations in TGFBR1 or TGFBR2. Nat Genet 2005;37:275–81.
20. Nicod P, Bloor C, Godfrey M, et al. Familial aortic dissecting aneurysm. J Am Coll Cardiol 1989;13:811–9.
21. Biddinger A, Rocklin M, Coselli J, et al. Familial thoracic aortic dilatations and dissections: a case control study. J Vasc Surg 1997;25:506–11.
22. Coady MA, Davies RR, Roberts M, et al. Familial patterns of thoracic aortic aneurysms. Arch Surg 1999;134:361–7.
23. Albornoz G, Coady MA, Roberts M, et al. Familial thoracic aortic aneurysms and dissections—incidence, modes of inheritance, and phenotypic patterns. Ann Thorac Surg 2006;82:1400–5.
24. Milewicz DM, Chen H, Park ES, et al. Reduced penetrance and variable expressivity of familial thoracic aortic aneurysms/dissections. Am J Cardiol 1998;82:474–9.
25. McKusick VA. Association of congenital bicuspid aortic valve and erdheim's cystic medial necrosis. Lancet 1972;1:1026–7.
26. Glick BN, Roberts WC. Congenitally bicuspid aortic valve in multiple family members. Am J Cardiol 1994;73:400–4.
27. Clementi M, Notari L, Borghi A, et al. Familial congenital bicuspid aortic valve: a disorder of uncertain inheritance. Am J Med Genet 1996;62:336–8.
28. Loscalzo ML, Goh DL, Loeys B, et al. Familial thoracic aortic dilation and bicommissural aortic valve: a prospective analysis of natural history and inheritance. Am J Med Genet A 2007;143:1960–7.
29. Glancy DL, Wegmann M, Dhurandhar RW. Aortic dissection and patent ductus arteriosus in three generations. Am J Cardiol 2001;87:813–5, A9.

30. Khau Van KP, Wolf JE, Mathieu F, et al. Familial thoracic aortic aneurysm/dissection with patent ductus arteriosus: genetic arguments for a particular pathophysiological entity. Eur J Hum Genet 2004; 12:173–80.

31. Pannu H, Fadulu V, Chang J, et al. Mutations in transforming growth factor-beta receptor type II cause familial thoracic aortic aneurysms and dissections. Circulation 2005;112:513–20.

32. Zhu L, Vranckx R, Khau Van KP, et al. Mutations in myosin heavy chain 11 cause a syndrome associating thoracic aortic aneurysm/aortic dissection and patent ductus arteriosus. Nat Genet 2006;38:343–9.

33. Guo DC, Pannu H, Papke CL, et al. Mutations in smooth muscle alpha-actin (ACTA2) lead to thoracic aortic aneurysms and dissections. Nat Genet 2007;39:1488–93.

34. Law C, Bunyan D, Castle B, et al. Clinical features in a family with an R460H mutation in transforming growth factor beta receptor 2 gene. J Med Genet 2006;43:908–16.

35. Tran-Fadulu VT, Pannu H, Kim DH, et al. Analysis of multigenerational families with thoracic aortic aneurysms and dissections due to TGFBR1 or TGFBR2 mutations. J Med Genet 2009;46:607–13.

36. Van Kien PK, Mathieu F, Zhu L, et al. Mapping of familial thoracic aortic aneurysm/dissection with patent ductus arteriosus to 16p12.2-p13.13. Circulation 2005;112:200–6.

37. Pannu H, Tran-Fadulu V, Papke CL, et al. MYH11 mutations result in a distinct vascular pathology driven by insulin-like growth factor 1 and angiotensin II. Hum Mol Genet 2007;16:3453–62.

38. Fatigati V, Murphy RA. Actin and tropomyosin variants in smooth muscles. Dependence on tissue type. J Biol Chem 1984;259:14383–8.

39. Guo DC, Papke CL, Tran-Fadulu V, et al. Mutations in smooth muscle alpha-actin (ACTA2) cause coronary artery disease, stroke, and moyamoya disease, along with thoracic aortic disease. Am J Hum Genet 2009;84:617–27.

Genetic Testing in Aortic Aneurysm Disease: CON

John A. Elefteriades, MD

KEYWORDS

- Genetic testing • Aortic aneurysm disease
- Linkage analysis • Marfan syndrome

Surgery on the thoracic aorta is challenging, dangerous, intricate, complex, demanding, and tremendously rewarding; it provides years of life, safety, and confidence to patients. However, it is *plumbing*, albeit delicate and intricate plumbing.

I expect, and hope, that 50 or 100 years from now, physicians and surgeons will look back at our current techniques and find them barbaric and ineffectual compared with the treatments of the future. Perhaps they will look with similar disdain on our techniques as present day medical professionals do on the electroshock treatment for aneurysms of the nineteenth century, which is depicted in **Fig. 1**.[1]

Therefore, the level of aortic care should be raised from the plane of plumbing. The key to this likely lies in understanding the molecular genetics of this disease. Understanding aortic diseases at the level of individual base pair mutations will elevate aortic care to a totally different, higher, plane. Such understanding promises to open the door to diagnosis and treatment of aortic diseases with an accuracy and effectiveness that can only be imagined now.

Some years ago, our group and Dr Milewicz's group recognized a hereditary pattern in many families with thoracic aortic aneurysm (**Fig. 2**).[2,3]

Multiple mendelian patterns were described, predominantly autosomal dominant inheritance with reduced penetrance. Most recently, our group identified segregation into 2 diseases based on association between proband and family member aneurysm sites. Specifically, probands with ascending aneurysm had family members with ascending aneurysm. However, probands with descending aneurysm most commonly tended to have family members with abdominal aortic aneurysm (**Fig. 3**).[4] This lends credence to a conception of 2 different diseases separated at the ligamentum arteriosum. Ascending aortic aneurysms are 1 genetic entity—highly familial, not linked to smoking and other arteriosclerotic risk factors, and without calcification or thrombus. Descending or abdominal aortic aneurysms, conversely, are strongly related to arteriosclerotic risk factors, have calcified walls, and are full of thrombus (**Fig. 4**).

Multiple investigators have identified in detail, over the last several decades, the specific genetic defects that produce the Marfan syndrome, and now more than 600 individual mutations involving the fibrillin 1 gene have been identified. Recently, the Loeys-Dietz syndrome has been identified and its molecular genetics clarified. [5]

Section of Cardiac Surgery, Department of Surgery, Yale University School of Medicine, Yale-New Haven Hospital, PO Box 208039, New Haven, CT 06520-8039, USA
E-mail address: john.elefteriades@yale.edu

Cardiol Clin 28 (2010) 199–204
doi:10.1016/j.ccl.2010.02.002
0733-8651/10/$ – see front matter © 2010 Elsevier Inc. All rights reserved.

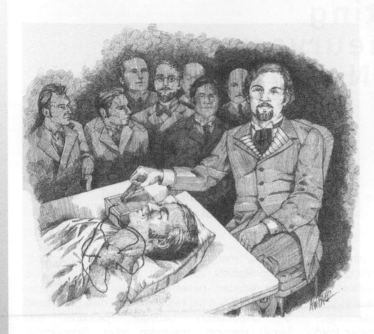

Fig. 1. Electroshock therapy for thoracic aortic aneurysm, circa 1850. Note trochar electrodes placed into the aneurysm and subsequently electrified. It was believed that a galvanic current would induce thrombosis and, thus, obliteration of thoracic and abdominal aortic aneurysms. (*Reprinted from* Elefteriades JA, editor. Acute aortic disease. New York: Informa Healthcare; 2007. p. ix; with permission.)

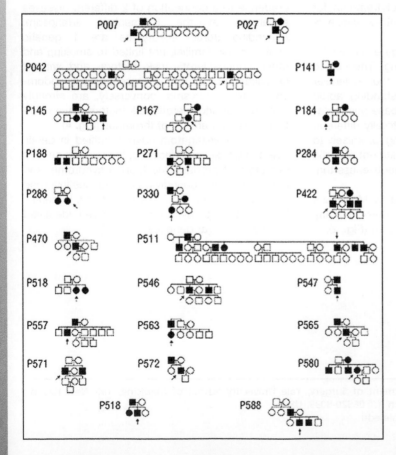

Fig. 2. Among the first 100 families constructed, 21 were positive for a family pattern. These 21 positive pedigrees are displayed here. Note a variety of genetic patterns, with autosomal dominance predominating. The 21% rate of positive family history was confirmed on later construction of 520 family pedigrees in patients with thoracic aortic aneurysm. (*Reprinted from* Coady MA, Davies RR, Roberts M, et al. Familial patterns of thoracic aortic aneurysms. Arch Surg 1999;134:364; with permission.)

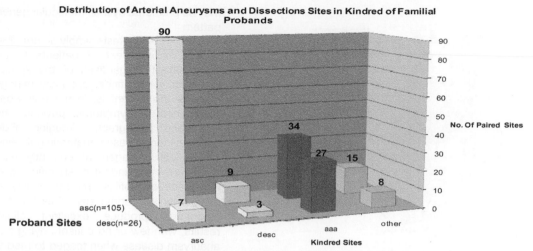

Distribution of Arterial Aneurysms and Dissections Sites in Kindred of Familial Probands

Fig. 3. Note that the location of the proband aneurysm influences the location of aneurysms in the family members. Note that probands with ascending aneurysms have family members with ascending aneurysm, whereas probands with descending thoracic aneurysm are more likely to have family members with abdominal aortic aneurysm. (*Reprinted from* Albornoz G, Coady MA, Roberts M, et al. Familial thoracic aortic aneurysms and dissections—incidence, modes of inheritance, and phenotypic patterns. Ann Thorac Surg 2006;82:1403; with permission.)

Dr Milewicz and colleagues[6–9] have gone on, via linkage analysis and genetic sequencing techniques, to identify specific mutations in patients with positive family histories but without Marfan disease or other major syndromes. These mutations include *TGFBR2* and *TGFBR1*, *MYH11*, and *ACTA2*. Dr Milewicz estimates that these genes together account for up to 20% of sporadic cases of thoracic aortic aneurysm and dissection.

Our own group, in collaboration with Applied Biosystems in California, has undertaken intensive efforts aimed toward identifying the specific genetic aberrations that underlie these family transmissions of aortic disease in the hope of developing a widely sensitive genetic screening test for thoracic aortic aneurysm. ***We studied expression patterns of 33,000 RNAs in the blood of patients with thoracic aortic aneurysm and compared them with control patients. It was found that a 41-SNP (single nucleotide polymorphism) panel could discriminate quite well between patients with and without aneurysm, from a blood test alone (**Fig. 5**).[10]

This "RNA Signature" is more than 80% accurate in determining from a blood test alone whether a patient harbors an aneurysm. It is hoped that this may eventuate in a screening test for family members or even for the general public. This level of accuracy far exceeds that of the prostate-specific antigen test used so commonly throughout the world to screen for prostate cancer.

In collaboration with colleagues at Celera Diagnostics in California, we have also performed genome-wide scans for DNA SNPs associated with thoracic aortic aneurysm and dissection. More than 500 Yale patients and their spousal controls were studied in this manner. Results are encouraging, with several SNPs strongly predicting the aneurysm disease. Replication studies from our European collection sites are currently underway.

As exciting and important as these genetic breakthroughs are, this section espouses the CON point of view vis-à-vis the usefulness of genetic testing in routine clinical practice. Specifically, the CON point of view is advocated for the following reasons:

- The diagnosis of Marfan syndrome remains a clinical endeavor, based on the recently modified Ghent criteria.[11] The diagnosis is usually made without difficulty by cardiologists or surgeons who deal commonly with aneurysm patients. Genetic sequencing is not required to make the diagnosis of Marfan syndrome, which depends on cardiac, ocular, and skeletal manifestations, as well as other systemic criteria. Also, some patients with identified Marfan mutations do not manifest clinical Marfan syndrome.[12] Moreover, some patients with clinical Marfan syndrome do not demonstrate any of the identified genetic mutations.[13,14]
- Loeys-Dietz is a rare syndrome in general aortic practice. For example, in 3000 patients with thoracic aortic aneurysm, even a single individual with the

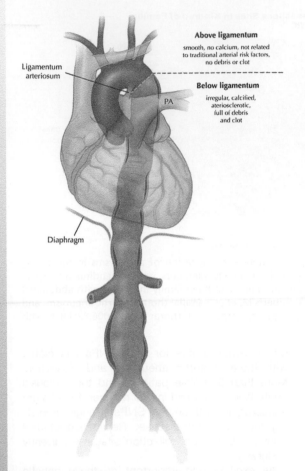

Above ligamentum
smooth, no calcium, not related
to traditional arterial risk factors,
no debris or clot

Ligamentum
arteriosum

Below ligamentum
irregular, calcified,
ateriosclerotic,
full of debris
and clot

PA

Diaphragm

Fig. 4. Note that thoracic aneurysm disease divides naturally into 2 patterns, separated at the ligamentum arteriosum. Above the ligamentum, the aorta is thin but not atherosclerotic; below the ligamentum, as with abdominal aortic aneurysms, heavy arteriosclerosis and calcification predominate. (*From* Elefteriades JA, Farkas E. Thoracic aortic aneurysm: clinically pertinent controversies and uncertainties. J Am Coll Cardiol 2010;55:841–57; with permission.)

characteristics of Loeys-Dietz has not been identified. So, genetic testing for this disorder is not a frequent clinical necessity.

- For the syndromes of TGFBR2 and TGFBR1, MYH11, and ACTA2, although some valuable clinical patterns have been identified (eg, rupture or dissection at relatively small sizes), the observed clinical patterns are based on a very small number of cases and an even smaller number of hard end points (rupture, dissection, death). So, the clinical observations can only be viewed as preliminary. The time will come when clinical behavior of patients' aortas

may be predicted by their molecular genetic pattern.

- Molecular genetic tests simply do not affect clinical management of patients to any great extent. Regardless of the specific molecular genetic findings, clinical management of the patient is, in the real world, determined by symptoms, physical findings, and radiographic imaging. Fairly good, evidence-based anatomic guidelines for clinical management currently exist, which are independent of specific molecular genetic profiles, relying mainly on symptoms and aortic size. These clinical algorithms produce excellent clinical results, with few or no patients dying from aneurysm disease when triaged to medical management (**Fig. 6**).[15]
- Molecular genetic testing for thoracic aortic aneurysm is not widely available for clinical purposes.
- Molecular genetic tests are complex (eg, >600 mutations in Marfan disease alone) and expensive.
- Molecular genetic tests do not affect clinical management of family members to any great extent. With few exceptions (eg, Marfan disease and the rare Loeys-Dietz syndrome), there is not enough confidence or experience with genetic patterns to exclude a family member from clinically requisite, regular radiographic imaging. As a key article indicates, "the key finding is that the prognosis of a patient depends on the clinical expression of the disease and not solely on the presence of a mutation in the TGRBR2 gene."[16]
- More genes need to be identified, as, at present, even with Dr Milewicz's pioneering work, known mutations explain only about 20% of cases of familial aortic aneurysm and dissection.

So, this section takes the CON point of view with a specific connotation: We do not contend that genetic testing is unimportant, for ours is a group of strong believers. Rather, we believe that routine genetic testing is not practical or clinically essential at the present time, that is, "*not yet.*" We eagerly look forward to a time in the near future when genetic testing is practical and clinically extremely valuable, helping us to exclude family members from regular radiographic screening and permitting our prediction of clinical course for specific aneurysm patients. This day is, we hope, right around the corner.

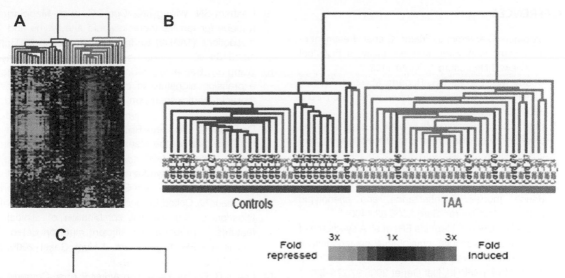

Fig. 5. The "RNA Signature" Test for thoracic aortic aneurysm. In the hierarchical cluster diagram on the left (*panel A*), each vertical line represents a patient and each horizontal line represents an RNA. In the grid (*panel A, C*), the lighter gray indicates underexpression and darker gray indicates overexpression. Note in the diagram on the left (*panel A*) how the overexpression and underexpression cluster, depending on phenotype. In the figure on the right (*panel B*), note that if all the lighter grays were together and all the darker grays were together, the test would have been 100% accurate. As it turns out, the overall accuracy was 82%. (*Reprinted from* Wang YY, Barbacioru CC, Shiffman D, et al. Gene expression signature in peripheral blood detects thoracic aortic aneurysm. PLoS ONE 2007;2(10):e1050; with permission.)

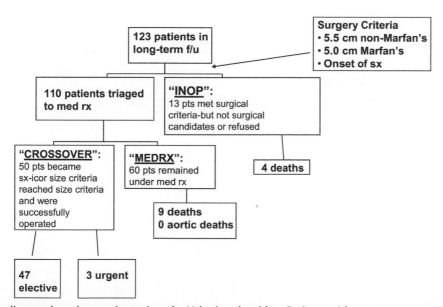

Fig. 6. Flow diagram based on patient triage by Yale size algorithm. Patients with aneurysms asymptomatic and less than 5 to 5.5 cm were treated medically. Note that no patient died on medical management. When patients were triaged to surgery and did not undergo such surgery (patient refusal, malignancy, overwhelming comorbidities), the aneurysm complication rates and death rates were high. Thus, the clinical algorithm worked well in the real world. (*From* Elefteriades JA, Farkas E. Thoracic aortic aneurysm: clinically pertinent controversies and uncertainties. J Am Coll Cardiol 2010;55:841–57; with permission.)

REFERENCES

1. Siddique K, Alvernia J, Fraser K, et al. Treatment of aneurysms with wires and electricity: a historical overview. J Neurosurg 2003;99:1102–7.
2. Coady MA, Davies RR, Roberts M, et al. Familial patterns of thoracic aortic aneurysms. Arch Surg 1999;134:361–7.
3. Biddinger A, Rocklin M, Coselli J, et al. Familial thoracic aortic dilatations and dissections: a case control study. J Vasc Surg 1997;25:506–11.
4. Albornoz G, Coady MA, Roberts M, et al. Familial thoracic aortic aneurysms and dissections—incidence, modes of inheritance, and phenotypic patterns. Ann Thorac Surg 2006;82:1400–5.
5. Loeys BL, Chen J, Neptune ER, et al. A syndrome of altered cardiovascular, craniofacial, neurocognitive, and skeletal development caused by mutations in TGFBR1 or TGFBR2. Nat Genet 2005;37:275–81.
6. Milewicz DM, Michael K, Fisher N, et al. Fibrillin-1 (FBN1) mutations in patients with thoracic aortic aneurysms. Circulation 1996;94:2708–11.
7. Putnam EA, Zhang H, Ramirez F, et al. Fibrillin-2 (FBN2) mutations result in the Marfan-like disorder, congenital contractural arachnodactyly. Nat Genet 1995;11:456–8.
8. Hasham SN, Lewin MR, Tran VT, et al. Nonsyndromic genetic predisposition to aortic dissection: A newly recognized, diagnosable, and preventable occurrence in families. Ann Emerg Med 2004;43:79–82.
9. Hasham SN, Willing MC, Guo DC, et al. Mapping a locus for familial thoracic aortic aneurysms and dissections (TAAD2) to 3p24-25. Circulation 2003; 107:3184–90.
10. Wang YY, Barbacioru CC, Shiffman D, et al. Gene expression signature in peripheral blood detects thoracic aortic aneurysm. PLoS One 2007;2(10): e1050.
11. De Paepe A, Devereux RB, Dietz HC. Revised diagnostic criteria for the Marfan syndrome. Am J Med Genet 1996;62:417–26.
12. Dean JC. Marfan syndrome: clinical diagnosis and management. Eur J Hum Genet 2007;15(7):724–33.
13. Stheneur C, Collod-Beroud G, Faivre L, et al. Identification of the minimal combination of clinical features in probands for efficient mutation detection in the FBN1 gene. Eur J Hum Genet 2009; 17:1121–8.
14. Loeys B, De Backer J, Van Acker P, et al. Comprehensive molecular screening of the FBN1 gene favors locus homogeneity of classical Marfan syndrome. Hum Mutat 2004;24:140–6.
15. Elefteriades JA, Farkas E. Thoracic aortic aneurysm: clinically pertinent controversies and uncertainties. J Am Coll Cardiol 2010;55:841–57.
16. Attias D, Stheneur C, Roy C, et al. Comparison of clinical presentations and outcomes between patients with TGFBR2 and FBN1 mutations in Marfan syndrome and related disorders. Circulation 2009; 120:2541–9.

Editorial Comment: Genetic Testing in Aortic Aneurysm Disease

John A. Elefteriades, MD

The article by Dr Dianna M. Milewicz's in this issue of *Cardiology Clinics* adds immensely to the understanding of aortic diseases. Dr John A. Elefteriades shows in his article that he is also a strong advocate for genetic investigations. They differ only in the assessment of whether routine testing is currently easy and advisable (**Table 1** and **Fig. 1**).

Table 1
Routine genetic screening in aneurysm patients

Pro: All Patients Should Be Screened (Milewicz)	Con: Most Patients Need Not Be Screened (Elefteriades)
Marfan genetics well elucidated.	Genetic testing is vitally important, but still predominantly a research tool.
Milewicz team has identified *TGFBR2, GFBR1, MYH11*, and *ACTA2* mutations, which may explain up to 20% of familial cases.	Genetic tests are complex and expensive.
Patients with Loeys-Dietz and some other specific defects seem likely to rupture or dissect at small aortic sizes.	Marfan is a clinical diagnosis (Ghent criteria).
Dr Milewicz recounts and explains genetic discoveries, rather than arguing strongly for immediate clinical application.	More than 600 individual mutations for Marfan alone.
	Pertinent tests not easily or widely available.
	New RNA test promising, perhaps on the horizon.
	Even if *TGFBR2, TGFBR1, MYH11*, or *ACTA2* mutations are identified, the clinical patterns to be expected are based on very small numbers of patients, that is, therapy unlikely to be affected by genetic information.

Section of Cardiac Surgery, Department of Surgery, Yale University School of Medicine, Yale-New Haven Hospital, PO Box 208039, New Haven, CT 06520-8039, USA
E-mail address: john.elefteriades@yale.edu

Cardiol Clin 28 (2010) 205–206
doi:10.1016/j.ccl.2010.02.007
0733-8651/10/$ – see front matter

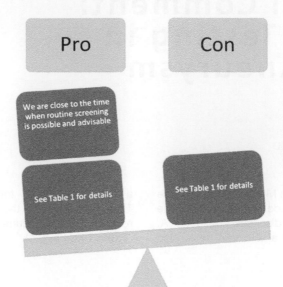

Fig. 1. We are certainly close to the point in time when routine screening is possible and advisable.

Biomarkers for Diagnosis in Thoracic Aortic Disease: PRO

Donald M. Botta Jr, MD

KEYWORDS

- Thoracic aortic aneurysm • Biomarkers
- Targeted imaging • Aortic size

According to the National Institutes of Health biomarker definitions working group, a biomarker is "A characteristic that is objectively measured and evaluated as an indicator of normal biological processes, pathogenic processes, or pharmacologic responses to a therapeutic intervention."[1] Identification of biomarkers for thoracic aortic aneurysm (TAA) disease is important because complications of TAAs are common. The population-based annual rate of thoracic aneurysmal rupture or dissection was 7.0 per 100,000[2] in one study; another study found a rate of rupture of 5.0 per 100,000.[3] The gravity of these occurrences is illustrated by the median survival of 3 days after aneurysmal dissection in the former study,[2] and 97% to 100% mortality after rupture in the latter.[3] The effect of this disease on public health can be brought into focus when one considers that, according to a recent National Hospital Discharge Survey, the mortality from human immunodeficiency virus infection in the United States was 5 per 100,000.[4] Preemptive operative repair of TAAs is effective in improving survival.[5] However, elective surgical repair for asymptomatic aneurysms remains a clinical decision that must be based on the patient's operative risk and the risk that a given TAA will rupture. Thus, it is vitally important to be able to identify which patients with TAAs are at the greatest risk for rupture or dissection.

The use of biomarkers can facilitate identification of at-risk patients. One normally thinks of biomarkers as circulating molecules that can be identified by blood test to predict the behavior of a certain pathologic process. This review focuses on the current state-of-the-art with respect to this type of biomarker. As late as 1995, a review of the literature revealed 294 articles on how to repair thoracic aneurysms, but only 7 articles on the natural history, or when to operate on TAAs.[6] Thus, not much literature has been devoted to biomarkers for TAA, circulating or otherwise.

The noncirculating biomarkers of aneurysm risk that have since been elucidated include aneurysm size and location, aneurysm growth rate, aneurysm symptoms, and family history.

The most commonly used noncirculating biomarker is aneurysm size. At the Yale Center for Thoracic Aortic Disease, the authors have been compiling an ongoing, cumulative database since 1995, including data and imaging studies on all patients that we treat for thoracic aortic disease. The database currently contains information on more than 1200 patients, with 3000 patient-years of follow-up and 3000 computerized imaging studies. Analysis of these data with specialized statistical methods that were developed and validated at our institution[7–9] has allowed us to quantify yearly rupture rates based on the diameter of the aneurysm, as well as annual aneurysmal expansion rates.[6]

Perhaps the simplest marker that portends ominous prognosis in patients with aneurysms is symptoms, especially among those with a strong family history of aneurysm-related complications.[10] When patients present with even moderately sized aneurysms and chest pain that is not attributable to another cause, operative repair is indicated.

Cardiac Surgery, Yale School of Medicine, PO Box 208039, New Haven, CT 06520-8039, USA
E-mail address: donald.botta@yale.edu

Cardiol Clin 28 (2010) 207–211
doi:10.1016/j.ccl.2010.01.009
0733-8651/10/$ – see front matter © 2010 Published by Elsevier Inc.

With regard to traditional biomarkers, or circulating biomarkers, great inroads are being made. Markers in clinical use and potential markers at the cellular, protein, and molecular level are discussed in the following sections.

MARKERS IN CLINICAL USE
D Dimers

Levels of D dimers have now been repeatedly shown to be sensitive for the presence of acute Stanford type A dissection. In addition, the D-dimer level on admission correlates with hospital survival in patients with acute type A dissection. This association is strong enough that D-dimer levels should be assessed on all individuals presenting with significant chest pain.[11] If the D-dimer level is increased, thoracic computed tomography should be performed to rule out type A dissection, as well as pulmonary embolism, which also may present with increased D-dimer levels.

Cellular Biomarkers

Two different cell types have been associated with the presence or progression of aneurysm disease. These include CD 28 null T cells and natural killer cells.

CD 28 null T cells are present in several inflammatory conditions, are relatively resistant to apoptosis, and are more commonly expressed with advancing age.[12–14] In 1 study, these cell types were present in greater numbers in the peripheral blood of those with aneurysms than in healthy controls. Ironically, those with smaller aneurysms had higher levels of these cells than those with larger aneurysms.[15] This raises the question as to whether these cells may be involved in the genesis of aneurysms.

Natural killer cells were shown to be present in greater numbers in a population of patients with abdominal aortic aneurysm (AAA) than in controls. These cells had greater cytotoxicity than normal natural killer cells, and this characteristic persisted even after extirpation of the aneurysm.[16]

Plasma and Serum Biomarkers

Changes in the levels of several plasma and serum elements have been associated with aneurysms. These can be broadly classified into markers of inflammation, markers of tissue turnover, and others.

The others include homocysteine, amyloid A,[17–19] osteopontin,[20] osteoprogerin,[21,22] and levels of plasmin/antiplasmin complexes.[23] Each of these has been associated with the presence of AAA,

diameter, or expansion, but has not been extensively studied.

Markers of inflammation have been more extensively studied, and aneurysm formation is now understood to be an inflammatory process. Many studies have identified associations between proinflammatory cytokines and AAA formation, expansion, or rupture. These cytokines include interleukin-1, interleukin-6, tumor necrosis factor alpha, interferon gamma, and cold reactive proteins.[24–27] Unfortunately, markers of inflammation are nonspecific and can be increased in several situations, so their usefulness as aneurysm markers is limited.

The matrix metalloproteinases (MMPs) deserve special mention. The MMPs are a group of zinc-dependent enzymes. The chief role of MMPs in physiologic and pathophysiologic states is to degrade the extracellular matrix.[28] MMPs are active in a wide array of disease processes, ranging range from periodontal disease[29] to congestive heart failure.[30–32] Experimentally, MMPs have been pharmacologically inhibited, resulting in improvement in disease processes, in animal[33–37] and human models.[38–41] Their activity in AAA disease is evident from animal studies, which have shown that MMP inhibition, either through targeted gene deletion[42] or pharmacologic inhibition,[43–46] results in decreased expansion of experimental AAAs. The importance of MMP activity in AAA disease has been reviewed by Kadoglou and Liapis.[47] With AAA, circulating levels of MMP-9 correlate directly to aortic wall levels of MMP-9.[48]

For thoracic aneurysms, recent work at our center[49] has noted an increased level of MMP-1 and MMP-9 in the walls of thoracic aortas that were either aneurysmal or dissected compared with controls. We also noted an increase in the MMP-9 to TIMP-1 ratio, which has been shown to favor proteolysis within the aortic wall[50] during AAA. The authors have also shown an extremely strong correlation between tissue and plasma levels of MMP-9 ($R^2 = 0.913$) (**Fig. 1**).[51] In agreement with this, several other studies have documented a strong correlation between MMP activity, especially MMP-9, and TAA formation and progression.[52–56] The relation between MMPs and aneurysm disease is now well enough established that large-scale clinical trials to verify a predictive biomarker relationship are warranted.

Molecular Biomarkers

Using RNA from circulating leukocytes, Elefteriades and colleagues[57] have been able to elucidate an expression profile that is present in most

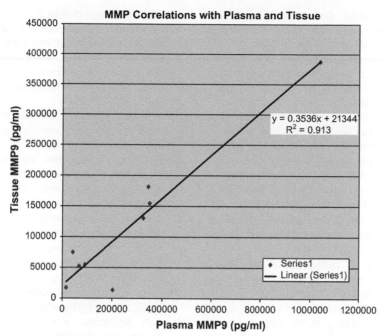

MMP Correlations with Plasma and Tissue

$y = 0.3536x + 21344$
$R^2 = 0.913$

Fig. 1. MMP correlations with plasma and tissue.

cases of sporadic aneurysm. In the initial validation trial, this RNA expression profile correctly identified patients with thoracic aneurysm with 78% accuracy.

In addition, a complementary DNA-based microarray study has identified some genes with over expression shared by TAAs and AAAs. These genes included those coding for intracellular adhesion molecule 1, v-yes-1 oncogene, mitogen-activated protein kinase 9, and MMP-9.[58]

Targeted Imaging

Possibly the most promising method of prognostication of the need for intervention in thoracic aneurysm disease is targeted imaging. The best example of this is activated MMP imaging. In an elegant study, Zhang and colleagues[59] used a molecular probe for activated MMPs to image vascular remodeling in a vascular injury model. Use of this or a similar imaging technique could describe not only the physical characteristics of the aneurysm but also the in situ activity of the pathologic process, and predict the likelihood of complications.

DISCUSSION

The authors have yet to encounter a perfect biomarker for any disease process. For myocardial infarction, the first well-described, circulating biomarker was aspartate aminotransferase.[60] This marker has since been supplanted by markers that are more specific to cardiac muscle necrosis. For TAA disease, the most well-described and broadly applicable biomarker is aortic size. Much progress has been made on circulating biomarkers, and the likelihood is that a panel of the currently available markers will be used to formulate a risk score predictive of aneurysm progression and complications. Much research is still required.

In addition, new molecular imaging techniques are showing promise of being able to not only image the size of aneurysms but also assess the activity of the pathologic processes that lead to complications. When these studies reach maturity, surgical decision making for TAA will be as precise as the operative repair techniques.

REFERENCES

1. Atkinson AJ, Colburn WA, & Biomarkers Definitions Working Group. Biomarkers and surrogate endpoints: preferred definitions and conceptual framework. Clin Pharmacol Ther 2001;69:89–95.
2. Clouse WD, Hallett JW Jr, Schaff HV, et al. Acute aortic dissection: population-based incidence compared with degenerative aortic aneurysm rupture. Mayo Clin Proc 2004;79(2):176–80.
3. Johansson G, Markstrom U, Swedenborg J. Ruptured thoracic aortic aneurysms: a study of incidence and mortality rates. J Vasc Surg 1995;21(6):985–8.

4. Centers for Disease Control and Prevention: National Center for Health Statistics, National Hospital Discharge Survey; 2001, Table 42.

5. Miller CC 3rd, Porat EE, Estrera AL, et al. Number needed to treat: analyzing of the effectiveness of thoracoabdominal aortic repair. Eur J Vasc Endovasc Surg 2004;28(2):154–7.

6. Elefteriades JA. Natural history of thoracic aortic aneurysms: indications for surgery, and surgical versus nonsurgical risks. Ann Thorac Surg 2002; 74(5):S1877–80 [discussion: S1892–8].

7. Rizzo JA, Coady MA, Elefteriades JA. Procedures for estimating growth rates in thoracic aortic aneurysms. J Clin Epidemiol 1998;51(9):747–54.

8. Rizzo JA, Coady MA, Elefteriades JA. Interpreting data on thoracic aortic aneurysms. Statistical issues. Cardiol Clin 1999;17(4):797–805.

9. Coady MA, Rizzo JA, Elefteriades JA. Developing surgical intervention criteria for thoracic aortic aneurysms. Cardiol Clin 1999;17(4):827–39.

10. Elefteriades JA, Tranquilli M, Darr U, et al. Symptoms plus family history trump size in thoracic aortic aneurysm. Ann Thorac Surg 2005;80(3): 1098–100.

11. Ohlman P, Faure A. Diagnostic and prognostic value of circulating D-Dimers in patients with acute aortic dissection. Crit Care Med 2006;34(5):1358–64.

12. Vallejo AN, Nestel AR, Schirmer M, et al. Aging-related deficiency of CD28 expression in CD4+ T cells is associated with the loss of gene-specific nuclear factor binding activity. J Biol Chem 1998; 273:8119–29.

13. Namekawa T, Snyder MR. Killer cell activating receptors function as costimulatory molecules on CD4+CD28null T cells clonally expanded in rheumatoid arthritis. J Immunol 2000;165:1138–45.

14. Speiser DE, Valmori D. CD28-negative cytolytic effector T cells frequently express NK receptors and are present at variable proportions in circulating lymphocytes from healthy donors and melanoma patients. Eur J Immunol 1999;29:1990–9.

15. Duftner C, Seiler R. High prevalence of circulating CD4+CD28- T-cells in patients with small abdominal aortic aneurysms. Arterioscler Thromb Vasc Biol 2005;25:1347–52.

16. Forester ND, Cruickshank SM. Increased natural killer cell activity in patients with an abdominal aortic aneurysm. Br J Surg 2006;93(1):46–54.

17. Rohde LE, Arroyo LH, Rifai N, et al. Plasma concentrations of interleukin-6 and abdominal aortic diameter among subjects without aortic dilatation. Arterioscler Thromb Vasc Biol 1999;19(7):1695–9.

18. Sofi F, Marcucci R, Giusti B, et al. High levels of homocysteine, lipoprotein (a) and plasminogen activator inhibitor-1 are present in patients with abdominal aortic aneurysm. Thromb Haemost 2005;94(5):1094–8.

19. Brunelli T, Prisco D, Fedi S, et al. High prevalence of mild hyperhomocysteinemia in patients with abdominal aortic aneurysm. J Vasc Surg 2000;32(3):531–6.

20. Golledge J, Muller J, Shephard N, et al. Association between osteopontin and human abdominal aortic aneurysm. Arterioscler Thromb Vasc Biol 2007;27(3):655–60.

21. Senzaki H, Chen CH, Ishido H, et al. Arterial hemodynamics in patients after Kawasaki disease. Circulation 2005;111:3119–25.

22. Hellenthal FA, Buurman WA, Wodzig WK, et al. Biomarkers of abdominal aortic aneurysm progression. Part 2: inflammation. Nat Rev Cardiol 2009; 6(8):543–52.

23. Lindholt JS, Jørgensen B, Fasting H, et al. Plasma levels of plasmin-antiplasmin-complexes are predictive for small abdominal aortic aneurysms expanding to operation-recommendable sizes. J Vasc Surg 2001;34(4):611–5.

24. Juvonen J, Surcel HM, Satta J, et al. Elevated circulating levels of inflammatory cytokines in patients with abdominal aortic aneurysm. Arterioscler Thromb Vasc Biol 1997;17(11):2843–7.

25. Dawson J, Cockerill GW, Choke E, et al. Aortic aneurysms secrete interleukin-6 into the circulation. J Vasc Surg 2007;45(2):350–6.

26. Norman P, Spencer CA, Lawrence-Brown MM, et al. C-reactive protein levels and the expansion of screen-detected abdominal aortic aneurysms in men. Circulation 2004;110(7):862–6.

27. Kosar F, Aksoy Y, Ozguntekin G, et al. C-reactive protein and aortic stiffness in patients with idiopathic dilated cardiomyopathy. Echocardiography 2007; 24(1):1–8.

28. Brinckerhoff CE, Matrisian LM. Matrix metalloproteinases: a tail of a frog that became a prince. Nat Rev Mol Cell Biol 2002;3(3):207–14.

29. Makela M, Salo T, Uitto VJ, et al. Matrix metalloproteinases (MMP-2 and MMP-9) of the oral cavity: cellular origin and relationship to periodontal status. J Dent Res 1994;73(8):1397–406.

30. Lee RT. Matrix metalloproteinase inhibition and the prevention of heart failure. Trends Cardiovasc Med 2001;11(5):202–5.

31. Spinale FG. Matrix metalloproteinases: regulation and dysregulation in the failing heart. Circ Res 2002;90(5):520–30.

32. Spinale FG. Matrix metalloproteinase gene polymorphisms in heart failure: new pieces to the myocardial matrix puzzle. Eur Heart J 2004;25(8): 631–3.

33. Islam MM, Franco CD, Courtman DW, et al. A nonantibiotic chemically modified tetracycline (CMT-3) inhibits intimal thickening. Am J Pathol 2003; 163(4):1557–66.

34. Sho E, Chu J, Sho M, et al. Continuous periaortic infusion improves doxycycline efficacy in

experimental aortic aneurysms. J Vasc Surg 2004; 39(6):1312–21.

35. Tronc F, Mallat Z, Lehoux S, et al. Role of matrix metalloproteinases in blood flow-induced arterial enlargement: interaction with NO. Arterioscler Thromb Vasc Biol 2000;20(12):E120–6.

36. Ramamurthy NS, McClain SA, Pirila E, et al. Wound healing in aged normal and ovariectomized rats: effects of chemically modified doxycycline (CMT-8) on MMP expression and collagen synthesis. Ann N Y Acad Sci 1999;30(878):720–3.

37. Carney DE, Lutz CJ, Picone AL, et al. Matrix metalloproteinase inhibitor prevents acute lung injury after cardiopulmonary bypass. Circulation 1999;100(4): 400–6.

38. Gapski R, Barr JL, Sarment DP, et al. Effect of systemic matrix metalloproteinase inhibition on periodontal wound repair: a proof of concept trial. J Periodontol 2004;75(3):441–52.

39. Preshaw PM, Hefti AF, Jepsen S, et al. Subantimicrobial dose doxycycline as adjunctive treatment for periodontitis. J Clin Periodontol 2004;31(9):697–707.

40. Emingil G, Atilla G, Sorsa T, et al. The effect of adjunctive low-dose doxycycline therapy on clinical parameters and gingival crevicular fluid matrix metalloproteinase-8 levels in chronic periodontitis. J Periodontol 2004;75(1):106–15.

41. Rudek MA, Figg WD, Dyer V, et al. Phase I clinical trial of oral COL-3, a matrix metalloproteinase inhibitor, in patients with refractory metastatic cancer. J Clin Oncol 2001;19(2):584–92.

42. Pyo R, Lee JK, Shipley JM, et al. Targeted gene disruption of matrix metalloproteinase-9 (gelatinase B) suppresses development of experimental abdominal aortic aneurysms. J Clin Invest 2000;105(11):1641–9.

43. Kaito K, Urayama H, Watanabe G. Doxycycline treatment in a model of early abdominal aortic aneurysm. Surg Today 2003;33(6):426–33.

44. Curci JA, Petrinec D, Liao S, et al. Pharmacologic suppression of experimental abdominal aortic aneurysms: a comparison of doxycycline and four chemically modified tetracyclines. J Vasc Surg 1998; 28(6):1082–93.

45. Prall AK, Longo GM, Mayhan WG, et al. Doxycycline in patients with abdominal aortic aneurysms and in mice: comparison of plasma levels and effect on aneurysm growth in mice. J Vasc Surg 2002;35(5): 923–9.

46. Curci JA, Mao D, Bohner DG, et al. Preoperative treatment with doxycycline reduces aortic wall expression and activation of matrix metalloproteinases in patients with abdominal aortic aneurysms. J Vasc Surg 2000;31(2):325–42.

47. Kadoglou NP, Liapis CD. Matrix metalloproteinases: contribution to pathogenesis, diagnosis, surveillance and treatment of abdominal aortic aneurysms. Curr Med Res Opin 2004;20(4):419–32.

48. Hovsepian DM, Ziporin SJ, Sakurai MK, et al. Elevated plasma levels of matrix metalloproteinase-9 in patients with abdominal aortic aneurysms: a circulating marker of degenerative aneurysm disease. J Vasc Interv Radiol 2000;11(10):1345–52.

49. Koulias GJ, Ravichandran P, Korkolis DP, et al. Increased tissue microarray MMP expression favors proteolysis in thoracic aortic aneurysms and dissections. Ann Thorac Surg 2004;78(6):2106–10 [discussion: 2110–1].

50. McMillan WD, Pearce WH. Increased plasma levels of metalloproteinase-9 are associated with abdominal aortic aneurysms. J Vasc Surg 1999;29(1): 122–7 [discussion: 127–9].

51. Botta DM, Elefteriades JA. Matrix metalloproteinases in thoracic aortic disease. Int J Angiol 2006; 15:1–8.

52. Sinha I, Bethi S, Cronin P, et al. A biologic basis for asymmetric growth in descending thoracic aortic aneurysms: a role for matrix metalloproteinase 9 and 2. J Vasc Surg 2006;43(2):342–8.

53. Taketani T, Imai Y, Morota T, et al. Altered patterns of gene expression specific to thoracic aortic aneurysms: microarray analysis of surgically resected specimens. Int Heart J 2005;46(2):265–77.

54. Koullias GJ, Ravichandran P, Korkolis DP, et al. Increased tissue microarray matrix metalloproteinase expression favors proteolysis in thoracic aortic aneurysms and dissections. Ann Thorac Surg 2004; 78(6):2106–10 [discussion: 2110–1].

55. Nataatmadja M, West M, West J, et al. Abnormal extracellular matrix protein transport associated with increased apoptosis of vascular smooth muscle cells in Marfan syndrome and bicuspid aortic valve thoracic aortic aneurysm. Circulation 2003; 108(Suppl 1):II329–34.

56. Segura AM, Luna RE, Horiba K, et al. Immunohistochemistry of matrix metalloproteinases and their inhibitors in thoracic aortic aneurysms and aortic valves of patients with Marfan's syndrome. Circulation 1998;98(Suppl 19):II331–7 [discussion: II337–8].

57. Wang Y, Barbacioru CC, Shiffman D, et al. Gene expression signature in peripheral blood detects thoracic aortic aneurysm. PLoS One 2007;2(10):e1050.

58. Absi TS, Sundt TM 3rd, Tung WS, et al. Altered patterns of gene expression distinguishing ascending aortic aneurysms from abdominal aortic aneurysms: complementary DNA expression profiling in the molecular characterization of aortic disease. J Thorac Cardiovasc Surg 2003;126(2): 344–57 [discussion: 357].

59. Zhang J, Nie Lei, Razavian M, et al. Molecular imaging of activated matrix metalloproteinases in vascular remodeling. Circulation 2008;118:1953–60.

60. Karmen A, Wróblewski F, LaDue JS. Transaminase activity in human blood. J Clin Invest 1955;34: 126–31.

Biomarkers for Diagnosis in Thoracic Aortic Disease: CON

Emily A. Farkas, MD

KEYWORDS

- Biomarker • Disease state • Disease trait
- Thoracic aortic aneurysm

Ambiguity is not commonplace among the ranks of medicine and science, and ambiguity may even be a direct contradiction to the methods of those disciplines. Yet, as the field of research known as "bioinformatics" rapidly expands, so do the vagaries surrounding the evidentiary process that links a candidate biomarker to a disease process or clinical outcome.

In 2001, an expert working group was convened by the National Institutes of Health that standardized the definition of a biomarker as "a characteristic that is objectively measured and evaluated as an indicator of normal biologic processes, pathogenic processes, or pharmacologic responses to a therapeutic intervention."[1] Because of the expectation that a biomarker enhances the ability of a clinician to optimally manage patients, a new biomarker is of clinical value only if it is accurate, reproducible, acceptable to the patient, easy to interpret, and has a high sensitivity and high specificity for the outcome it is expected to identify. Further, the biomarker should explain a reasonable proportion of the clinical outcome (independently of established predictors) consistently in multiple studies; and most importantly, there must be data to suggest that knowledge of biomarker levels independently alters clinical management (**Box 1**).[2]

Protocols for the introduction of new candidate markers have been offered that suggest rigorous evaluation of every step from discovery, qualification, verification, research assay standardization, clinical validation, and commercial use.[3,4] Although these guidelines have not been uniformly respected, they should be systematically applied to evaluate the use of biomarkers in the clinical care of patients. In reference to aortic aneurysm disease, this requires examination in the context of three distinct clinical scenarios: (1) biomarkers as indicators of disease trait (risk); (2) disease state (pathogenesis); and (3) disease rate (progression).[2,5]

BIOMARKERS AND DISEASE TRAIT

Named genetic syndromes that predispose to aortic pathology have been extensively studied. Marfan syndrome has been related to mutations in the FBN1 gene coding for fibrillin, and mutations in the TGFBR2 gene coding for transforming growth factor-β receptors have been associated with overlapping phenotypes, familial thoracic aortic aneurysms, and Loeys-Deitz syndrome (characterized by arterial aneurysms, arterial tortuosity, marfanoid habitus, and unusual craniofacial features).[6] The diagnosis of these disorders, however, cannot be based on molecular analysis alone because of limited availability, imperfect mutation detection, and the fact that not all FBN1 and TGBR2 mutations are associated with Marfan and related syndromes.[7] Despite the vast amount of information assembled about biomarkers for these connective tissue disorders, Marfan and related syndromes are diagnosed instead based on clinical criteria using the Ghent nosology (which focuses mainly on skeletal and ophthalmologic features in combination with anthropometric data and family history).[8] Identifying a given mutation is also of limited value in establishing a phenotype or providing a prognosis

Department of Surgery, Cardiothoracic Surgery, Saint Louis University School of Medicine, 3635 Vista Avenue, 8th Floor Des Loges Towers, St Louis, MO 63110, USA
E-mail address: efarkas@slu.edu

Cardiol Clin 28 (2010) 213–220
doi:10.1016/j.ccl.2010.01.018

because of the large number of unique mutations (>500 fibrillin gene mutations) reported, and because of the clinical heterogeneity among individuals with the same mutation.[9] Furthermore, in December 2009, a review of the largest reported group of patients with the TGFBR2 gene mutations (N = 71) was published, comparing them with age- and gender-matched control subjects and patients harboring FBNI mutations. This large-scale multi-institutional trial concluded that clinical outcomes were not significantly different between patients with TGFBR2 and FBN1 mutations and also that the "key finding is that the prognosis of a patient depends on the clinical expression of the disease and not solely on the presence of a mutation in the TGRBR2 gene."[10] The determination of the genetic biomarkers for Marfan and overlapping syndromes provides marginal use for the diagnosis, prognosis, or intention to treat in relationship to these disorders.

Foresight regarding the nonsyndromic, familial variant of aortic aneurysm disease by molecular diagnosis seems more advantageous at first glance. Yet even leading molecular geneticists in this field suggest that meaningful information is limited by a phenotype that has a variable age of onset and clinical presentation, genetic heterogeneity resulting in more than one gene leading to this familial disease, and also decreased penetrance with the inheritance and presence of a defective gene not always resulting in realized aortic disease.[11,12] Aortic aneurysm is a complex human disease that results from the inputs of both genetic and environmental factors, making its molecular basis different from mendelian inheritance because the underlying mutation induces only a subtle alteration in the protein functions or the levels of gene expression.[13] Genetic mapping and linkage analysis continue to enumerate various categories of mutations, but no predictive model currently exists. Regardless, there is little

doubt that a genetic diagnosis of the aneurysm diathesis will continue to be fervently pursued.

Science aside, what is the emotional cost of knowledge of an aneurysm diathesis? Familial aggregation studies have confirmed a wide range in age of initial diagnosis of aortic disease, ranging from 1 to 87 years of age.[14] Should a child and his or her parents be burdened with the knowledge and anxiety of a potentially lethal problem when the average age of the affected individual is approximately 50 years? Will patients and families begin demanding preemptive surgery far earlier than the recommended indications when faced with this knowledge? In comparison, women who are informed that they harbor one of the breast cancer gene mutations (BRCA) have pursued prophylactic treatment as dramatic as bilateral mastectomy and bilateral oophorectomy to minimize yet not eliminate their risk of developing breast cancer; certainly there is no analogous procedure that provides similar protection throughout the length of the aorta.

Finally, confirmation of the aneurysm diathesis does not obviate the need for aortic imaging, and might prompt excessive radiologic surveillance over many years, imparting its own unique and additive morbidity. Current conventional clinical guidelines can direct appropriate imaging for relatives of familial aortic aneurysm patients and for patients with heritable connective tissue syndromes at risk for aortic pathology; the presence of a disease trait biomarker would not significantly alter this need for surveillance or change the indications for intervention based on extent (aortic diameter) and progression of aortic dilation.

BIOMARKERS AND DISEASE STATE

Unraveling the pathogenesis of thoracic aortic aneurysm has been an elusive goal. Investigators have measured circulating concentrations of an expansive number of markers that presumably reflect aortic wall destruction and inflammatory activity. Much of this work has been predicated on previous studies examining the vascular biology of abdominal aortic aneurysm (AAA), although this concept is fundamentally flawed; the histopathologic characteristics of medial degeneration most common in an aneurysm of the ascending aorta differ markedly from the typical inflammatory and atherosclerotic AAA. Embryology, mechanical elastic properties, and biochemical composition are distinct between the ascending and descending thoracoabdominal aorta. This was confirmed by a recent molecular characterization of disparate patterns of gene expression distinguishing ascending aortic aneurysm from AAA.[15] The premise for targeting similar biomarkers as indicators of disease state in these heterogeneous molecular environments is not conceptually sound.

Regardless, this body of investigation was stimulated by examination of aortic biopsies from patients undergoing open AAA repair, demonstrating a paucity of vascular smooth muscle cells, an accumulation of macrophages and lymphocytes, elastin fragmentation, high concentrations of proteolytic enzymes and cytokines, and laminated thrombus.[16–18] The role of multiple candidate biomarkers has been hypothesized on the basis of these pathologic features, but perhaps most attention has been directed to a group of enzymes called "matrix metalloproteinases" (MMPs) and their tissue inhibitors (TIMPs). The balance between these two sets of enzymes results in degradation of the extracellular matrix, which consists predominantly of macromolecules, such as elastin and collagen, and serves many functions that are essential for vessel homeostasis.[19] Circulating concentrations of MMP-9 have been investigated most frequently, but the findings have not been completely consistent (**Table 1**).[20–25] Two out of six of the most recent studies on the issue, including the largest, found no association between circulating levels of MMP-9 in patients with AAA compared with control patients.[21,22] Concentrations of MMP-9 are higher in serum than in plasma because of platelet degranulation, but the negative association studies involved assessments of plasma in one instance and serum in the other, suggesting that the inconsistent findings are not explained by differences in sampling alone.[18]

Another disparity surrounds whether circulating values that could potentially be obtained in a peripheral blood sample as biomarker are actually reflective of the local pathologic process in the aortic wall. One recent study comparing the circulating concentrations of MMP-1, MMP-2, MMP-3, MMP-9, TIMP-1, and TIMP-2 directly with intraoperative specimens found no correlation for any MMP or TIMP.[26] Furthermore, correlation between MMP-9 levels in the aneurysm wall and aneurysm diameter was negative ($r = -0.42$; $P = 0.019$).[26] Similarly, even studies that confirm a higher level of plasma MMP-9 in patients with AAA when compared with controls have found no correlation between MMP-9 plasma levels and AAA size.[19,24] Perhaps the most meaningful end point would assess whether or not MMPs could predict AAA expansion or progression. A recent 2009 study did not find a correlation between plasma levels of MMP-9 and annual expansion of AAA in 208 patients, which is nearly six times the sample size of earlier studies asserting an ability to predict size using the very same assay.[27,28]

These contradictory results suggest that although initially encouraging, the measurement of MMPs will likely not be able satisfactorily to predict aneurysm size, expansion rate, or complications, and does not meet the criteria of a satisfactory biomarker that influences treatment significantly. Although many other potential markers exist, MMPs were regarded as the most promising. The conflicting results surrounding the use of MMPs and TIMPS are likely to be representative of disparities that will be uncovered with similar candidate biomarkers of this complex aneurysm pathogenesis.

BIOMARKERS AND DISEASE RATE

The ability to predict expansion rate and acute decompensation is closely related in aortic pathology. Two features of aneurysm disease make the need for such prediction compelling: most patients experience rupture or dissection as their very first clinical manifestation of

Table 1
Circulating levels of matrix metalloproteinase-9 in patients with abdominal aortic aneurysm versus controls

Author, Year (ref)	AAA/Controls, N	AAA/Controls, MMP-9 Concentration
Watanabe et al, 2006[20]	53/26	$622 \pm 400.2/282.6 \pm 158.5$ $P<.001$
Eugster et al, 2005[21]	95/83	$353 \pm 252/455 \pm 499$ NS
van Laake et al, 2005[22]	22/12	$61 \pm 49/51 \pm 28$ NS
Sangiorgi et al, 2001[23]	45/10	$30.9 \pm 17.1/8.9 \pm 2.5$ $P<.05$
Hovsepian et al, 2000[24]	25/20	$99.4 \pm 17.4/45.4 \pm 9.1$ $P<.05$
McMillan and Pearce, 1999[25]	22/17	$85.6 \pm 11.6/19.5 \pm 3.1$ $P<.001$

Abbreviations: AAA, abdominal aortic aneurysm; MMP, matrix metalloproteinase.

aneurysm disease, and a high degree of lethality surrounds these acute aortic events. The search is ongoing for a molecular signature that detects a critical change in aneurysm characteristics immediately before an acute event, or one that confirms the frequently challenging diagnosis during those crucial first moments and hours.

One approach to achieve this is by pursuing a biomarker that could serve as a surrogate end point for the clinical outcome of an acute aortic event. The National Institutes of Health working group on biomarkers has raised many concerns regarding the use and interpretation of biomarkers in this context, but as more platforms for genetic evaluation become readily available, this practice only expands.[1] Hybridizing samples of RNA and DNA in solution to short nucleotide sequences that form arrays is not a novel technique; array technology, however, has expanded enormously over the last decade of rapid advancement in bio-instrumentation. Through a whole-genome gene expression profiling analysis in thoracic aneurysm patients and controls, a 41-gene signature has been identified in peripheral blood cells that distinguishes aneurysm patients from controls with a 78% ± 6% overall classification accuracy.[29] The initial focus was to develop a blood-based gene expression test to detect an aneurysm diathesis as a screening tool. With further clinical testing, however, the authors hope that this might set the stage for a peripheral blood test that could be surveyed over time, with any "blip" in the profile heralding the onset of an acute aortic event and prompting pre-emptive surgery, or potentially assisting in the management of a patient presenting to the emergency room with chest pain to uncover the possibility of an aneurysm-related complication.[30]

Another major area of focus has been on interleukins, which are a large group of cytokines hypothesized to be vital in the progression and rupture of aneurysms.[31–35] Only interleukin-1B and interleukin-6 have been investigated as predictors of AAA expansion[36] and the level of neither of these interleukins has correlated with aneurysm expansion in patients with AAAs between 33 and 66 mm in diameter.[37] A recent study published in 2009 also failed to find a correlation between plasma concentration of interleukin-6 and AAA progression.[27]

In regard to identification of acute aortic events, however, the biomarker that has received the most attention involves the D-dimer value as an indicator of aortic dissection.[38] D dimers are fibrin degradation products representing an indirect demonstration of the activation of the coagulation cascade leading to fibrin formation. Multiple studies have reported close to 100% sensitivity for D dimer in excluding aortic dissection, although many discrepancies limit the reproducibility of these results: inclusion bias exists with poorly defined eligible patient populations; the reported time from symptom onset ranges from 1 to 120 hours; heterogeneity exists for the lower limit of detection among the different studies (0.1–0.9 μg/mL); and multiple different assays are used to obtain the values (**Table 2**).[39–46]

Despite the lack of consistency in the literature, there are still some authors who suggest that the D dimer may be used as the singular testing modality to rule out an acute aortic dissection. The International Registry of Acute Aortic Dissection Substudy on Biomarkers Experience was a recently completed prospective multicenter trial enrolling 220 patients initially suspected of having aortic dissection. Their data revealed that the lack of false lumen patency resulted in lower D-dimer levels, presumably from the decreased likelihood of stimulating the clotting cascade compared with those patients with luminal extension.[44] This has been emphasized in the literature with confirmation of false-negative D-dimer results.[47–49] A 2009 publication also cautions clinicians regarding the negative predictive value following their finding that 18% (11 of 61) of patients enrolled in their study with confirmed aortic dissection had D-dimer values below 0.4 μg/mL, which could be interpreted as a negative result excluding the diagnosis.[43] It has similarly been shown that intramural hematoma, a variant of aortic dissection that lacks communication with the aortic lumen, may not show elevations in the D-dimer concentrations.[50] Finally, D-dimer levels may remain falsely elevated in chronic aortic dissection because of the thrombotic process in the false lumen, obscuring the acute cause of an unrelated episode of chest pain.[43]

Relying solely on the D dimer as a biomarker that can definitively rule out aortic dissection seems like a gamble with potentially catastrophic consequences. Even studies highlighting 100% sensitivity recommend obtaining imaging regardless of a negative D-dimer assay if there is a high degree of clinical suspicion for aortic dissection,[44] and experts in the field emphasize that appropriate imaging is always required for definitive diagnosis and confirmation.[43]

Data such as these beg the question regarding the actual use of the D-dimer test. It has been suggested that D dimer could be used to triage patients in a smaller community center without access to imaging,[43] although one could question the decision to delay at all in a facility incapable of definitive imaging or treatment. In a tertiary or

Table 2
Disparities among recent D-dimer studies

Author, Year, (ref)	N	D-Dimer Sens. % (95% CI)	Cutoff, μg/mL	False Neg (%)	D-Dimer Assay Type
Retrospective studies					
Wiegand et al, 2007[41]	25	88 (67.7–96.8)	0.5	3 (12)	Immunoassay (Diagnostica Stago, Parsippany, NJ, USA)
Hazui et al, 2006[40]	113	92 (85–96.1)	0.4	9 (8)	Latex agglutination (Roche diagnostic, Tokyo, Japan)
Ohlmann et al, 2006[42]	94	99 (93.3–99.9)	0.4	1 (1)	Immunoassay (Diagnostica Stago, Parsippany, NJ, USA)
Prospective studies					
Paparella et al, 2009[43]	61	82	0.4	11 (18)	Immuno-turbidimetric assay (Auto-Dimer; Trinity Biotech, Wicklow, Ireland)
Suzuki et al, 2009[44]	220	96.6 (90.3–99.3)	0.5	3 (1)	Immunoassay/Triage D-Dimer (Biosite, San Diego, CA, USA)
Sbarouni et al, 2007[45]	18	94 (70.6–99.7)	0.7	1 (<1)	ELISA (Vidas D-Dimer; BioMerieux, Marcy l'Etoile, France)
Sodeck et al, 2007[46]	65	86 (74.8–93.1)	0.9	9 (14)	STA –Latex agglutination (Roche Diagnostic, Tokyo, Japan)
Akutsu et al, 2005[39]	30	100 (85.9–100)	0.5	0	Rapid bedside cardiac assay (Roche)

quaternary referral center, would D dimer help stratify the patient with chest pain more favorably than clinical impression alone? If the D-dimer assay is quantified as negative, the clinician is faced with the risks addressed previously in accepting this stand-alone diagnostic tool. If the D-dimer concentration is considered positive, the clinician is obliged to obtain the same imaging to confirm an aortic dissection (as opposed to other pathology that elevates D dimers, such as pulmonary embolism), which would have been required without awaiting the D-dimer assay. Any unnecessary delay is especially poignant in such a disease as an ascending aortic dissection, which incurs a cumulative 1% to 2% hourly mortality in the first 24 hours.[39,47] Finally, it is hard to imagine a scenario wherein a positive D-dimer assay streamlines the pathway to the operating room, because few surgeons would commit to such treatment without radiographic confirmation of the presence, location, extent, and specific complications of aortic dissection.

SUMMARY

Fundamental requirements for a meaningful biomarker have not been met in the prediction of the aneurysm trait, the progression of the aneurysm disease state, or the prevention of catastrophic aortic complications. Of particular pertinence in today's health care climate, any test that does not change disease management and does not improve patient outcome is unlikely to be cost effective. Aortic aneurysm is a worthy opponent on all fronts, and clinicians should continue actively to evaluate all potential diagnostic and therapeutic adjuncts with high levels of scientific scrutiny and rigor, so that the understanding and management of this disease process evolves in a complementary rather than duplicative manner. In the meantime, proteomics, genomics, and metabolomics continue to represent a muse of sorts in scientific circles, but clinicians are responsible for verifying the relevance and meaningful application of its postulates as they apply to individual patients within the context of efficient and effective global health care delivery.

REFERENCES

1. Downing G. Biomarkers and surrogate endpoints: preferred definitions and conceptual framework. Biomarkers definitions working group. Clin Pharmacol Ther 2001;69(3):49–95.
2. Vasan RS. Biomarkers of cardiovascular disease: molecular basis and practical considerations. Circulation 2006;113(19):2335–62.
3. Dotsenko O, Chackathayil J, Jeetesh V, et al. Candidate circulating biomarkers for the cardiovascular disease continuum. Curr Pharm Des 2008;14(24):2445–61.
4. Lee JW, Figeys D, Vasilescu J. Biomarker assay translation from discovery to clinical studies in cancer drug development: quantification of emerging protein biomarkers. Adv Cancer Res 2007;96:269–98.
5. Fox N, Growdon JH. Biomarkers and surrogates. Neuro Rx 2004;1:181.
6. Loeys BL, Chen J, Neptune ER, et al. A syndrome of altered cardiovascular, craniofacial, neurocognitive, and skeletal development caused by mutations in TGFBR1 or TGFBR2. Nat Genet 2005;37:275–81.
7. Dean JC. Marfan syndrome: clinical diagnosis and management. Eur J Hum Genet 2007;15(7):724–33.
8. De Paepe A, Devereux RB, Dietz HC. Revised diagnostic criteria for the Marfan syndrome. Am J Med Genet 1996;62:417–26.
9. Montgomery RA, Geraghty MT, Bull E. Multiple molecular mechanisms underlying subdiagnostic variants of Marfan syndrome. Am J Hum Genet 1998;63:1703–11.
10. Attias D, Stheneur C, Roy C, et al. Comparison of clinical presentations and outcomes between patients with TGFBR2 and FBN1 mutations in Marfan syndrome and related disorders. Circulation 2009;120:2541–9.
11. Guo D, Hasham S, Kuang SQ, et al. Familial thoracic aortic aneurysms and dissections: genetic heterogeneity with a major locus mapping to 5q13-14. Circulation 2001;103:2461–8.
12. Hasham SN, Willing MC, Guo DC, et al. Mapping a locus for familial thoracic aortic aneurysms and dissections (TAAD2) to 3p24-25. Circulation 2003;107:3184–90.
13. Milewicz, et al. Genetic basis of thoracic aortic aneurysms and dissections. In: Elefteriades JA, editor. Acute aortic disease. New York: Informa Healthcare; 2007. p. 99–124.
14. Hasham SN, Lewin MR, Tran VT, et al. Nonsyndromic genetic predisposition to aortic dissection: a newly recognized, diagnosable, and preventable occurrence in families. Ann Emerg Med 2006;7:11–20.
15. Absi TS, Sundt TM, Tung WS. Altered patterns of gene expression distinguishing ascending aortic aneurysms from abdominal aortic aneurysms: complementary DNA expression profiling in the molecular characterization of aortic disease. J Thorac Cardiovasc Surg 2003;126:344–57.
16. Golledge J, Muller J, Daugherty A, et al. Abdominal aortic aneurysm: pathogenesis and implications for management. Arterioscler Thromb Vasc Biol 2006;26:2605–13.

17. Golledge J, Wolanski P, Parr A, et al. Measurement and determinants of infrarenal aortic thrombus volume. Eur Radiol 2008;18:1987–94.

18. Golledge J, Tsao PS, Dalman RL, et al. Circulating markers of abdominal aortic aneurysm presence and progression. Circulation 2008;118:2382–92.

19. Hellenthal FA, Buurman WA, Wodzig WK, et al. Biomarkers of AAA progression. Part 1: extracellular matrix degeneration. Nat Rev Cardiol 2009;6:464–74.

20. Watanabe T, Sato A, Sawai T, et al. The elevated level of circulating matrix metalloproteinase-9 in patients with abdominal aortic aneurysms decreased to levels equal to those of health controls after an aortic repair. Ann Vasc Surg 2006;20:317–21.

21. Eugster T, Huber A, Obeid T, et al. Aminoterminal propeptide of type III procollagen and matrix metalloproteinases-2 and -9 failed to serve as serum markers for abdominal aortic aneurysm. Eur J Vasc Endovasc Surg 2005;29:378–82.

22. van Laake LW, Vainas T, Dammers R, et al. Systemic dilation diathesis in patients with abdominal aortic aneurysms: a role for matrix metalloproteinase-9? Eur J Vasc Endovasc Surg 2005;29:371–7.

23. Sangiorgi G, D'Averio R, Mauriello A, et al. Plasma levels of metalloprotienases-3 and -9 as markers of successful abdominal aortic aneurysm exclusion after endovascular graft treatment. Circulation 2001;104(Suppl):I/288–95.

24. Hovespian DM, Ziporin SJ, Sakurai MK, et al. Elevated plasma levels of matrix metalloproteinase-9 in patients with abdominal aortic aneurysms: a circulating marker of degenerative aneurysm disease. J Vasc Interv Radiol 2000;11:1345–52.

25. McMillan WD, Pearce WH. Increased plasma levels of metalloproteinase-9 are associated with abdominal aortic aneurysms. J Vasc Surg 1999;29:122–7.

26. Wilson WR, Choke EC, Dawson J, et al. Plasma matrix metalloproteinase levels do not predict tissue levels in abdominal aortic aneurysm suitable for elective repair. Vascular 2008;16(5):248–52.

27. Karlsson L, Bergqvist D, Lindback J, et al. Expansion of small-diameter abdominal aortic aneurysms is not reflected by the release of inflammatory mediators IL-6, MMP-9 and CRP in plasma. Eur J Vasc Endovasc Surg 2009;37:420–4.

28. Lindholt JS, Vammen S, Fasting H, et al. The plasma level of matrix metalloproteinase-9 may predict the natural history of small abdominal aortic aneurysms: a preliminary study. Eur J Vasc Endovasc Surg 2000;20:281–5.

29. Wang Y, Barbacioru CC, Shiffman D, et al. Gene expression signature in peripheral blood detects thoracic aortic aneurysm. PLoS One 2007;2(10): e1050.

30. Elefteriades JA. Future prospects: molecular diagnosis, enhanced imaging, molecular-based conventional drugs, and gene therapy. In: Elefteriades JA, editor. Acute aortic disease. New York: Informa Healthcare; 2007. p. 347–51.

31. Treska V, Topolcan O, Pecen L. Cytokines as plasma markers of abdominal aortic aneurysm. Clin Chem Lab Med 2000;38:1161–4.

32. Sun J, Sukhova GK, Yang M, et al. Mast cells modulate the pathogenesis of elastase-induced abdominal aortic aneurysms in mice. J Clin Invest 2007; 117:3359–68.

33. Walton LJ, Franklin IJ, Bayston T, et al. Inhibition of prostaglandin E2 synthesis in abdominal aortic aneurysms: implications for smooth muscle cell viability, inflammatory processes, and the expansion of abdominal aortic aneurysms. Circulation 1999;100:48–54.

34. Swartbol P, Truedsson L, Norgren L. Adverse reactions during endovascular treatment of aortic aneurysms may be triggered by interleukin 6 release from the thrombotic content. J Vasc Surg 1998;28: 664–8.

35. Jones KG, Brull DJ, Brown LC, et al. Interleukin-6 (IL-6) and the prognosis of abdominal aortic aneurysms. Circulation 2001;103:2260–5.

36. Hellenthal FA, Buurman WA, Wodzig WH, et al. Biomarkers of abdominal aortic aneurysm progression. Part 2: inflammation. Nat Rev Cardiol 2009;6: 543–52.

37. Juvonen J, Surcel HM, Satta J, et al. Elevated circulating levels of inflammatory cytokines in patients with abdominal aortic aneurysm. Arterioscler Thromb Vasc Biol 1997;17:2843–7.

38. Suzuki T. Cardiovascular diagnostic biomarkers: the past, present and future. Circ J 2009;73:806–9.

39. Akutsu K, Sato N, Yamamoto T, et al. A rapid bedside D-dimer assay (cardiac D-dimer) for screening of clinically suspected acute aortic dissection. Circ J 2005;69:397–403.

40. Hazui H, Nishimoto M, Hoshiga M, et al. Young adult patients with short dissection length and thrombosed false lumen without ulcer-like projections are liable to have false-negative results of D-dimer testing for acute aortic dissection based on a study of 113 cases. Circ J 2006;70:1598–601.

41. Wiegand J, Koller M, Bingisser R. Does a negative D-dimer test rule out aortic dissection? Swiss Med Wkly 2007;137:462.

42. Ohlmann P, Faure A, Morel O, et al. Diagnostic and prognostic value of circulating D-dimers in patients with acute aortic dissection. Crit Care Med 2006; 34:1358–64.

43. Paparella D, Malvindi PG, Scrascia G. D-dimers are not always elevated in patients with acute aortic dissection. J Cardiovasc Med 2009;10: 212–4.

44. Suzuki T, Distante A, Zizza A, et al. Diagnosis of acute aortic dissection by D-dimer. The International Registry of Acute Aortic Dissection Substudy on

Biomarkers (IRAD-Bio) experience. Circulation 2009;119:2702–9.

45. Sbarouni E, Georgiadou P, Marathias A, et al. D-dimer and BNP levels in acute aortic dissection. Int J Cardiol 2007;122:170–2.

46. Sodeck G, Domanovits H, Schillinger M. D-dimer in ruling out aortic dissection: a systematic review and prospective cohort study. Eur Heart J 2007; 28(24):3067–75.

47. Sutherland A, Escano J, Coon TP. D-dimer as the sole screening test for acute aortic dissection: a review of the literature. Ann Emerg Med 2008;52:339–43.

48. Eggebrecht H, Naber C, Bruch C. Value of plasma fibrin D-dimers for detection of acute aortic dissection. J Am Coll Cardiol 2004;44: 804–9.

49. Hazui H, Fukumoto H, Negoro N, et al. Simple and useful tests for discriminating between acute aortic dissection of the ascending aorta and acute myocardial infarction in the emergency setting. Circ J 2005;69:677–82.

50. Evangelista A, Mukherjee D, Mehta RH, et al. Acute intramural hematoma of the aorta: a mystery in evolution. Circulation 2005;111:1063–70.

Editorial Comment: Biomarkers for Diagnosis in Thoracic Aortic Disease

John A. Elefteriades, MD

The article by Dr Donald J. Botta Jr in this issue of *Cardiology Clinics* paints a picture of great promise for biomarkers of thoracic aortic disease (**Table 1**). D-dimer is clinically relevant even at the present time. D-dimer assay detects the dissection, however, after it occurs. The key is to detect aneurysmal deterioration before dissection or rupture. Biomarkers that predict aneurysmal behavior are still in the development stage.

Dr Emily J. Farkas brings us a reality check in her article, pointing out how preliminary the search is for effective biomarkers (**Fig. 1**).

Table 1
Effective biomarkers for thoracic aortic disease

Pro: We Do Have Effective Biomarkers (Botta)	Con: We Do Not Have Effective Biomarkers (Farkas)
D-dimer is extremely sensitive for aortic dissection and is in current clinical use as a biomarker	A biomarker should • Detect disease • Detect diathesis to disease (eg, genetically) • Predict outcome/complications
Cellular biomarkers (of inflammation) hold promise	Current biomarkers for aortic diseases do not satisfy these criteria
Among serum biomarkers, MMPs hold the most promise and are entering clinical use	D-dimer is fraught with issues (upper limit of normal, misses IMH, etc.)
Among molecular biomarkers, a new RNA signature test holds promise	MMPs in serum do not correlate with tissue
Targeted imaging promises to combine molecular probes with imaging technologies to permit visualization of the molecular state of the aortic wall	The promise of MMPs has not been realized
	Other biomarkers have been less promising than MMPs
	RNA signature screening test still needs to be refined and studied

Abbreviations: IMH, intramural hematoma; MMP, matrix metalloproteinase.

Section of Cardiac Surgery, Department of Surgery, Yale University School of Medicine, Yale-New Haven Hospital, PO Box 208039, New Haven, CT 06520-8039, USA
E-mail address: john.elefteriades@yale.edu

Cardiol Clin 28 (2010) 221–222
doi:10.1016/j.ccl.2010.02.017

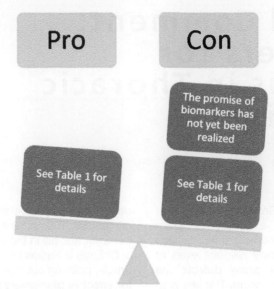

Fig. 1. Final impression: much promise, not yet realized.

Routine Screening of Young Athletes for Aneurysm: PRO

John A. Elefteriades, MD

KEYWORDS
- Weight lifting • Aortic dissection • Exertion
- Strength training

Several years ago, our aortic nurse (Maryann Tranquilli) noticed that we had operated on several young weightlifters, all ostensibly healthy, within a short period of time, all for type A aortic dissection. Review of our records revealed 5 such patients and resulted in our initial report of a connection between weightlifting and aortic dissection.[1]

After that report was published, we received unsolicited documentation of similar cases from around the country.

CASE VIGNETTE

A hospital president called, greatly distressed, but resolved to inform our team about his son's case to help others in the future. His son was on the football team at a well-known college. The young man went to the gym early on a Saturday morning to perform an extra personal workout. This workout was not required but was an indication of the young man's dedication and desire to do even better for his team. The young man developed chest pain and was seen in the college infirmary. The diagnosis was a sprain of the pectoral muscles. The father was contacted but was told that there was no concern and that there was no need for him to travel to the state in which the college was located. The young man continued to complain of pain; he told multiple caregivers that he was going to die.No one on the patient care team suspected any serious cardiac problem in such a young, healthy man. About 6:30 PM on the day of pain, a cardiac echo was ordered. The echocardiogram showed a type A aortic dissection, with intrapericardial rupture. A helicopter was called, but the young man died before the helicopter arrived.

This case vignette demonstrates vividly the great tragedy involved in the loss of these promising young athletes due to exertion-related aortic dissection. It is imperative that the physicians treating on the front lines understand the relationship of exertion to aortic dissection .

Thanks to the generosity and courage of families who called and wrote from around the country to describe similarly tragic stories regarding their loved ones, we compiled a group of 31 such events, which permitted us to formulate some substantive observations regarding the relationship between exertion and aortic dissection (**Table 1**).[2]

The affected individuals were almost entirely men. Athletic activity was involved in many cases, and in others, a severe straining effort at work or in the course of daily activities led to the acute aortic dissection. All affected individuals had previously unknown aortic enlargement, usually in the range of 4 to 5 cm. About 88% of cases involved the ascending aorta, and the remainder the descending. The single case affecting the descending aorta occurred in a cardiac surgeon, who immediately recognized the course of events. The event precipitating the aortic dissection was usually strength training or similar straining, not usually aerobic type of exercise. In many cases, because of the

Section of Cardiac Surgery, Department of Surgery, Yale University School of Medicine, Yale-New Haven Hospital, PO Box 208039, New Haven, CT 06520-8039, USA
E-mail address: john.elefteriades@yale.edu

Cardiol Clin 28 (2010) 223–228
doi:10.1016/j.ccl.2010.01.015
0733-8651/10/$ – see front matter © 2010 Published by Elsevier Inc.

Table 1
Relationship between exertion and aortic dissection

No.	Occupation	Age	Sex	Treated At	Family History	Activity	Aortic Size (cm)	Type of Dissection	Surgery	Outcome
1	Student	24	M	Yale	Yes	Weight lifting	5.5	Asc	Yes	Alive
2	Student	19	M		No	Weight lifting	5.0	Asc	No	Dead[a]
3	Salesman	53	M	Yale	No	Weight lifting	4.0	Asc	Yes	Alive
4	Policeman	37	M	Yale	No	Push-ups	5.0	Asc	Yes	Alive
5	Security	52	M		No	Push-ups		Asc	No	Dead[b]
6	Attorney	68	M		No	Weight lifting (175 lb)	Dilated	Asc	Yes	Dead
7	Signalman	55	M		No	Lifting generator (80 lb)	3.0	Asc	Yes	Dead
8	Repairman	44	M		No	Lifting tank (400 lb)	7.8	Asc	Yes	Alive
9	Professor	49	M		No	Weight lifting	6.3	Asc	Yes	Alive
10	Writer	43	M		No	Weight lifting (300 lb)		Asc	No	Dead[b]
11	Social worker	42	M		No	Weight lifting	4.0	Asc	Yes	Alive
12	Surgeon	63	M		Yes	Weight lifting	3.8	Desc	Yes	Alive
13	Mason	34	M		No	Lifting concrete blocks (150 lb)	4.0	Desc	No	Alive
14	Priest	56	M		No	Weight lifting (250 lb)	3.0	Asc	Yes	Alive
15	Businessman	40	M		No	Weight lifting	6.9	Asc	Yes	Alive
16	Journalist	50	M		No	Weight lifting (500 lb)		Asc	Yes	Alive
17	Surgeon	43	M		No	Intense swimming	4.0	Asc	Yes	Alive
18	Mason	75	M	Yale	No	Intense swimming	6.0	Asc	Yes	Alive

#	Occupation	Age	Sex	School	Prior	Event	Size	Location	Imaging	Status
19	Clerk	49	F	Yale	No	Pulling hard against large dog	4.3	Asc	Yes	Alive
20	Professor	74	M	Yale	No	Intense tennis	4.0	Desc	Yes	Alive
21	Mailman-ret	76	M	Yale	No	Moving heavy boxes	4.3	Desc	Yes	Alive
22	Unemployed	35	M	Yale	No	Exercising	3.1	Asc	Yes	Alive
23	Computers	50	M	Yale	No	Changing storm windows	6.0	Asc	Yes	Dead
24	Security guard	48	M	Yale	No	Intense swimming	4.9	Asc	Yes	Alive
25	Businessman	35	M	Yale	No	Intense racquetball	4.1	Asc	Yes	Alive
26	Machinist	50	M	Yale	No	Shoveling snow		Asc	Yes	Alive[c]
27	Mechanic	51	M	Yale	Yes	Weight lifting	6.0	Asc	Yes	Alive[c]
28	-	37	M		No	Weight lifting		Asc	No	Dead[b]
29	Construction	35	M		No	Lifted power washer from truck	4.1	Asc	No	Dead[b]
30	Mover	38	M		No	Carried freezer 2 flights (700 lb)	4.3	Asc	No	Dead[b]
31	Engineer	43	M		No	Weight lifting	4.0	Asc	Yes	Dead

Abbreviations: Asc, ascending; Desc, descending; M, male.

[a] Diagnosis made by imaging (echocardiogram or computed tomography), but patient not transferred in time for surgery.
[b] Diagnosis not made during life. Postmortem confirmatory.
[c] Prior type B dissection.

inability to reach attention in time, the outcome was lethal.

These observations spurred further clinical investigations. Our residents and students interviewed all patients and their family members treated at Yale University for acute aortic dissection. The pain of aortic dissection is usually so severe that patients and families remember exactly what they were doing at the instant that the pain occurred. It was found (**Fig. 1**) that in nearly two-thirds of cases, patients or family members remembered either a severe exertion or a severe emotional event immediately preceding the onset of dissection pain.[3] Emotional events included being told of a cancer diagnosis, disruption of a marriage, bad business meetings, and loss of loved ones.

These findings prompted us to perform some physiologic investigations. We measured blood pressure during weightlifting in ourselves, using an apparatus developed at our institution that could record instantaneous blood pressure without an arterial line.[4] We found that weight lifting was accompanied by extraordinary elevations of blood pressure (**Fig. 2**), maximal during the effort cycle of the lift. Pressures can easily exceed 300 mm Hg (even higher in professionals), a degree of hypertension simply not seen in other settings, even in intensive care unit environments.

These observations improved our conception of the inciting events leading to acute aortic dissection. We used to believe that the onset of an acute aortic dissection was random. We now believe that this is far from a random process, specifically, that a particular sequence of events leads up to an acute aortic dissection, and explains its choice of a particular date and time to occur (**Fig. 3**). Specifically, a genetic predisposition might lead to destruction of the aortic wall components, at least

partially through excess activity of the lytic matrix metalloproteinases. This description of the events underlying the pathophysiology of aortic dissection, oversimplified for purposes of illustration, is beyond the scope of thisarticle, but is detailed elsewhere.[5] This pathologic sequence of events leads to dilatation of the aorta, which increases mechanical stress.[6] Then, a particular exertion or emotional event, via transient severe hypertension, overwhelms the strength of the aortic wall, leading to an intimal tear and a consequent aortic dissection.

A diagram from in vivo studies of the mechanical properties of the human aorta illustrates vividly how hypertension in the setting of an enlarged aorta can easily exceed the inherent tensile strength of the aortic wall (**Fig. 4**).

The evidence discussed earlier indicates that young athletes with unknown moderate enlargement of the ascending aorta are prone to aortic dissection during exertion. These data strongly suggest a link to transient, severe hypertension during the intense athletic effort. Promising young athletes are dying from this phenomenon. It is for this reason that we suggest routine echocardiographic examination of young athletes. If aortic dilatation is detected, needless death of these young people can be prevented. It is worth noting that the Olympic Committee now requires an echocardiogram before any athlete participates in the Olympic Games. (This recommendation, of course, is made for the detection of not only aneurysms but also cardiomyopathy and idiopathic hypertrophy, which also make the athletes vulnerable).

The counter-argument is that exercise-related aortic dissection is a rare phenomenon in young athletes. This argument is true, but even one such death represents a preventable tragedy. Opponents point out the enormous social

Inciting events for acute aortic dissection

65/90 (66.6%) reported physical/ emotional inciting events:

24/90 (26.6%) physical

36/90 (40%) emotional

Fig. 1. Emotional or exertional events immediately preceding the onset of the pain of acute aortic dissection. (*From* Elefteriades, JA. Thoracic aortic aneurysm: reading the enemy's playbook. Yale J Biol Med 2008;81(4):175–86; with permission.)

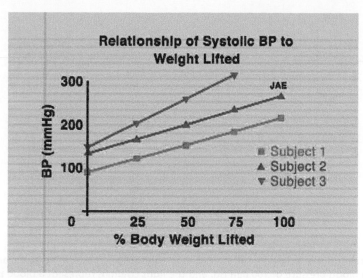

Fig. 2. Even in healthy individuals, blood pressure can soar to astronomic values, exceeding 300 mm Hg, during weightlifting. Subject 1: healthy 16-year-old athlete. Subject 2: the author, who has performed weightlifting since early adolescence. Subject 3: anesthesiologist, former athlete, now sedentary. (*From* Elefteriades, JA. Thoracic aortic aneurysm: reading the enemy's playbook. Yale J Biol Med 2008;81(4):175–86; with permission.)

and evaluation of athletes, which are valid, important considerations. However, in the overall context, echocardiography can be done at a low cost in screening programs like those performed in shopping malls. For professional athletes, the cost of an echocardiogram is miniscule compared with the amount involved in salaries and team costs. Especially for basketball players, an echocardiogram would be important, as the extreme height and joint flexibility that characterize connective tissue disease often make for great basketball players. Even for college and high school athletes, the cost of an echocardiogram would be less than that of high-end athletic shoes for a particular sport, which can cost more than $400 per pair.

The socio-economic objections are therefore cogent. However, even a single preventable death of a young athlete is tragic. We hope that by communicating the connection of exertion with aortic dissection to the general public, awareness can be raised, which would eventuate in at least

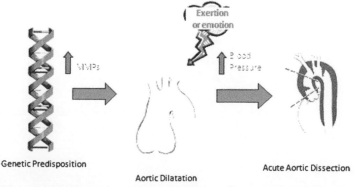

Fig. 3. Overall schematic understanding of how aortic dissection picks a specific time to occur. Note role of acute hypertension from exertion or emotion. (*From* Elefteriades JA, editor. Acute aortic disease. New York: Informa Healthcare; 2007. p. 186; with permission.)

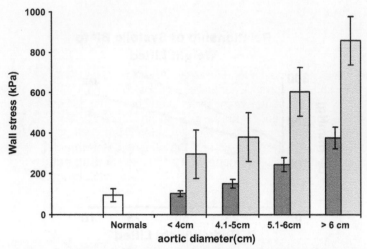

Fig. 4. Exponential relationship between wall stress and aneurysm size in ascending aortic aneurysms. The dark columns represent a blood pressure of 100 mm Hg, and the light columns represent a blood pressure of 200 mm Hg. The lines at 800–1000 kPa represent the range of maximum tensile strength of the human aorta. Note that a patient with a 6-cm aorta will "flirt" with the ultimate tensile strength of the aorta anytime during the course of a day when his blood pressure exceeds 200 mm Hg. (*From* Koullias G, Modak R, Tranquilli M et al. Mechanical deterioration underlies malignant behavior of aneurysmal human ascending aorta. J Thorac Cardiovasc Surg 2005;130:681; with permission.)

some of the athletic population at risk being screened proactively.

REFERENCES

1. Elefteriades JA, Hatzaras I, Tranquilli M, et al. Weight lifting and rupture of silent aortic aneurysms. JAMA 2003;290:2803.
2. Hatzaras I, Tranquilli M, Coady M, et al. Weight lifting and aortic dissection: more evidence for a connection. Cardiology 2007;107:103–6.
3. Hatzaras IS, Bible JE, Koullias GJ, et al. Role of exertion or emotion as inciting events for acuteaortic dissection. Am J Cardiol 2007;100:1470–2.
4. Elefteriades JA. Beating a sudden killer. Sci Am 2005; 293(2):64–71.
5. Elefteriades JA. Thoracic aortic aneurysm: reading the enemy's playbook. Curr Probl Cardiol 2008;33: 203–77.
6. Koullias G, Modak R, Tranquilli M, et al. Mechanical deterioration underlies malignant behavior of aneurysmal human ascending aorta. J Thorac Cardiovasc Surg 2005;130:677–83.

Routine Screening of Young Athletes for Aneurysm: CON

Jaime Gerber, MD[a,b,*], Michael Arcarese, MD[a]

KEYWORDS
- Echocardiography • Acute aortic syndrome
- Screening program • Marfan syndrome

The death of a young athlete is a particularly devastating moment in any society because these individuals represent our strengths and physical prowess as human beings. For this reason, the concept of preparticipation screening has captured attention. This article examines the scope of the problem from the perspective of acute aortic syndrome and aortic death, and reviews ways, if any, to systematically screen the population to help eradicate this wanton killer of gifted young athletes.

WHAT ARE THE CHARACTERISTICS OF A SUCCESSFUL SCREENING PROGRAM?

A routine screening program applied nonselectively to a particular population in the hopes of reducing morbidity and mortality from a disease must meet certain criteria to be useful. First, the disease must be sufficiently common to justify the cost and effort involved with screening. Second, the testing modality must show the characteristics of reliability, validity, yield, and acceptance.[1] In the case of thoracic aortic disease there is general agreement that the tools that are available, predominantly transthoracic echocardiography, are reliable and valid in documenting the presence of aortic, valvular, and ascending aortic pathology.[2] Compared with transesophageal echocardiography, newer modalities such as magnetic resonance imaging and multidetector computed tomography show a pooled sensitivity of 98% to 100% and a specificity of 95% to 98%.[3] Although these imaging techniques show great promise for enhanced diagnostic accuracy in the setting of complications of aortic disease, such as dissection or aortic rupture, they are not suitable for screening at this point because of the attendant cost, complexity, and the irradiation they entail. The expected yield of the screening program of echocardiography in detecting individuals at risk for aortic dissection or rupture during athletics is low. Finally, effective therapeutic interventions, including medical therapy, surgical repair, or avoidance of sports activities, must be at hand to improve outcomes of the disease being screened. Consistent data showing the effectiveness of medical therapy to prevent aortic complications are lacking at this point in time.[4]

WHAT ARE THE COST AND LEGAL RAMIFICATIONS OF A SCREENING PROGRAM TO REDUCE SUDDEN AORTIC DEATH?

A cost-sensitive environment that serves as a brake on the implementation of imaging-based screening programs exists globally. Considering not just aortic disease but the full spectrum of cardiovascular disorders that may result in sudden cardiac death (SCD), the cost per life-year saved by screening high school athletes alone is estimated to be in excess of $20,000; with a national cost of conducting echocardiographic screening estimated to be $245 million.[5] This national cost is not supportable for a single program. False-positive results will occur that may lead to untoward

a Section of Cardiology, Yale University School of Medicine, 333 Cedar Street, New Haven, CT 06510, USA
b Cardiology Associates of New Haven, 1591 Boston Post Road, Guilford, CT 6437, USA
* Corresponding author. Section of Cardiology, Yale University School of Medicine, 333 Cedar Street, New Haven, CT 06510.
E-mail address: jgerber@ca-nh.com

Cardiol Clin 28 (2010) 229–236
doi:10.1016/j.ccl.2010.01.010

emotional consequences and unwarranted restrictions on some athletes. Further, the costs associated with additional evaluation of these individuals will be substantial (**Table 1**).

Medicolegal concerns may arise within the scope of implementation of a screening program.[6] Currently, the United States cardiology community does not have a consensus regarding the preparticipation screening of athletes against the risk of sudden aortic death or other causes of SCD. This health issue must now be discussed with each individual athlete and reviewed as a matter of policy by each athletic governing body on a local level. The establishment of consensus guidelines may have the effect nationally of creating expectations of a standard of care that may not be fulfilled. This point needs to be carefully considered in the context of the health care system's ability to provide the requisite screening tools, and shoulder the cost of that screening as well as provide unfettered access to further evaluation should that become necessary. The medical delivery system seems inadequate to this charge at the current time.

Socioeconomic and racial disparities in access to care further complicate the implementation of screening programs and the interpretation of worldwide results. The Italian experience and other non-US publications largely reflect the experience of populations far more homogeneous than the Unites States experience, where more than 100 million minorities reside and 40% of the elite athletes who encounter field deaths are nonwhite.[7,8]

WHAT IS THE INCIDENCE OF SUDDEN AORTIC DEATH IN THE ATHLETE?

A potentially lethal entity, acute aortic syndrome is an exceedingly rare phenomenon in young athletes. Selection and reporting bias diminish the accuracy of published reports, although recent efforts provide some guidance.

The US National Registry of Sudden Death reviewed 1866 SCDs (including resuscitated events) in young athletes over a 27-year period from 1980 to 2006. The incidence of SCD was determined to be 0.61 per 100,000 athlete-years. There is a significant gender bias, with 89% of the SCDs occurring in young men, and a racial bias, with a disproportionate number among African American athletes. A structurally normal heart was found in the majority (53%) of cases during postmortem evaluation, with death therefore believed to be caused by arrhythmia.[7] Among the deaths attributed to a structural cardiac anomaly, only 3.3% were determined to be of acute aortic origin. The largest proportion was attributable to hypertrophic cardiomyopathy (36%), coronary artery anomalies (17%), and congenital aortic stenosis (2.7%). Further, underscoring the gender gap, a study from Eckart found that only 15 sudden deaths occurred in 852,300 women military recruits during 1977 to 2001. In[9] this series, 81% of the deaths were deemed likely to be from a cardiac cause, with no cases of acute aortic pathology reported.

How do these data compare with those obtained in other parts of the world? SCD in

Table 1
Costs and characteristics of preparticipation screening programs of high school athletes

Parameters	AHA-Specific CV History and Physical	12-Lead ECG	2-D Echo
Sensitivity	6%	70%	80%
Specificity	97.8%	84.3%	100%
Cost to screen 700,000 HSA annually	$0	$7 million	$245 million
Cost to evaluate abnormal responses annually	$7.7 million	$40.2 million	$0 dollars
Total cost to screen 700,000 HSA annually	$77 million	$47.2 million	$245 million
Total amount of life gained from 700,000 HSA screened annually	92 y	1080 y	1232 y
Cost per year of life saved	$84,000	$44,000	$200,000

Abbreviations: 2-D, 2-dimensional; AHA, American Heart Association; CV, cardiovascular; ECG, electrocardiogram; HSA, high school athlete.
   Data from Fuller CM. Cost-effectiveness analysis of screening of high school athletes for risk of sudden cardiac death. Med Sci Sports Exerc 2000;32(5):887–90.

athletes from the Veneto region in Italy, initially reported from 1979 to 1999, appeared to be higher than in the United States, with a reported incidence of 2.1 per 100,000 athlete-years. The proportion of attributed acute aortic deaths was similar to the United States experience at approximately 2% of events. This low incidence of acute aortic pathology in the young athlete is confirmed in the Norwegian experience[10] in which there were no acute aortic deaths reported among the 0.9 SCDs per 100,000 athlete-years. Additional series from Sweden and Australia included the nonathlete and older subjects, and revealed slightly higher rates of acute aortic pathology consistent with the role of atherosclerosis and hypertension in the development of acute aortic dissection.

Therefore, the incidence of SCD in the athletes is low and the segment of deaths attributable to acute aortic pathology is in the range of 2% to 3% of all cardiac events; both observations limiting the applicability of routine echocardiographic screening.

Although there are no systematic studies of echocardiographic screening of the young athlete at this time, some lessons from the Italian experience using electrocardiographic screening may be considered. The impact of electrocardiographic screening has been studied[11] in the Veneto region of Italy, where it has been mandatory since 1982. Of the 33,735 young athletes screened, only 8.9% were referred for echocardiography based on abnormal physical examination, family history, or abnormal electrocardiographic findings. Of these 3002 patients referred for echocardiography, only 22 (0.6%) were found to have evidence of hypertrophic cardiomyopathy. No cases of aortic pathology were reported. An assessment in the racially dissimilar United States population

estimates that approximately 10% of high school athletes would require echocardiography based on an initial screening with physical examination, electrocardiography, and family history.[5] **Fig. 1** compares the incidence of SCD in the athletes in Minnesota with that of the athletes in Veneto.

The impact of the reduced sudden death rates in this region is notable, and has led to calls for increased screening of all athletes. The reasons for this reduction are not clear but may include an excess of early deaths in the Italian experience caused by arrhythmogenic right ventricular dysplasia in the Veneto region. Subsequently the incidence of athletic sudden death in the Italian population has declined to parity with that in the United States experience.[8] Notable in both these experiences is the paucity of deaths caused by acute aortic syndrome, with the cause of sudden death in the athletes in both populations predominantly being cardiomyopathies, myocarditis, congenital coronary artery anomalies, Brugada or long QT syndrome, and congenital aortic stenosis. No deaths during the reporting period were caused by acute aortic pathology. In summary, it seems that screening with echocardiography would not be useful in reducing death from acute aortic syndrome in that the rate of SCD in the young athlete is low, with aortic pathology being responsible for a vanishingly small number of those events.

WHAT ARE THE CAUSES OF ACUTE AORTIC SYNDROME AND SUDDEN AORTIC DEATH?

Sudden aortic death occurs as a result of a complication of aortic disease, either acute aortic dissection or rupture of the aorta. This complication may occur in the setting of a thoracic aneurysm or equally frequently in those with normal-sized

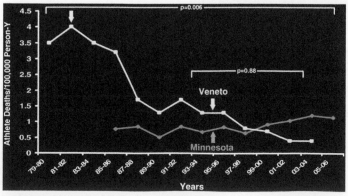

Fig. 1. The incidence of SCD in athletes in Minnesota versus Veneto. (*From* Maron BJ, Haas TS, Doerer JJ, et al. Comparison of US and Italian experiences with sudden cardiac deaths in young competitive athletes and implications for preparticipation screening strategies. Am J Cardiol 2009;104(2):276–80; with permission.)

aortas on echo. Most cases of aortic dissection do not occur during physical activity,[12] with a predilection for dissection during the morning hours. Though dramatic and notable, sudden deaths during competition are rare.[12] Spontaneous aortic dissection has been reported to occur during participation in basketball, football, swimming, and weight lifting.[13,14] The rheological forces and biochemical milieu induced during maximal effort are suspected to play a role in inducing aortic dissection or rupture in susceptible individuals.

Most aortic dissections are caused by acquired diseases. Chronic hypertension is present in 75% of all subjects with aortic dissection.[15] Intramural hematoma, a complication of atherosclerotic disease of the aorta,[16] occurs more frequently in older patients and progresses to dissection in 16% of cases. Cocaine use, trauma, deceleration injuries, prior thoracic vascular surgery, or cardiac percutaneous intervention may also be associated with acute aortic syndrome. These subjects are those who would fall out of our consideration for screening for athletic participation because of their age and detectable comorbidities. **Fig. 2** shows a characteristic image of Type A aortic dissection.

Heritable disorders of the aorta would be targeted when screening for athletic participation. The classic heritable disorder is Marfan syndrome (**Fig. 3**), an autosomal dominant trait characterized by a mutation in the fibrillin-1 (*FBN1*) gene located on chromosome 15 that encodes for extracellular matrix protein.[4] Marfan syndrome is a multisystem disorder primarily involving the musculoskeletal, cardiovascular, and ocular systems, and is

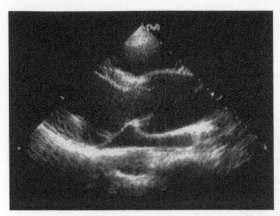

Fig. 3. Echocardiographic image typical of Marfan involvement of the aortic root showing dilatation at the root level, effacement of the sinotubular junction, absence of calcifications, and the normal appearing aortic valve insertion and leaflets. (*From* Kornbluth M, Schnittger I, Eyngorina I, et al. Clinical outcome in the Marfan syndrome with ascending aortic dilatation followed annually by echocardiography. Am J Cardiol 1999;84(6):753–5; with permission.)

diagnosed through application of the Ghent criteria documenting 3-organ involvement, including assessment of aortic size in suspected individuals. The incidence of Marfan syndrome in the general population is estimated at 1 in 100,000, with as many as 80% of those subjects manifesting aortic dilatation at presentation. The clinical criteria, if met, have a 95% concordance rate for mutation in *FBN1*.[17] Other heritable diseases that may lead to acute aortic syndrome are bicuspid aortic valve with aneurysm, Ehlers-Danlos syndrome, Turner syndrome, familial aortic dissection, and annuloaortic ectasia.[18] Common among the pathophysiology of these conditions are medial degeneration, activation of matrix metalloproteinases, and decreased fibrillin-1 activity leading to weakening of the aortic wall and an increased risk of dissection. These chemical abnormalities may allow the future development of biomarkers to detect those at risk of aortic dissection.

CAN SCREENING ECHOCARDIOGRAPHY IDENTIFY THOSE AT RISK FOR SUDDEN AORTIC DEATH?

The incidence of aortic dissection increases as a function of the size of the aorta.[19] This may occur at the aortic root, sinotubular junction, sinuses of Valsalva, or ascending aorta level.[20] This is not to say that only those subjects with enlarged aortas are at risk for aortic complications. Approximately half of the individuals who suffer aortic dissection

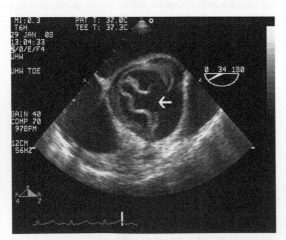

Fig. 2. Characteristic image of a Type A aortic dissection showing intimal flap. (*From* Morimoto N, Okada K, Okita Y. Aortic regurgitation and coronary malperfusion secondary to intimo-intimal intussusception into the left ventricle in acute aortic dissection. Eur J Cardiothorac Surg 2009;36:189–90; with permission.)

do not have significantly dilated aortas. According to currently accepted criteria for replacement (5.5 cm), most patients presenting with acute aortic dissection would not meet current published criteria for elective aortic replacement surgery based on the size of their aorta alone.[20,21] Gender differences also exist whereby in one study, 12% of women with aortic dissection were found to present with an aortic size less than 4.0 cm[22,23] The presence of a family history of aortic dissection along with aortic symptoms constitutes a significant risk setting for aortic syndrome, perhaps more predictive than aortic size alone.[24] Therefore, the presence of a normal-sized aortic root or ascending aorta on echocardiographic study does not confer a risk of dissection similar to background risk. The areas of involvement in Type A and Type B dissection are shown in **Fig. 4**.

WHAT CONSTITUTES NORMAL AORTIC SIZE?

The determination of normal aortic size, and by extension, the delineation of accurate thresholds for high-risk aortic size are based on scant data.[25] This was recently revisited, allowing nomograms to be constructed based on age, gender, and body surface area.[26] The observations of this study, that ascending aortic dimensions greater than or equal to 4.6 cm (men) and greater than or equal to 4.3 (women) are abnormal, contradicts the notion that aortic complications can be predicted with any assurance based on aortic size alone. Observations from the pediatric literature[27] propose a ratio between the aortic root and the descending thoracic aorta as a more accurate determinant of dissection risk in Marfan syndrome. The aortic index as a predictor of rupture risk is also proposed for the adult

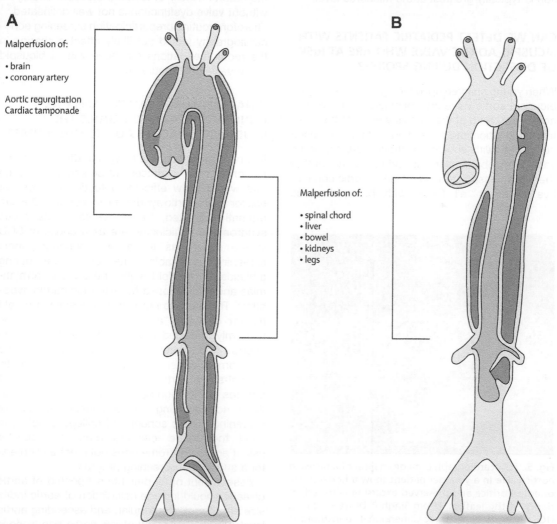

A

Malperfusion of:

• brain
• coronary artery

Aortic regurgitation
Cardiac tamponade

B

Malperfusion of:

• spinal chord
• liver
• bowel
• kidneys
• legs

Fig. 4. Areas of involvement in Type A and Type B dissection. (*From* Golledge J, Eagle KA. Acute aortic dissection. Lancet 2008;372:55–66; with permission.)

population,[28] thus correcting the raw aortic measurement for body surface area. Therefore, there is no single or consolidated criterion on which to base echocardiographic preparticipation screening for sudden aortic syndrome, as normal aortic size is poorly defined and dissection may occur in an ostensibly normal-sized aorta.

The most common[29] hereditable cardiac condition is bicuspid aortic valve (**Fig. 5**) with aneurysm, and it is associated with risk for aortic dissection and rupture. The incidence of bicuspid aortic valve is reported to range between 0.46% (echocardiographic studies) and 1.37% (autopsy results),[30,31] and may be associated with ascending aortic aneurysm on initial echo. Up to 37% of children evaluated show aortic enlargement on initial echocardiogram. The morphology differs somewhat from patients with Marfan syndrome, in that dilatation is typically greatest at the midaortic level.[32]

CAN WE DETECT PEDIATRIC PATIENTS WITH BICUSPID AORTIC VALVE WHO ARE AT RISK OF DISSECTION DURING SPORTS?

When young children up to the age of 19 years with bicuspid aortic valve are considered, the average aortic size, both at the root as well as at the sinotubular junction and ascending aorta, is increased compared with subjects without bicuspid aortic valve, This observation supports the concept that there is an associated defect in the aortic connective tissue in all those with bicuspid aortic

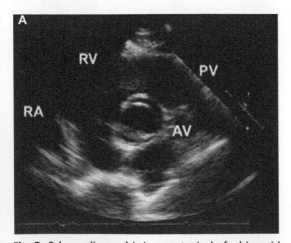

Fig. 5. Echocardiographic images typical of a bicuspid aortic valve in a younger patient show a horizontally oriented orifice and preserved excursion with redundancy of the leaflets. (*From* Singh P, Dutta R, Nanda NC. Live/real time three-dimensional transthoracic echocardiographic assessment of bicuspid aortic valve morphology. Echocardiography 2009;26:478–80; with permission.)

valve.[33,34] However, most of those children have aortic measurements within the normal range for their age as determined by nomogram. Therefore an echocardiographic screening program would have difficulty separating those subjects with aortic involvement in bicuspid aortic disease and be expected to miss some who are at risk for dissection. Associated aortic valve dysfunction is common in bicuspid aortic valve. Whether the degree of aortic enlargement and, by association, the risk of aortic dissection or rupture is affected by valvular dysfunction is an unsettled question.[35,36] The incidence of aortic dissection is increased in individuals with a bicuspid aortic valve, believed by some to be a situation similar to that of the patient with Marfan syndrome, although the data on patients with bicuspid aortic aneurysm without valve dysfunction are scant and the natural history of isolated bicuspid aneurysm without valve dysfunction is not well delineated.[31] Therefore routine preparticipation screening echocardiography would not likely effect a change in the recommendations for those with a bicuspid aortic valve and aneurysm.

WHAT MEASURES CAN WE APPLY AS CLINICIANS TODAY TO REDUCE THE INCIDENCE OF ACUTE AORTIC SYNDROME?

It can be seen from the foregoing discussion that the criteria for a successful screening program that would allow efficient detection of those at risk for acute aortic syndrome are not met. Despite dramatic, isolated, tragic events, acute aortic syndrome is sufficiently rare as a cause of SCD in the athlete as to make echocardiographic screening untenable. The SCD rate during athletics is manyfold higher because of arrhythmias and undiagnosed hypertrophic cardiomyopathy.[8] The data do not help one identify a herald marker of risk of aortic dissection that can be uniformly identified among those participating in sports, and many persons with acute aortic syndromes suffer dissections with apparently normal-sized aortas. The cost of screening all athletes on the high school level alone is prohibitive,[5] not including the additional expense of screening middle school and college athletes. In short, the routine echocardiogram to screen for risk of aortic syndrome does not meet any criteria for a successful screening program.

Assessment of all patients suspected of aortic disease should include calculation of aortic index size at the root, sinotubular, and ascending aortic levels. Simple reporting of raw aortic size alone is not sufficient to predict risk of aortic syndrome. Medical management of aortic dilatation in Marfan syndrome should at this time include routine use of β-blockers, with atenolol being the agent most studied.[4] The effectiveness of β-blockers in non-Marfanoid aortic dilatation has not been validated, although this agent is commonly used in the hope of reducing hemodynamic stress within a dilated aorta. The routine use of angiotensin II blockers such as losartan[37] holds promise and is under systematic study. Individuals with hypertension and aortic enlargement should be considered for these agents primarily as first-line treatment for hypertension.

Participation in athletics by individuals with aortic dilatation must be assessed on an individual basis. Recommendations to avoid competitive athletics requiring maximal effort, particularly weight lifting that entails achievement of lifting single repetition maximal weight, seems prudent. Moderate degrees of aerobic activity[38,39] maintaining 50% of maximal predicted heart rate have been suggested.

WHAT ARE THE DIRECTIONS FOR RESEARCH?

It seems that the answer to the question of preventing acute aortic syndromes and aortic deaths does not lie in the routine use of imaging studies alone. A targeted multidisciplinary evaluation of the athlete including an accurate family history, screening for hypertension and Marfan syndrome by physical examination, auscultation for murmurs, and selected use of electrocardiography seems to be a firm foundation for screening procedures. Individuals with underlying cardiovascular or metabolic disturbances will need additional attention before participation in competitive sports is allowed. Opportunity clearly exists to more accurately define the morphologic characteristics of the aorta at risk for dissection. The application of reduced-cost ultrasound technologies may also be explored, using handheld machines and trained noncardiologist screeners in selected populations; and a cost analysis study of a novel system of care delivery is timely.

The biochemical commonality among the diseases of the aorta holds promise because inflammatory markers, matrix metalloproteinase, and chromosomal abnormalities have all been described in patients at risk for aortic dissection. Development of serum biomarker assays, along with genetic testing, may allow precise detection of those at risk for this sudden killer. Finally, definitive demonstration of effective medical therapy in reducing mortality and dissection rates in those at risk should ignite much enthusiasm to search systematically for the danger that lurks.

REFERENCES

1. Rutstein DD, Craige E. Screening tests in mass surveys and their use in heart disease case finding. Circulation 1951;4(5):659–65.
2. Cheitlin MD, Alpert JS, Armstrong WF, et al. ACC/AHA guidelines for the clinical application of echocardiography: a report of the American College of Cardiology/American Heart Association Task Force on Practice Guidelines (Committee on Clinical Application of Echocardiography) developed in collaboration with the American Society of Echocardiography. Circulation 1997;95(6):1686–744.
3. Shiga T, Wajima Z, Apfel CC, et al. Diagnostic accuracy of transesophageal echocardiography, helical computed tomography, and magnetic resonance imaging for suspected thoracic aortic dissection: systematic review and meta-analysis. Arch Intern Med 2006;166(13):1350–6.
4. Keane MG, Pyeritz RE. Medical management of Marfan syndrome. Circulation 2008;117(21):2802–13.
5. Fuller CM. Cost effectiveness analysis of screening of high school athletes for risk of sudden cardiac death. Med Sci Sports Exerc 2000;32(5):887–90.
6. Myerburg RJ, Vetter VL. Electrocardiograms should be included in preparticipation screening of athletes. Circulation 2007;116(22):2616–26.
7. Maron BJ, Shirani J, Poliac LC, et al. Sudden death in young competitive athletes: clinical, demographic, and pathological profiles. JAMA 1996;276(3):199–204.
8. Maron BJ, Haas TS, Doerer JJ, et al. Comparison of U.S. and Italian experiences with sudden cardiac deaths in young competitive athletes and implications for preparticipation screening strategies. Am J Cardiol 2009;104(2):276–80.
9. Eckart RE, Scoville SL, Shry EA, et al. Causes of sudden death in young female military recruits. Am J Cardiol 2006;97(12):1756–8.
10. Solberg EE, Gjertsen F, Haugstad E, et al. Sudden death in sports among young adults in Norway. Eur J Cardiovasc Prev Rehabil 2009. [Epub ahead of print].
11. Corrado D, Basso C, Pavei A, et al. Trends in sudden cardiovascular death in young competitive athletes after implementation of a preparticipation screening program. JAMA 2006;296(13):1593–601.
12. Mehta RH, Manfredini R, Hassan F, et al. Chronobiological patterns of acute aortic dissection. Circulation 2002;106(9):1110–5.
13. Hatzaras I, Tranquilli M, Coady M, et al. Weight lifting and aortic dissection: more evidence for a connection. Cardiology 2007;107(2):103–6.
14. Uchida K, Imoto K, Yanagi H, et al. Acute aortic dissection occurring during the butterfly stroke in

a 12-year-old boy. Interact Cardiovasc Thorac Surg 2009;9(2):366–7.

15. Golledge J, Eagle KA. Acute aortic dissection. Lancet 2008;372(9632):55–66.

16. Evangelista A, Mukherjee D, Mehta RH, et al. Acute intramural hematoma of the aorta: a mystery in evolution. Circulation 2005;111(8):1063–70.

17. Loeys BL, Schwarze U, Holm T, et al. Aneurysm syndromes caused by mutations in the TGF-beta receptor. N Engl J Med 2006;355(8):788–98.

18. Caglayan AO, Dundar M. Inherited diseases and syndromes leading to aortic aneurysms and dissections. Eur J Cardiothorac Surg 2009;35(6):931–40.

19. Davies RR, Goldstein LJ, Coady MA, et al. Yearly rupture or dissection rates for thoracic aortic aneurysms: simple prediction based on size. Ann Thorac Surg 2002;73(1):17–28.

20. Meijboom LJ, Timmermans J, Zwinderman AH, et al. Aortic root growth in men and women with the Marfan syndrome. Am J Cardiol 2005;96(10):1441–4.

21. Neri E, Barabesi L, Buklas D, et al. Limited role of aortic size in the genesis of acute type A aortic dissection. Eur J Cardiothorac Surg 2005;28(6):857–63.

22. Parish LM, Gorman JH III, Kahn S, et al. Aortic size in acute type A dissection: implications for preventive ascending aortic replacement. Eur J Cardiothorac Surg 2009;35(6):941–6.

23. Pape LA, Tsai TT, Isselbacher EM, et al. Aortic diameter > = 5.5 cm is not a good predictor of type a aortic dissection: observations from the International Registry of Acute Aortic Dissection (IRAD). Circulation 2007;116(10):1120–7.

24. Elefteriades JA, Tranquilli M, Darr U, et al. Symptoms plus family history trump size in thoracic aortic aneurysm. Ann Thorac Surg 2005;80(3):1098–100.

25. Vasan RS, Larson MG, Levy D. Determinants of echocardiographic aortic root size: the Framingham Heart Study. Circulation 1995;91(3):734–40.

26. Biaggi P, Matthews F, Braun J, et al. Gender, age, and body surface area are the major determinants of ascending aorta dimensions in subjects with apparently normal echocardiograms. J Am Soc Echocardiogr 2009;22(6):720–5.

27. Kemna MS, Murphy DJ, Silverman NH. Screening for aortic root dilation in Marfan syndrome using the ratio of the aortic root to descending aortic diameters in children. J Am Soc Echocardiogr 2009; 22(10):1109–13.

28. Davies RR, Gallo A, Coady MA, et al. Novel measurement of relative aortic size predicts rupture of thoracic aortic aneurysms. Ann Thorac Surg 2006;81(1):169–77.

29. Nistri S, Basso C, Marzari C, et al. Frequency of bicuspid aortic valve in young male conscripts by echocardiogram. Am J Cardiol 2005;96(5):718–21.

30. Roberts WC. The congenitally bicuspid aortic valve: a study of 85 autopsy cases. Am J Cardiol 1970; 26(1):72–83.

31. Basso C, Boschello M, Perrone C, et al. An echocardiographic survey of primary school children for bicuspid aortic valve. Am J Cardiol 2004;93(5): 661–3.

32. Cecconi M, Nistri S, Quarti A, et al. Aortic dilatation in patients with bicuspid aortic valve. J Cardiovasc Med 2006;7(1):11–20.

33. Ward C. Clinical significance of the bicuspid aortic valve. Heart 2000;83(1):81–5.

34. Tadros TM, Klein MD, Shapira OM. Ascending aortic dilatation associated with bicuspid aortic valve: pathophysiology, molecular biology, and clinical implications. Circulation 2009;119(6):880–90.

35. Della Corte A, Romano G, Tizzano F, et al. Echocardiographic anatomy of ascending aorta dilatation: correlations with aortic valve morphology and function. Int J Cardiol 2006;113(3):320–6.

36. Warren AE, Boyd ML, O'Connell C, et al. Dilatation of the ascending aorta in paediatric patients with bicuspid aortic valve: frequency, rate of progression and risk factors. Heart 2006;92(10):1496–500.

37. Habashi JP, Judge DP, Holm TM, et al. Losartan, an AT1 antagonist, prevents aortic aneurysm in a mouse model of Marfan syndrome. Science 2006;312: 117–21.

38. Braverman AC. Exercise and the Marfan syndrome. Med Sci Sports Exerc 1998;30:S387–95.

39. Maron BJ, Chaitman BR, Ackerman MJ, et al. Recommendations for physical activity and recreational sports participation for young patients with genetic cardiovascular diseases. Circulation 2004; 109:2807–16.

Editorial Comment: Routine Screening of Young Athletes for Aneurysm

John A. Elefteriades, MD

In his article in this issue of *Cardiology Clinics*, Dr Jaime Gerber makes an excellent, well-reasoned case that all sudden cardiac deaths are extremely rare in young athletes and that aortic-related deaths are a very small subgroup of sudden deaths (**Table 1**). He recognizes that echocardiography is very effective at imaging the aorta but indicates that exactly what constitutes aortic enlargement is not totally clear. He makes the case that the cost of screening is unjustifiable.

The article by Dr John A. Elefteriades establishes the link of strength training–type exercise with hypertension. He links hypertension with high wall tension in the human aorta. He makes an emotional plea for routine, low-cost, mass echo screening.

The weight of evidence is on the con side of the argument, as shown in **Fig. 1**.

Table 1 Routine echo screening of young athletes for aortic aneurysms	
Pro: Athletes Should be Screened (Elefteriades)	**Con: Athletes Need Not be Screened (Gerber)**
Aortic dissection does occurs in young athletes with unsuspected moderate aortic enlargement (4–5 cm)	Sudden death of young athletes is not sufficiently common to justify screening (1866 cases over 27 years in the United States)
This senseless loss of promising young lives needs to be stopped	Of those deaths, more than 50% were judged to be because of arrhythmia, as there was no structural cardiac abnormality. Only 3.3% were caused by acute aortic disease
The link between exercise and extreme instantaneous hypertension has been demonstrated	
Aortic wall tension "flirts" with the ultimate tensile strength of the aorta in patients with moderate aortic enlargement and moderate hypertension	
Although there are socio-economic issues, the cost of a mass echo is less than that of high-end sports shoes	

Section of Cardiac Surgery, Department of Surgery, Yale University School of Medicine, Yale-New Haven Hospital, PO Box 208039, New Haven, CT 06520-8039, USA
E-mail address: john.elefteriades@yale.edu

Cardiol Clin 28 (2010) 237–238
doi:10.1016/j.ccl.2010.02.009
0733-8651/10/$ – see front matter

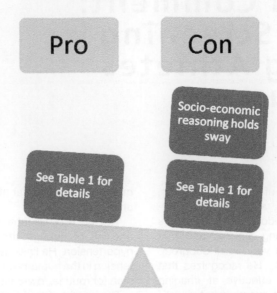

Fig. 1. Although the emotional impact of the needless loss of the life of a promising young athlete is strong, socio-economic reasoning (especially vis-à-vis the rarity of exercise-related sudden aortic death) holds sway.

Physicians Should be Legally Liable for Missing an Atypical Aortic Dissection: PRO

Moses Lebovits, BA, JD

KEYWORDS
- Legal • Liability • Standard of care • Diagnosis

Any discussion of the potential legal exposure of a health care provider for the failure to diagnose and treat a medical condition is premised on multiple considerations. The legal profession must ask (1) does the case have merit, (2) what harm was caused by the act of omission or commission, (3) what damages were suffered as a result of that conduct, and (4) what are the chances of success and the economic reality of pursuing the claim. A meritorious claim may well be declined by attorneys or not brought at all because of economics. The unfortunate and unnecessary death of an elderly patient may be declined simply because the hard reality of economics is that it could cost as much to prosecute the claim as the potential verdict that may be achieved.

As a result of many competing factors, including economics, medical malpractice claims since the year 2000 are down 45%, medical malpractice premiums are less than one-half of 1% of the country's overall health care costs, and medical malpractice claims are a mere one-fifth of 1% of health care costs. Yet medical malpractice insurer profits are higher than the rest of the property casualty industry.[1] Most statistics lend no credence to the claim that there is substantial frivolous litigation within the medical malpractice system. In fact, contingency fees and the prevalence of medical errors make the pursuit of "meritless" lawsuits bad business.[2–4] "Previous research has established that the great majority of patients who sustain a medical injury as a result of negligence do not sue."[2,5,6] Studdert and colleagues[2] found that claims that lack evidence of the error are not uncommon, but most are denied compensation, and that the overall claims not involving errors accounted for only 13% to 16% of the system's total monetary cost.[7] "The malpractice system performs reasonably well in its function of separating claims without merit from those with merit and compensating the latter. In a sense, the author's findings lend support to this view that three-quarters of the litigation outcomes were concordant with the merits of the claim."[2]

THE MALPRACTICE SYSTEM: COMMISSION OF A TORT

So if the malpractice system performs reasonably well, why? The author submits it does so because ultimately the tort system that employs expert testimony and jury trials works well. Malpractice is a subset of torts. "Tort" comes from the Latin word "tortus" or twisted. So is a tort a conduct that is twisted or wrong? One definition of a tort, over 100 years old, is "an act or omission, not a mere breach of contract, and producing injury to another, in the absence of any existing lawful relation of which such act or omission is a natural outgrowth or incident."[8] Therefore, whether a physician commits a tort (malpractice) for an atypical presentation is based on his or her conduct. In modern parlance; did he or she breach the standard of care, did that breach cause harm, and what is the extent and severity of the injuries?

Daniels, Fine, Israel, Schonbuch & Lebovits, LLP, 1801 Century Park East, Ninth Floor, Los Angeles, CA 90067, USA

E-mail address: lebovits@dfis-law.com

Cardiol Clin 28 (2010) 239–244
doi:10.1016/j.ccl.2010.01.004
0733-8651/10/$ – see front matter © 2010 Elsevier Inc. All rights reserved.

The question of whether a physician should be legally liable for missing an atypical aortic dissection, recognizing that more than half of the cases are not suspected antemortem, is answered by various definitions of negligence and standard of care.

STANDARD OF CARE

In California (and almost all states have similar definitions), professional negligence is defined as a negligent act or omission to act by a health care provider in the rendering of professional services which act or omission is the legal cause of the personal injury or wrongful death, provided that such services were within the scope of services for which the provider was licensed and not within any restriction imposed by the licensing agency or hospital.[9] The California Supreme Court has supported the broad interpretation of the concept of professional negligence.[10]

The standard of care for physicians and surgeons requires that they exercise that degree of skill, knowledge, and care ordinarily possessed and exercised by other members of the profession acting under similar conditions and circumstances.[11] If a treatment proves unsuccessful or if the natural course of the patient's disease or condition resulted in their death, it does not raise the presumption of liability.[12] Typically, standard of care is provided by the opinion testimony of a medical expert. In California, *Evidence Code* Section 801(b) addresses this and in the Federal Court the Federal Rules of Evidence 702, 703, and 705 do the same.

To prove that a physician is legally liable for missing an atypical aortic dissection the plaintiff must prove (1) the physician owed a legal duty of care to that plaintiff or that individual's family (typically that is not an issue when a physician is caring for a patient in a hospital setting); (2) there was an act of commission or omission by the defendant, that is, the breach of the duty or breach of the standard of care; (3) that there is injury, damage, or death to the individual; and (4) that the physician's breach of duty was the legal cause of that injury, damage, or death.[13]

Is there a breach of the standard of care for the failure to diagnose an atypical presentation of an aortic dissection? As noted above, California Evidence Code section 801(b) and Federal Rules of Evidence 702, 703, and 705 require the opinion testimony of a medical expert as to whether there was a breach of the standard of care; or, as stated previously, did the physician or surgeon, whether it be the internist, emergency room physician, or cardiothoracic surgeon, exercise that degree of skilled care, learning, and knowledge ordinarily possessed and exercised by other members acting under similar conditions?

The question regarding standard of care requires an understanding of the circumstances under which the failure to recognize the atypical presentation occurred. Did it occur in an office setting? Did it occur in an emergency room? Was it in a large metropolitan center, whether in Los Angeles, St Louis, or Miami; or was it in a small regional institution? The author would argue that smaller regional institutions, if they offer an emergency room and provide surgical care, should be held to the same standard as any major metropolitan hospital including those with a major university. Each of these institutions is mandated by its hospital accreditations to set out various protocols and procedures, many in writing, and manuals for the operation of their emergency room, catheterization laboratories, and other departments. Those procedures and protocols will set out, for example, the order set in the emergency department for chest pain and catheterization laboratory, acute myocardial infarction (AMI) diagnosis, and treatment. The vast majority of these institutions require stat laboratory tests to include troponin, complete blood count, basic metabolic panel, lipid panel, portable chest radiograph, and further cardiac studies if there is indeed chest pain. **Fig. 1** is an example of such a protocol in a large metropolitan center.

Department Order Set: E.D. CHEST PAIN/ Cath Lab AMI			
Date & Door Time:	Please use a ballpoint pen and press firmly.		
Delete those orders denoted by an "X" over the number. Check appropriate box where choice indicated			
File original in chart, and send copy to Pharmacy			
Emergency Dept. CHEST PAIN		Time completed	Initials
1.	STAT 12-Lead ECG (CI chest pain) § Code AMI called at:_____		
2.	Cardiac monitor		
3.	STAT Labs/Tests:Troponin, Basic Metabolic Panel, Lipid Panel, Portable Chest X-ray, A/P now (CI chest pain)		
4.	Additional Labs/Tests:		

Fig. 1. Department order set: Emergency Department. Chest pain/catheterization laboratory AMI.

Furthermore, many institutions will have specific policies for admission for AMI, which would include a physical examination targeted to exclude the well-known mimics of AMI, including aortic dissection. **Fig. 2** is an example of a protocol for Code A.M.I. in a large metropolitan center.

A lawyer examining the question of whether there was a failure to follow the standard of care should look to see if such protocols existed and whether in fact they were followed. He or she should determine, if the protocols were not followed, whether that breach was a "legal" cause of the harm suffered by the patient.

MEDICAL LITERATURE AND EXPERT TESTIMONY INFORMS THE STANDARD OF CARE

When attorneys are confronted with the question of whether the failure to diagnose and treat an atypical presentation of a disease process, whether an aortic dissection or otherwise, led to the damage or death, they will turn to medical literature, textbooks, and articles to educate themselves about the standard of care. Attorneys will use that literature in their discussions with their consultants, and ultimately, with their expert witnesses. Lawyers will argue that standards found in the medical literature determine what doctors should do, what conditions they should suspect, and what diagnostic tools they should

employ; these parameters determine the standard of care.

There is substantial literature that addresses the standard of care for a doctor. It has been reported that up to 30% of patients later found to have aortic dissection are initially suspected to have other conditions, such as acute coronary syndrome, nondissecting aneurysm, pericarditis, pulmonary embolism, aortic stenosis, or even cholecystitis. Consequently, acute aortic dissection should always be considered in patients presenting with unexplained syncope, chest pain, back pain, abdominal pain, stroke, acute onset of congestive heart failure, pulse differential, or malperfusion syndrome of extremities or viscera.[14]

It has been stated that acute aortic dissection is the most frequently fatal condition in the spectrum of chest pain syndromes.[15]

Over the last 4 decades, advances in medical and surgical therapy have improved survival of aortic dissection from 16% to more than 90% within 30 days when optimal management is provided.[16]

The most prevailing symptom in clinical presentation of acute aortic dissection is typically severe pain, which is dramatically present in more than 90% of cases. However, there are many circumstances whereby only atypical signs are present, so although characteristically associated with a chest pain syndrome, aortic dissection should, as a general rule, always be considered in the differential diagnosis thought process for any

Subject: CODE A.M.I. (ACUTE MYOCARDIAL INFARCTION)	
Effective Date: 10/03	Category: Policy
Supersedes: 01/01/02	Number C-15

PURPOSE

To facilitate and ensure the care rendered to the acute myocardial infarction patient falls within the guidelines of the American Heart Association and the American College of Cardiology.

The two specific areas we will focus on will be the hospital admission process and time to reperfusion therapy.

GENERAL INSTRUCTIONS

Admission:

   Initial evaluation of acute myocardial infarction should be accomplished within 10 minutes of the recognition of a chest pain patient in the emergency department and should include a complete history and a 12-lead electrocardiogram (ECG).

   Physical examination should be targeted to exclude the well-known mimics of acute myocardial infarction: aortic dissection, acute pericarditis, spontaneous pneumothorax, and acute pulmonary embolism.

Fig. 2. Protocol for Code A.M.I. in a large metropolitan center.

patient with unexplained syncope, stroke, congestive heart failure, acute limb or abdominal ischemia, or abnormal mediastinal silhouette on chest radiograph, even when the pain is not the dominant presenting symptom.[16]

Acute aortic dissection of the ascending aorta is lethal, with mortality ranging between 1% and 2% per hour early after symptom onset. Symptoms such as instantaneous onset of severe chest (85%) or back (46%) pain are characteristic; however, abdominal pain (22%), syncope (13%), and stroke (6%) are common as well.[17]

As Nienaber[17] has said, "The challenge in managing acute aortic syndrome, especially dissection, is an appropriate clinical suspicion and action in pursuing rapid diagnosis and therapy. Typical features of aortic dissection are the acute onset of chest or back pain, of blunt, severe, and sometimes radiating and migrating nature. "Yet up to 20% of patients with acute aortic dissection may present with syncope without a history of typical pain or neurologic findings."[17]

Nienaber outlines the steps that should be taken for initial diagnosis and decisions. Although a routine chest radiograph is abnormal in 60% to 90% of cases of suspected aortic dissection,[17] Nienaber concludes by stating "a high index of suspicion for the problem is more important than the type of test used."

If acute aortic dissection is suspected, patients should be transferred to a center with interventional and surgical backup. Each institution should establish pathways for diagnosis, early treatment, and eventual transfer to definitive care.[17] Why? Because the condition is lethal if not caught and treated. Nienaber concludes by saying that diagnostic pitfalls currently are less of a problem than delays in the diagnostic pathway.[18]

Arun Raghupathy and Kim Eagle, contributors to Elefteriades' excellent book, *Acute Aortic Diseases*, write that establishing the correct diagnosis is essential because treatment of acute coronary syndrome, that is, anticoagulation and cardiac catheterization, may have catastrophic consequences in the presence of aortic dissection.[19]

Today a doctor cannot hide behind the notion that "aortic dissection is the great masquerader," given that dissection is the most frequent fatal condition in the spectrum of chest pain syndrome, and given that it is now possible simply and safely to differentiate dissection from other chest pain syndromes. Computed tomography (CT), magnetic resonance imaging (MRI), and transesophageal electrocardiography (TEE) are all acceptable imaging modalities for the diagnosis of aneurysm and dissection, and in ambiguous cases dual modalities should be employed. Aneurysms cause more deaths in the United States than human immunodeficiency virus–related disease, so it is not as if we are dealing with a rare disease.[19]

Raghupathy and Eagle write in *Acute Aortic Disease*,

It is imperative for the clinician to recognize patients who are more likely to present atypically and aggressively and pursue the diagnosis of an acute aortic condition in any patient who presents with unexplained hypoperfusion to an end organ or extremity. Symptoms consistent with end-organ malperfusion may include abdominal pain, neurological deficit due to ischemia of the spinal cord, limb ischemia, and renal failure. In IRAD (the Internal Registry of Acute Aortic Dissection, up to 6.4% of patients denied any pain on presentation, consistent with the 5% to 15% incidence, reported in the literature. When compared to patients who describe pain on presentation, these patients are significantly more likely to have syncope, congestive heart failure, stroke, and in-hospital death. Patients presenting without pain had a median time of 29 h for diagnosis vs. 10 h for those who presented with typical pain. Another atypical presentation is that of acute aortic dissection manifesting in a patient who presents with a primary or isolated complaint of abdominal pain. This challenging presentation was reported in approximately 5% of patients in IRAD, and each patient was ultimately diagnosed with acute Type B aortic dissection.

Although easily available and commonly ordered for the emergency room, chest x-ray has limited value in confirming the diagnosis of aortic dissection, and the sensitivity and specificity of chest radiography are only 64 and 86 percent.[20]

and

Although the classic radiographic finding of widened mediastinum or abnormal aortic contour is seen in up to 75 percent of subjects with acute dissection, it is important to realize that the chest x-ray is completely normal in up to 15 percent of these patients.[20]

These investigators conclude that an unremarkable chest radiograph should never dissuade the clinician from pursuing confirmatory testing in any patient suspected of having acute aortic syndrome, given that the utmost priority is to obtain a rapid and accurate diagnosis. The routine chest radiograph should probably be replaced by a first-line, more highly sensitive modern aortic imaging modality.[21]

ARGUMENT FOR BREACH OF THE STANDARD OF CARE FOR FAILURE TO RECOGNIZE AN ATYPICAL PRESENTATION OF AORTIC DISSECTION

Armed with the medical knowledge outlined earlier, one can now address the question of whether the physician should be responsible for the failure to diagnose and treat an atypical presentation of an acute aortic syndrome.

The first question is: Did the standard of care require the physician to have the appropriate clinical suspicion and action in pursuing rapid diagnosis and therapy? Aortic dissection of the ascending aorta is lethal. A high index of suspicion for the problem is more important than the type of test used, and the wrong diagnosis, and therefore wrong treatment, can indeed kill the patient. For example, anticoagulation and cardiac catheterization often has catastrophic consequences in the presence of an aortic dissection. As such, it is imperative for physicians to follow the guidelines and protocols of their hospital, obtain the portable chest radiograph, obtain the echocardiogram, and obtain more sophisticated cardiac examinations when there is an atypical presentation, thereby aggressively pursuing the diagnosis, or the exclusion, of an acute aortic condition in their differential diagnosis.

Putting it another way, if an individual presents to an emergency room with an atypical presentation, such as no onset of severe chest pain, but rather abdominal pain, or syncope, or stroke, with no particular supporting history that is otherwise explained, a normal chest radiograph, or an abnormal mediastinal silhouette on chest radiograph but without chest pain, and the physician did not consider aortic dissection, is he or she liable?

Clearly the medical literature supports that the standard of care be that the physician should suspect and consider atypical aortic dissection. The standard of care is for the physician to know that 64% of patients deny pain on presentation and are significantly more likely to have syncope or stroke; that 5% of presenting patients have severe abdominal pain, otherwise unexplained; that it takes more time (29 hours vs 10 hours) to make the diagnosis in an atypical presentation, time that permits the "luxury" of obtaining a CT or MRI; that 15% of patients present with a normal chest radiograph; and that presentation can occur with congestive heart failure otherwise unexplained. The failure to suspect an atypical presentation in the spectrum of diseases will be lethal to the patient. The medical literature, the author submits, supports the argument that the failure to consider the atypical presentation of aortic dissection in the differential diagnosis, to take action to rule aortic dissection in or out, is below the standard of care.

Although the physician should suspect an atypical presentation and the failure to do so may well be below the standard of care, the question still remains: is that failure a legal cause of death? Put another way, even with the correct diagnosis, what was the patient's risk of morbidity and mortality? Recall that there are multiple elements that are required to establish liability, such as duty, breach, actual and legal cause, and damages. The discussion above only addresses duty and breach, specifically, standard of care and its breach.

The medical literature is not markedly helpful on the issue of causation. Patients and physicians may use the statistics about morbidity and mortality based on age, gender, and disease presentation. Whether the breach of duty, the conduct that fell below the standard of care, caused harm to the patient will predominantly be based on the expert (medical) analysis of the patient, the presenting complaints, health, condition, age, and multiple other factors. The conclusion could be that notwithstanding the failure to meet the standard of care, the patient's morbidity or mortality was so great that the expert is compelled to say that the probable outcome would not have changed. Without that element, legal cause, the patient or family cannot establish the prima facie case. As such, there may well be a breach of the standard of care but no ultimate liability.

SUMMARY

The author submits that failure to consider the atypical presentation is below the standard of care, given that the ability to isolate this disease has become simple and relatively innocuous. CT, MRI, and TEE are acceptable and easily employable, and their application will prevent an unnecessary death. The liability of the health care provider does not rest on the "will" of the attorney. It is not a claim "without error." Rather, it is a claim based on error that is derived from the breach of the standard of care, the standard described in the medical literature, and by the retained expert witness. Yet whether the physician is ultimately liable for the poor outcome will depend not just on the breach of the standard of care, but whether it was a legal cause of the poor outcome. A poor outcome in and of itself does not create legal liability.

As Dr Isselbacher so simply stated: one cannot make a diagnosis that one does not consider. Given the highly lethal nature of an acute aortic dissection, it is imperative (and the standard of care requires) that the physician recognizes patients who are more likely to present atypically, and aggressively pursue the diagnosis of acute aortic dissection. Any other course is unacceptable.

REFERENCES

1. True risk: medical liability, malpractice insurance and healthcare. Americans for Insurance Reform 2009;2, 4, 5, 12.
2. Studdert DM, Mello MM, Gawande AA, et al. Claims errors and compensation payments in medical malpractice litigation. N Engl J Med 2006;354(19): 2025–31.
3. Keeton WP, Dobbs DB, Keeton RE, et al. The truth about medical malpractice, trial. Available at: http://www.atla.ort/medmal/prez.aspx. April 2002. Accessed April 14, 2006.
4. Baker T. The medical malpractice myth. Chicago: University of Chicago Press; 2005.
5. Localio AR, Lawthers AG, Brennan TA, et al. Relation between malpractice claims and adverse events due to negligence: results of the Harvard Medical Practice Study III. N Engl J Med 1991;325:245–51.
6. Studdert DM, Thomas EJ, Burstin HR, et al. Negligent care and malpractice claiming behavior in Utah and Colorado. Med Care 2000;38:250–60.
7. Studdert DM, Mello MM, Gawande AA, et al. Claims, errors, and compensation payments in medical malpractice litigation. N Engl J Med 2006;354(19): 2024–33.
8. Cooke A. Proposed new definition of a tort, 1899, 12. Harv Law Rev 335, 336.
9. Business & Professions Code Section 6146(c)(3).
10. Headland v. Superior Court (1983) 34 Cal.3d 695, 700–704.
11. Landros v. Flood (1976) 17 Cal.3d 399, 408; Brown v. Colm (1974) 11 Cal.3d 639, 642–643.
12. BAJI 6.00.1 –"Physician and surgeon have a duty to use reasonable diligence and his or her best judgment in the exercise of skill in the application of learning and the exercise of skill, and the application of learning and the duty to use the care and skill ordinarily exercised in like cases by reputable members of the profession practicing in the same or similar locality under similar circumstances. The failure to perform any of these duties is negligence".
13. Hoyan v. Manhattan Beach City District (1978) 22 Cal.3d 508, 513–514; Civil Code Section 1714(a) and 3333.
14. Nienaber CA. Aortic dissection and related syndromes. p. 33.
15. Nienaber CA, Fattori R. Diagnosis and treatment of aortic diseases; 1999. p. 5.
16. Nienaber CA, Fattori R. Diagnosis and treatment of aortic diseases; 1999. p. 14.
17. Baliga RR, Nienaber CA, Isselbacher EM, et al. Aortic dissection and related syndromes, 2007. p. 26, 32, 35.
18. Baliga RR, Nienaber CA, Isselbacher EM, Eagle KA. Aortic dissection and related syndromes;2007, p. 36.
19. Elefteriades J. Acute aortic disease. New York: Informa Healthcare; 2007. p. 73.
20. Elefteriades J. Acute aortic disease. New York: Informa Healthcare; 2007. p. 71, 74.
21. Elefteriades J. Acute aortic disease. New York: Informa Healthcare; 2007. p. 40–3.

Physicians Should Be Legally Liable for Missing an Atypical Aortic Dissection: CON

John A. Elefteriades, MD

KEYWORDS

- Legal • Aortic aneurysm • Screening
- Differential diagnosis

We recently published an analysis of 33 legal cases involving thoracic aortic aneurysm and dissection. Ninety percent of the adverse outcomes prompting legal action involved death, and 10% involved stroke or paraplegia. Most cases centered on delay in diagnosis or surgical treatment, with only a few concerning surgical technique. Emergency physicians were especially vulnerable, as were others on the front line of assessment, including cardiologists (**Table 1**). In two-thirds of these litigated cases, our panel found bona fide evidence of suboptimal care contributing to adverse outcome; in the remainder, we believed that outcome was suboptimal despite fully appropriate care. Because of the virulence of these diseases, adverse outcome can readily ensue. We learned from a review of these cases that it is critical for emergency physicians to include aortic aneurysm and dissection in their differential diagnosis. Such inclusion will lead to diagnostic tests to exclude an aortic catastrophe. We urged liberal imaging of the aorta (by computer tomographic [CT] scan, echocardiography, or magnetic resonance imaging scan). We believed that CT scan was especially useful because of its "triple rule-out" capabilities, namely, a CT scan can rule out the 3 most threatening potential causes of death in patients with chest symptoms: coronary artery disease, pulmonary embolism, and aortic dissection (**Fig. 1**). We emphasized

the use of D dimer as an initial screen: if the D dimer is not elevated, the patient simply does not have an aortic dissection. (D dimer is extremely sensitive, but not specific for aortic dissection.)

Based on this analysis, litigation in thoracic aortic aneurysm was described as "a tempest in the malpractice maelstrom." Because aortic dissection can result in occlusion of any branch of the aorta, from coronary arteries to iliacs, dissection can result in ischemia of any organ (**Fig. 2**). For this reason, dissection can mimic a primary problem in any organ, such as brain, heart, kidneys, intestines, and extremities. Because of this broad potential presentation, thoracic aortic dissection is "the great masquerader," making physicians especially vulnerable in diagnosing and treating this disease.

In this article, some pertinent medical literature on the accuracy of diagnosis and treatment in acute aortic dissection is also reviewed. The difficulty of diagnosis of aortic dissection has been well documented in the scientific literature. Nearly 20% of affected patients present without typical signs and symptoms (ie, without chest pain, malperfusion phenomena, cerebral disturbances, or signs of cardiac compromise).[1–4] Furthermore, clinical studies have documented that the diagnosis of aortic dissection is frequently missed on initial evaluation and not made until postmortem examination in 27% to 55% of patients.[4–8] In

Section of Cardiac Surgery, Department of Surgery, Yale University School of Medicine, Yale-New Haven Hospital, PO Box 208039, New Haven, CT 06520-8039, USA
E-mail address: john.elefteriades@yale.edu

Cardiol Clin 28 (2010) 245–252
doi:10.1016/j.ccl.2010.02.001
0733-8651/10/$ – see front matter © 2010 Published by Elsevier Inc.

Table 1
Individual nontraumatic thoracic aortic cases reviewed

Patient	Age (Decile)	Sex	Aneurysm or Dissection (Plus Location)	Onset of Symptoms	Malpractice Claim	Alive or Dead	Meritorious
01	50s	M	Type A dissection	Lifting heavy device on job	Failure to exclude from hazardous duty	D	No
02	70s	F	Thoracoabdominal aneurysm	Ruptured in operating room holding area, after case cancellation	Delay in surgery	D	No
03	50s	M	Type A dissection	Doing morning push-ups	Failure to diagnose (not until postmortem)	D	Yes
04	40s	F	Type A dissection	Developed abdominal symptoms (nausea, vomiting, pain, anorexia)	Failure to diagnose on 2 emergency room visits (not until postmortem, chest radiograph misread)	D	Yes
05	50s	M	Type A dissection	Stress at work, chest and abdominal symptoms	Delay in diagnosis (CT scan eventually demonstrated dissection, but patient died on transfer to tertiary facility)	D	No
06	60s	M	Descending aneurysm (9 cm)	Surgery performed	Failure to prevent paraplegia	A	No
07	40s	M	Type B dissection	Subacute presentation (thoracic back pain)	Delay in diagnosis	D	Yes
08	50s	M	Aortic rupture (descending)	Iatrogenic perforation during intra-aortic balloon pump placement	Surgical error, intra-aortic balloon pump placed during cardiac arrest resuscitative efforts	D	No
09	60s	M	Aortic rupture (descending)	Weeks of chest and back pain	Delay in diagnosis (missed on CT scan)	D	Yes
10	20s	M	Type A dissection	One week of back pain, abdominal pain, bloody diarrhea	Failure to diagnose (not until postmortem)	D	Yes

11	Teens	M	Type A dissection	Chest pain after training	Delay in diagnosis (died before transfer to tertiary facility)	D	Yes
12	30s	F	Coarctation	Presented with congestive heart failure	Failure to prevent paraplegia	A	No
13	50s	M	Type B dissection (prior type A repair)	Sudden-onset chest pain	Delay in surgery, ruptured awaiting catheterization	D	No
14	50s	F	Type A dissection	Pain watching television	Failure to diagnose (chest radiograph misread)	D	Yes
15	50s	M	Type A dissection	Pain on job	Failure to diagnose (arrested during cardiac catheterization)	D	Yes
16	70s	M	Type A dissection	Atypical chest pain	Delay in surgery for symptomatic aneurysm, 6.8-cm aorta ruptured	D	Yes
17	70s	M	Thoracoabdominal aneurysm	Abdominal pain	Delay in surgery, aneurysm diagnosed, repeated CT scans looking for signs of rupture, patient's 7-cm aneurysm ruptured after being heparinized for atrial fibrillation	D	Yes
18	70s	M	Ascending aneurysm (iatrogenic dissection)	Operated urgently, aortic replacement	Improper postoperative care	D	Yes
19	40s	M	Type A dissection (status post aortic valve replacement twice)	Abdominal symptoms (nausea, vomiting), pancreatitis by enzymes	Failure to diagnose (not until postmortem)	D	Yes

(continued on next page)

Table 1
(continued)

Patient	Age (Decile)	Sex	Aneurysm or Dissection (Plus Location)	Onset of Symptoms	Malpractice Claim	Alive or Dead	Meritorious
20	30s	F	Type A dissection	Chest pain 6 days postpartum, bicuspid aortic valve	Failure to diagnose (not until postmortem), repeated rule out pulmonary embolism, unaware of phenomenon of peripregnancy dissection	D	Yes
21	60s	M	Thoracoabdominal aneurysm	Gut ischemia after difficult operation (atheroembolism)	Improper conduct of operation	D	No
22	30s	M	Type A dissection	Acute gastrointestinal symptoms	Failure to diagnose	D	Yes
23	40s	M	Type A dissection	Syncope, chest pain, bradycardia	Failure to diagnose (not until postmortem)	D	Yes
24	Teens	M	Type A dissection (following prior aortic root operation)	Chest pain on exertion	Inadequate preoperative care, died on operating room table	D	No
25	20s	F	Type A dissection	Chest pain 2 days after delivery of child	Failure to diagnose (not until postmortem), treated for flu	D	Yes
26	50s	M	Type A dissection	Iatrogenic dissection during coronary angioplasty	Improper surgical conduct (ligated innominate artery)	A	Yes
27	70s	F	Ascending aneurysm	Postoperative aortic insufficiency, requiring early reoperation, subsequent death	Improper surgical conduct (causing early aortic insufficiency)	D	Yes

#	Age	Diagnosis	Sex	Presentation	Comment		Outcome
28	30s	Ascending aneurysm	M	Months of feeling unwell, with heartburn	Two-month delay in cardiology consultation to follow-up on diastolic murmur, died of apparent rupture between echocardiogram/catheterization and surgical consultation	D	Yes
29	20s	Type A dissection	M	Two weeks of nausea, vomiting, feeling ill, no chest pain	Delay in diagnosis (repeated emergency department visits, diagnosed as asthma, bronchitis), massive cardiomegaly when chest radiograph ultimately done, dissection of 10-cm aorta and massive aortic insufficiency found, died of pulmonary edema	D	Yes
30	40s	Type A dissection	F	Sudden onset of abdominal pain/ nausea/vomiting	Failure to make diagnosis (until postmortem), CT scan misread	D	Yes
31	30s	Type A dissection	F	Sudden onset of severe chest pain	Failure to diagnose	D	Yes
32	50s	Type A dissection	M	Sudden onset of severe chest pain	Delay in diagnosis (minimal)	D	No
33	60s	Type A dissection	M	One week of chest pain	Improper surgical conduct	D	No

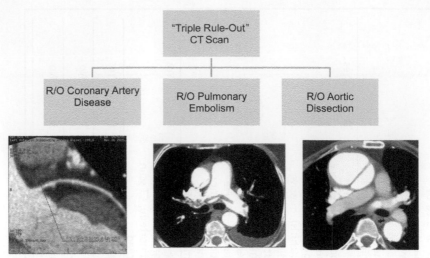

Fig. 1. The "triple rule-out" CT scan that may be so useful in diagnosing or ruling out the "big three" conditions that threaten the life of the patient with chest pain: coronary artery disease, pulmonary embolism, and aortic dissection. We strongly recommend its use. (*From* Elefteriades JA, Barrett PW, Kopf GS: Litigation in nontraumatic aortic diseases—a tempest in the malpractice maelstrom. Cardiology 2008;109:263-72; with permission from S. Karger AG, Basel.)

fact, the diagnosis of aortic dissection is often made incidentally on an imaging study done for another reason.[6]

To determine what must legally be expected of physicians, it is prudent to examine the definition of a medical "standard of care." Wikipedia provides the following definition:

The level at which an ordinary, prudent professional having the same training and experience in good standing in a same or similar community would practice under the same or similar circumstances. An "average" standard would not apply because in that case at least half of any group of practitioners would not qualify.

In the case of thoracic aortic aneurysm and dissection, where atypical presentation and failure to diagnose are common, the concept of malpractice in failing to diagnose aortic dissection becomes intrinsically suspect, especially when the accepted definition of malpractice indicated earlier is applied. This definition indicates that even an average level is too much to expect, because half of the physicians must, of necessity, be below average. The evidence cited in the paragraph before the definition argues for a high degree of leniency in the physician's favor in determining departure from the standards of care in thoracic aortic diseases. In fact, difficulty in diagnosis, delayed diagnosis, or failure to diagnose are so common as to approach the norm for this disease, even in the best hands, rather than the

exception. Put succinctly, the legal system cannot expect correct diagnosis of a disease that thwarts diagnosis nearly one-half the time in the recorded literature. The centers represented in literature articles, moreover, usually have special interest and expertise in aortic diseases.

This all is not to say that the medical diagnosis and management of aortic diseases are optimal. They are not. The legal attention to these diseases makes that clear. Even in the series that we analyzed, a panel of medical experts reviewing the cases for the purpose of our article concluded that level of care was below optimal in two-thirds of cases. We were looking from a medical, not a legal perspective. Clearly, much has to be improved in our medical systems vis-à-vis aortic aneurysm and dissection. Improvement can be instigated by encouraging physicians on the front lines to

- Include aortic diseases in the differential diagnosis of all cases of chest pain or unexplained abdominal pain or hypotension.
- Use D dimer liberally as a screening tool for aortic dissection (100% sensitive).
- Image liberally (a "triple rule-out" CT will exclude the 3 major killers: myocardial infarction, pulmonary embolism, and acute aortic dissection).

Most current lawsuits concern physicians at the front lines, who see a vast array of cases. Even in patients with chest pain, aortic dissection is uncommon compared with other causes. In fact, it has been estimated that on the front lines, a physician will, on average, see 80 patients with

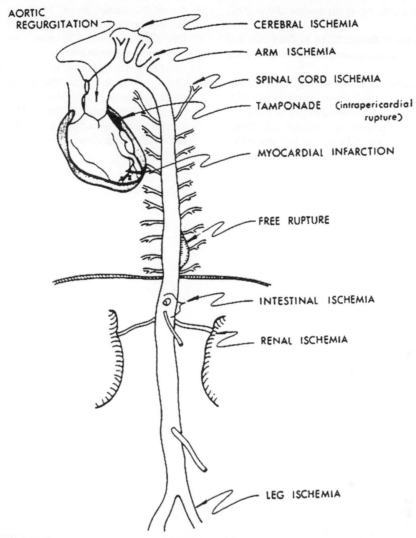

AORTIC REGURGITATION

CEREBRAL ISCHEMIA

ARM ISCHEMIA

SPINAL CORD ISCHEMIA

TAMPONADE (intrapericardial rupture)

MYOCARDIAL INFARCTION

FREE RUPTURE

INTESTINAL ISCHEMIA

RENAL ISCHEMIA

LEG ISCHEMIA

Fig. 2. Aortic dissection can affect virtually any branch and any organ of the body, leading to potentially protean manifestations and justifying its reputation as "the great masquerader." (*From* Elefteriades JA, Barrett PW, Kopf GS: Litigation in nontraumatic aortic diseases—a tempest in the malpractice maelstrom. Cardiology 2008; 109:263–72; with permission from S. Karger AG, Basel.)

acute coronary syndrome before encountering a single patient with aortic dissection.[5]

It is unfair to hold specific physicians on the front lines to a standard that exceeds what can currently be expected of their peers. Always considering aortic dissection, always ruling this disorder out, and making a correct diagnosis of aortic dissection in a large majority of cases currently exceeds the reasonable expectations of a peer group, as vividly illustrated in the 27% to 55% rate of failure to diagnose documented in the literature.

Through education, via articles and lectures, as well as increased attention in lay media, specialists in aortic care aim to increase the consideration of aortic diseases in differential diagnosis by front-line physicians. In the near future, the baseline level of consideration and diagnosis of acute aortic dissection is likely to improve. Then, by the definition of standard of care, higher expectations may be required of front-line physicians by the legal system.

REFERENCES

1. Elefteriades JA, Barrett PW, Kopf GS. Litigation in nontraumatic aortic diseases—a tempest in the malpractice maelstrom. Cardiology 2008;109: 263–72.
2. Hagan PG, Nienaber CA, Isselbacher EM, et al. The International Registry of Acute Aortic Dissection

(IRAD): new insights into an old disease. JAMA 2000; 283:897–903.

3. Erbel R, Alfonso F, Boileau C, et al. Diagnosis and management of aortic dissection. Eur Heart J 2001; 22:1642–81.

4. Ohlmann P, Faure A, Morel O, et al. Diagnostic and prognostic value of circulating D dimers in patients with acute aortic dissection. Crit Care Med 2006;34:1358–64.

5. Von Kodolitsch Y, Schwartz AG, Nienaber CA. Clinical prediction of acute aortic dissection. Arch Intern Med 2000;160:2977–82.

6. Spittell PC, Spittell JA Jr, Joyce JW, et al. Clinical features and differential diagnosis of aortic dissection: experience with 236 cases (1980–1990). Mayo Clin Proc 1993;68:642–51.

7. Von Kodolitsch Y, Nienaber CA, Dieckman C, et al. Chest radiography for the diagnosis of acute aortic syndrome. Am J Med 2004;116:73–7.

8. Fradet G, Jamieson WRE, Janusz MT, et al. Aortic dissection:current expectations and treatment: experience with 258 patients over 25 years. Can J Surg 1990;33:465–9.

Editorial Comment: Legal Liability in Atypical Aortic Dissection

John A. Elefteriades, MD

In his article in this issue of *Cardiology Clinics*, Attorney Moses Lebovits makes a thoughtful, logical case that emergency and cardiac physicians and surgeons should be manifestly aware of the possibility of atypical presentation for aortic dissection—with the corollary that they be held liable if they have not investigated this possibility. Mr Lebovits' reasoning, from definition of legal concepts through pertinent aortic medicine to logical conclusions, is highly cogent (**Fig. 1**, **Table 1**).

The article by Dr John A. Elefteriades points that the standard of practice required by law is, by definition, not even as high as that of the "average" physician, because to use the average as the standard implies that half of doctors fell below the standard. So, a lower-than-average standard is required, namely that of "an ordinary, prudent professional." So, if in this disease, 50% or more of cases are incorrectly diagnosed premortem, how can a physician be held liable? Dr. Elefteriades argues for a high degree of leniency in favor of physicians in cases involving aortic dissection. He makes the case for liberal use of the triple rule-out CT scan, which can exclude the 3 major causes of death in patients with chest symptoms: coronary artery disease, pulmonary embolism, and acute aortic dissection.

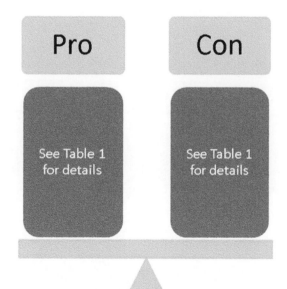

Fig. 1. The debate ends in a stalemate, depending on one's point of view.

Section of Cardiac Surgery, Department of Surgery, Yale University School of Medicine, Yale-New Haven Hospital, PO Box 208039, New Haven, CT 06520-8039, USA
E-mail address: john.elefteriades@yale.edu

Cardiol Clin 28 (2010) 253–254
doi:10.1016/j.ccl.2010.02.012
0733-8651/10/$ – see front matter © 2010 Elsevier Inc. All rights reserved.

Table 1
Legal liability in atypical aortic dissection

Pro: Physician Should be Liable (Lebovits)	Con: Physician Should not be Liable (Elefteriades)
Definition of malpractice: • Was standard of care breached? • Was there harm? • What is the extent of injury?	Aortic dissection really is "the great masquerader"
Today, all physicians must keep acute aortic dissection in their differential diagnosis	20% of Cases have atypical presentation
All physicians should be aware of potential atypical presentation of aortic dissection	More than 50% of cases are not correctly diagnosed premortem; so, how can the standard of care be for correct diagnosis?
Aortic dissection is easily ruled out by imaging studies	

Does Medical Therapy for Thoracic Aortic Aneurysms Really Work? Are β-Blockers Truly Indicated? PRO

John A. Elefteriades, MD

KEYWORDS
- β-blockers • Thoracic aortic aneurysm
- Aortic dissection • Type B dissection

Upon critical review, the widespread use of β-blockers for chronic thoracic aortic aneurysms can fairly be questioned. One wonders how strong the evidence is for this therapy that has quietly become standard practice. Similarly, one may ask how strong is the evidence for the use of β-blocker–based therapy for acute aortic dissection. This article examines the supporting evidence.

HISTORY OF "ANTI-IMPULSE" THERAPY FOR ACUTE AORTIC DISSECTION: TALES OF TURKEYS AND TYGON TUBING

The groundbreaking work in medical management of type A aortic dissection grew out of the classic studies by Wheat and colleagues[1] more than forty years ago. Most of the modern medical management of aortic dissection is a result of an ex vivo model: artificial constructs by Wheat and colleagues[1] on artificial "aortas" constructed from Tygon tubing coated internally with rubber cement (**Fig. 1**).[1,2] The two primary goals of pharmacological therapy, reduction of blood pressure and diminution of left ventricular ejection force (dp/dt), were established by Wheat and colleagues'[1] experiments (**Fig. 2**). Some of the theories were also tested on isolated (ex vivo) canine aortas, but the many decades of medical management of aortic dissection were established primarily without testing in living animal or human models.

The thrust of the studies by Wheat and colleagues[1] was that the contractile force of the myocardium, expressed as the change in pressure over time (dp/dt), plays a major role in initiation and propagation of acute aortic dissection. The dp/dt is expressed in the initial upstroke of the arterial pressure curve (**Fig. 3**). In Wheat and colleagues'[1] in vitro studies, neither high pressure alone nor high blood flow alone caused aortic dissection to progress; rather, it was the strength of pulsation that led to progression of the aortic dissection.

Historically, the most effective animal model for aortic dissection is a broad-breasted white turkey. Although it is not generally appreciated, these birds are quite prone to aortic dissection. Whole populations of turkeys can be rendered exceptionally dissection prone, via iatrogenic induction of lathyrism, so that the majority of the animals die from acute aortic dissection. β-aminopropionitrile, an inhibitor of lysyl oxidase (found in concentrated form in certain types of peas), was used to effect medial degeneration by interfering with the formation of elastin and collagen cross-links.[3] These studies looked at the effects of chronic

Section of Cardiac Surgery, Department of Surgery, Yale University School of Medicine, Yale-New Haven Hospital, PO Box 208039, New Haven, CT 06520-8039, USA
E-mail address: john.elefteriades@yale.edu

Cardiol Clin 28 (2010) 255–260
doi:10.1016/j.ccl.2010.02.016

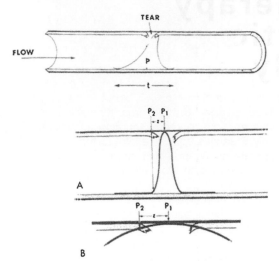

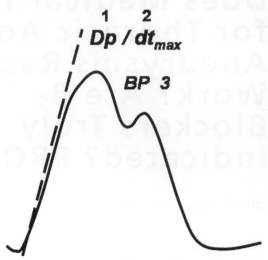

Fig. 1. (*Top*) Tygon tubing utilized by Wheat in 1960s. A lining of rubber cement was placed within the Tygon tubing. A tear was created in the rubber cement to mimic the intimal tear of aortic dissection. P, pressure wave; t, time. (*Bottom*) Comparison of the pressure gradient between the intima and the adventitia (rubber and Tygon) in two conditions. (*A*) A normal or increased pulse pressure. (*B*) A pharmacologically blunted pulse wave. When the pressure curve is flattened (as with β-blockade), the pressure differential ΔP becomes less. The ΔP is thought to drive the process of dissection. P, pressure applied to the adventitia at point P1; P2, pressure applied to the adventitia at point P2; Z, length of the torn intima. (*Reprinted from* Wheat MW Jr, Palmer RF, Barley TD, et al. Treatment of dissecting aneurysms of the aorta without surgery. J Thorac Cardiovasc Surg 1965;50:364; with permission.)

Fig. 3. In the aortic pressure curve, the tangent (*dashed line*) of the steepest portion of the ascending limb indicates the maximum pressure change (dp/dt). Bp; blood pressure. (*Reprinted from* Sanz J, Einstein A, Fuster V. In: Acute aortic dissection anti-impulse therapy. Elefteriades J, editor. Acute Aortic Disease. New York: Informa Healthcare 2007; with permission.)

administration of various drugs on the risk of aortic rupture in turkeys. B-blockers were found to decrease the incidence of aortic rupture.[4]

It is important to note that blood pressure management alone does not suffice to control aortic dissection (**Fig. 4**). Nitroprusside was successful in controlling the arterial hypertension, but could not halt the progress of the dissection. Propranolol alone was also insufficient in controlling or limiting propagation of dissection. The best results were obtained with a combination of nitroprusside and propranolol, or with trimethaphan (an autonomic ganglion blocker with effects on both contractility and vascular resistance).[5] Vasodilators as sole therapy drop the peak systolic pressure but may actually increase dp/dt, reflecting reflex sympathetic discharge in response to the drop in blood pressure, with attendant chronotropic and inotropic stimulation. This phenomenon is demonstrated in the leftmost curve in **Fig. 4**. The increase in dp/dt from sole vasodilator therapy has been associated with increase in rupture of the dissected aorta.[6] On the other hand, β-blocker therapy, while producing a smaller drop in blood pressure, decreases chronotropy and inotropy, with attendant fall in dp/dt. This decrease in dp/dt from β-blocker therapy is depicted in the rightmost curve in **Fig. 4**. It is the combination of vasodilator therapy with sympathetic control via β-blockade that constitutes effective "anti-impulse therapy" for acute aortic dissection.

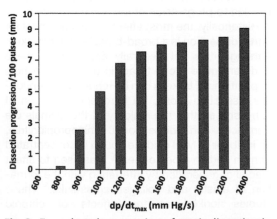

Fig. 2. Exacerbated progression of aortic dissection in relation to increasing dp/dt. In this experimental setting, no progression occurs until a threshold level of dp/dt is exceeded. (*Reprinted from* Prokop EK, Palmer RF, Wheat MW Jr. Hydrodynamic forces in dissecting aneurysms: in-vitro Studies in a Tygon model and in dog aortas. Circ Res 1970;27;121–7; with permission.)

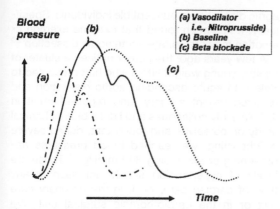

Fig. 4. Aortic pressure curves under various conditions. Curve (a), the administration of a vasodilator agent such as nitroprusside; curve (b), the baseline state, curve (c), β-blockade administration. Note the significant decrease in blood pressure and acceleration in heart rate, at the expense of a steeper slope of the ascending portion of the curve (representing increased dp/dt). Although the degree of pressure lowering is usually smaller, the characteristic negative chronotropy and inotropy result in a blunted upstroke of the blood pressure curve, representing decreased impulse and dp/dt. (*Reprinted from* Sanz J, Einstein A, Fuster V. In: Acute aortic dissection anti-impulse therapy. Elefteriades J, editor. Acute Aortic Disease. New York: Informa Healthcare 2007; with permission.)

Some human studies have been performed as well. One study in Marfan patients showed propranolol to be less effective in presence of a dilated aortic root than had been hoped, as its intravenous use failed acutely to reduce dp/dt.[7]

Based on these historical studies, aggressive reductions in dp/dt, as well as blood pressure, have come to constitute the basis for medical therapy of acute aortic syndromes. These treatments, developed many decades ago (predominantly in nonliving preparations) have continued to represent the standard of care even in modern times.

Cornerstone in the medical management of hypertensive and most normotensive patients with suspected acute aortic dissection is anti-impulse therapy and blood pressure control. The initial therapeutic goal is elimination of pain and reduction of systolic blood pressure to 100 to 120 mm Hg (mean arterial pressure of 60 to 75 mm Hg) or the lowest level compatible with adequate vital organ perfusion.[8,9] This is done with β-blockers and intravenous vasodilators (especially nitroglycerine and nitroprusside).

It is imperative to realize that drugs with arterial vasodilator properties, while successful in lowering the arterial pressure, also stimulate arterial baroreceptors, which, in a reflex sympathetic response, cause a paradoxical increase in dp/dt and thus increase the risk of aortic wall rupture.[10]

MEDICAL MANAGEMENT OF CHRONIC THORACIC AORTIC ANEURYSM

Here, the author considers the effectiveness of β-blockers in the treatment of chronic thoracic aortic aneurysms. The promising concept of using angiotensin receptor blockers for control of thoracic aortic aneurysms is covered in elsewhere in this issue.

The main work cited by proponents of β-blockers is the Shores and colleagues[11] study from Johns Hopkins. In this study, 70 predominantly young patients with Marfan disease were randomized to treatment with or without a β-blocker and followed for a mean of 10 years. Beneficial findings included a reduced rate of aortic growth and improved avoidance of a combined endpoint, including death, congestive heart failure, aortic regurgitation, aortic dissection, or cardiovascular surgery (**Fig. 5**). This study, with a small number of patients but long follow-up, represents the cornerstone of justification for use of β-blockers in aortic diseases. Of course, it

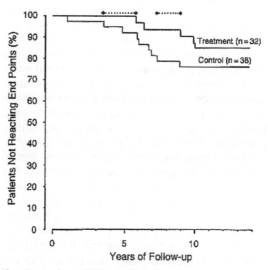

Fig. 5. Kaplan-Meier survival analysis based on the clinical endpoints in the study (death, congestive heart failure, or aortic regurgitation, aortic dissection, or cardiovascular surgery). The dashed lines at the top indicate the periods when the 90% confidence limits for the difference between the curves did not include zero. The curves diverge the most in the middle years but do not intersect at any point. (*Reprinted from* Shores J, Berger KR, Murphy EA, et al. Progression of aortic dilatation and the benefit of long-term beta-adrenergic blockade in Marfan's syndrome. N Engl J Med 1994;330(19):1335–41; with permission.)

does represent a considerable leap of faith to transfer this data to patients without Marfan disease, who make up a much larger proportion of the aneurysm population.

A number of other articles provide some support for the use of β-blockers in thoracic aortic aneurysms.

Marfan Disease

Rossi-Foulkes and colleagues[12] also found a beneficial impact of β-blockers on aortic growth in Marfan patients. Yetman and colleagues,[13] however, found no benefit of β-blockers in Marfan patients. Multiple studies looking at aortic elastic properties in patients with Marfan syndrome have yielded mutually contradictory results, with some showing improved elastic properties and some showing deterioration in aortic distensibility.[5,14–18]

Acute Type B Dissection

Kodama and colleagues[19] found that patients with tighter rate control with β-blockers (to pulse < 60) had fewer early and late complications (rupture, extension, expansion, organ ischemia, or need for surgery) than patients with looser control. This suggests a beneficial effect of β-blockers in this setting.

Although suggestive, the studies cited above do not give an unequivocal message of benefit and strong indication for use of β-blockers in thoracic aortic aneurysm. Yet, use of β-blockers in patients with thoracic aortic aneurysm has achieved widespread application—becoming, so to speak, standard practice. The reason likely has to do with the fact that it makes strong intuitive sense to keep blood pressure and the strength of cardiac contraction well controlled in aneurysm patients.

Along those lines, one recent finding that is theoretically supportive of use of β-blockers has to do with the inciting factors for occurrence of acute dissection in a chronic thoracic aortic aneurysm. One may consider the following question: How does aortic dissection pick a specific date and time to occur in a susceptible individual (eg, one with connective tissue disease or thoracic aortic aneurysm)? It used to be thought that this was random. It is interesting that aortic dissection has long been known to occur in circadian and diurnal patterns, with a preponderance of instances in the winter months and in the early morning hours. The reasons behind these patterns are unknown, but these characteristics correlate with the season and time of day when blood pressure is known to be highest.

Studies at Yale have added another interesting dimension to our understanding of the timing of aortic dissection in susceptible individuals. Specifically, it has been found that extreme exertion or emotion may precipitate acute aortic dissection.[20]

A few years ago, the author noticed a cluster of healthy young weight lifters who had presented to Yale with acute ascending aortic dissection and required urgent surgery (and reported on it in JAMA[21]). My colleagues and I did a biomechanical study on ourselves and found that, during severe weight lifting, we reached blood pressures approaching or exceeding 300 mmHg.[21] These are levels of hypertension simply not seen in any type of cardiac care, be it in the coronary care unit or in the cardiothoracic surgical unit. We hypothesized that extreme elevation of blood pressure during lifting was a factor in the cluster of dissections we had treated in weight lifters. After publication of our original report, we received cases from around the country. We did a follow-up report enumerating 31 similar cases of acute aortic dissection in the setting of weight lifting or severe straining activity.[22] Nearly all of these dissections occurred in young men with previously unknown moderate aortic enlargement (4 to 5 cm). Based on this evidence, we recommended routine screening of all athletes embarking on weight lifting or other heavy athletic activity. We saw this as the only means to protect these young athletes from needless death. It is interesting and reassuring that the International Olympic Committee now requires an echocardiogram for every athlete competing in the Olympics. We would like to see this prescription extended to college and high school athletes.

The author and colleagues[20] subsequently did another study in which we contacted each patient or family member we had treated for acute aortic dissection at Yale University. This investigation implicated emotion as well as exertion as a causal factor in the acute onset of aortic dissection. Specifically, we found that a majority of patients could recall a specific episode of severe emotional upset (notification of a cancer diagnosis, losses at the casino, illness in a loved one) or extreme exertion at the time of their dissection (**Fig. 6**).

These studies, looking at aneurysm and dissection from multiple viewpoints—clinical, biologic, genetic (Mendelian and molecular), mechanical, epidemiologic—permit formulation of a schema for the onset of acute aortic dissection in a specific individual at a specific time.

The susceptibility to aortic aneurysm and dissection is set from birth by genetics. The aorta is destroyed over time, at least in part by excess proteolysis by the matrix metalloproteinases. The aorta enlarges as its wall is damaged. As the aorta enlarges, the mechanical properties deteriorate,

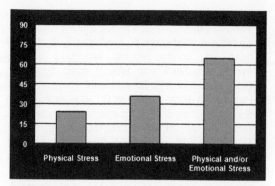

Fig. 6. Emotional or exertional events immediately preceding the onset of the pain of acute aortic dissection. Sixty-five of 90 patients (66%) reported physical/emotional inciting events: 24/90 (26.6%) physical and 36/90 (40%) emotional. (*Reprinted from* Hatzaras IS, Bible JE, Koullias GJ, et al. Role of exertion or emotion as inciting events for acute aortic dissection. Am J Cardiol 2007;100:1470–2; with permission.)

with loss of distensibility and imposition of excess wall tension. An acute hypertensive event supervenes—usually emotional or exertional—and exceeds the tensile limit of the aortic wall, producing an acute aortic dissection.

In this context, with the understanding that an acute blood pressure spike from exertion or emotion may well precipitate aortic dissection, it again makes intuitive sense that β-blockers may be indicated in thoracic aneurysm patients—specifically for the purpose of blunting the blood pressure spike seen in response to severe exertion or emotion.

SUMMARY
Acute Aortic Dissection

Much of the original work that underlies current treatment protocols for acute Type A aortic dissection was conducted on Tygon-tubing mock aortas or on the aortas of aneurysm-prone turkeys. Yet, the principles of anti-impulse therapy for acute dissection have stood the test of time. The very consideration of medical management for acute Type A dissection represents a "back to the future" paradigm shift reminiscent of the earliest recommendations for dissection treatment many decades ago before surgical therapy was feasible or safe.

Chronic Thoracic Aortic Aneurysm

The study on a small number of Marfan patients followed at Johns Hopkins for many years set the stage for use of β-blockers in patients with chronic thoracic aortic aneurysms. Although evidence subsequent to this study is far from conclusive, such therapy has

continued as standard practice. Recent findings that acute exertion or emotion trigger aortic dissection add credence to the use of β-blockers because this therapy may blunt the severity of the pressure spikes with acute exertion or emotion.

REFERENCES

1. Wheat MW Jr, Palmer RF, Barley TD, et al. Treatment of dissecting aneurysms of the aorta without surgery. J Thorac Cardiovasc Surg 1965;50:364.
2. Palmer RF, Wheat MW Jr. Treatment of dissecting aneurysms of the aorta. Ann Thorac Surg 1967;4:38–52.
3. Simpson CF, Boucek RJ. The B-aminopropionitrile fed turkey: a model for detecting potential drug action on arterial tissue. Cardiovasc Res 1983;17(1):26–32.
4. Boucek RJ, Gunja-Smith J, Noble L, et al. Modulation by propranolol of the lysyl cross-links in elastin and collagen of the aneurysm-prone turkey. Biochem Pharmacol 1983;32:275–80.
5. Yin FC, Brin KP, Ting CT, et al. Arterial hemodynamics indexes in Marfan's syndrome. Circulation 1989;79(4):854–62.
6. Fuster V, Andrews P. Medical treatment of the aorta. Cardiol Clin 1999;17(4):697–715.
7. Moran JF, Derkac WM, Conkle DM. Pharmacologic control of acute aortic dissection in hypertensive dogs. Surg Forum 1978;29:231–4.
8. Erbel R, Alfonso F, Boileau C, et al. Diagnosis and management of aortic dissection: task force on aortic dissection, European society of cardiology. Eur Heart J 2004;22(18):1642–81.
9. Elefteriades JA, Geha AS, Cohen LS. Acute aortic emergencies. House officer guide to ICU care. 2nd edition. New York: Lippincott-Raven; 1994.
10. Beaven DW, Murphy EA. Dissecting aneurysms during methonium therapy: a report on nine cases treated for hypertension. Br Med J 1956;49(58):77–80.
11. Shores J, Berger KR, Murphy EA, et al. Progression of aortic dilatation and the benefit of long-term beta-adrenergic blockade in Marfan's syndrome. N Engl J Med 1994;330(19):1335–41.
12. Rossi-Foulkes R, Roman MJ, Rosen SE, et al. Phenotypic features and impact of beta blocker or calcium antagonist therapy on aortic lumen size in the Marfan syndrome. Am J Cardiol 1999;83:1364–8.
13. Yetman AT, Bournemeier RA, McCrindle BW, et al. Usefulness of enalapril versus propranolol or atenolol for prevention of aortic dilatation in patients with the Marfan syndrome. Am J Cardiol 2005;95:1125–7.
14. Nollen GJ, Westerhof BE, Groenink M. Aortic pressure-area relation in Marfan patients with and without beta blocking agents: a new non-invasive approach. Heart 2004;90:314–8.

15. Haouzi A, Berglund H, Pelikan PC, et al. Heterogeneous aortic response to acute beta-adrenergic blockade in Marfan syndrome. Am Heart J 1997; 133(1):60–3.

16. Groenink M, de Roos A, Mulder BJ, et al. Changes in aortic distensibility and pulse wave velocity assessed with magnetic resonance imaging following beta-blocker therapy in the Marfan syndrome. Am J Cardiol 1998;82:203–8.

17. Meijboom LJ, Westerhof BE, Noilen GJ, et al. Beta-blocking therapy in patients with the Marfan syndrome and entire aortic replacement. Eur J Cardiothorac Surg 2004;26:901–6.

18. Rios AS, Silber EN, Bavishi N, et al. Effect of long-term beta-blockade on aortic root compliance in patients with Marfan syndrome. Am Heart J 1999; 137:1051–61.

19. Kodama K, Nishigami K, Sakamoto T, et al. Tight heart rate control reduces secondary adverse events in patients with Type B aortic dissection. Circulation 2008;118(Suppl I):S167–70.

20. Hatzaras IS, Bible JE, Kallias GJ, et al. Role of exertion or emotion as inciting events for acute aortic dissection. Am J Cardiol 2007;100:1470–2.

21. Elefteriades JA, Hatzaras I, Tranquilli MA, et al. Weight lifting and rupture of silent aortic aneurysms. JAMA 2003;290:2803.

22. Hatzaras I, Tranquilli M, Coady MA, et al. Weight lifting and aortic dissection: More evidence for a connection. Cardiology 2006;107(2):103–6.

Does Medical Therapy for Thoracic Aortic Aneurysms Really Work? Are β-Blockers Truly Indicated? CON

Steve L. Liao, MD[a,b], Sammy Elmariah, MD[b],
Sarina van der Zee, MD[b], Brett A. Sealove, MD[b],
Valentin Fuster, MD, PhD[b,c],*

KEYWORDS

• Aortic aneurysm • Medical therapy • β-Blockers

Thoracic aortic aneurysms (TAA) often represent the final manifestation of hereditary or degenerative disease processes. TAA are primarily caused by age-related degenerative changes, although many other factors may play a role. The pathogenesis of TAA is characterized by an imbalance in the regulatory mechanisms that normally act to stabilize aortic wall integrity, and is triggered or accelerated by hereditary factors and atherosclerotic risk factors such as smoking, hypertension, age, and male gender. Once an aneurysm develops, anatomic and hemodynamic features contribute to its expansion.[1]

Although recent data support inhibition of the renin-angiotensin system in delaying and even reversing aortic dilatation, other medical therapies have shown less convincing efficacy in TAA. In this article, the authors highlight the most common pathophysiologic mechanisms responsible for TAA formation (**Fig. 1**) and review the paucity of evidence supporting the spectrum of medical therapies for TAA other than renin-angiotensin inhibition.

ANEURYSM FORMATION

Homeostasis of the aortic wall is maintained by several enzymes and growth factors that include transforming growth factor (TGF)-β, matrix metalloproteinases (MMPs), and tissue inhibitors of matrix metalloproteinases (TIMPs). The TGF-β family of growth factors regulates cell survival, proliferation, differentiation, tissue morphogenesis, and cellular response to injury, whereas MMPs process or degrade numerous extracellular substrates.[2,3] Almost all types of vascular cells, including endothelial cells, vascular smooth muscle cells (VSMCs), and adventitial fibroblasts, secrete MMPs in normal conditions. The relative concentration of active MMPs and TIMPs determines net proteolytic activity.[3,4]

Aging, environmental factors, and connective tissue abnormalities compromise the ability of the aorta to withstand high pressure.[5] The first degenerative change noted in the aging aorta is cystic medial degeneration (CMD), an accumulation of mucopolysaccharide cysts within the aortic

[a] James J. Peters Veteran Affairs Medical Center, Cardiovascular Division, Department of Medicine, Bronx, NY, USA
[b] The Zena and Michael A. Wiener Cardiovascular Institute, The Marie-Josee and Henry R. Kravis Center for Cardiovascular Health, The Mount Sinai School of Medicine, One Gustave L. Levy Place, Box 1030, New York, NY 10029, USA
[c] Centro Nacional de Investigaciones Cardiovasculares, Madrid, Spain
* Corresponding author. The Zena and Michael A. Wiener Cardiovascular Institute, The Marie-Josee and Henry R. Kravis Center for Cardiovascular Health, The Mount Sinai School of Medicine, One Gustave L. Levy Place, Box 1030, New York, NY 10029.
E-mail address: valentin.fuster@mssm.edu

Cardiol Clin 28 (2010) 261–269
doi:10.1016/j.ccl.2010.01.002
0733-8651/10/$ – see front matter. Published by Elsevier Inc.

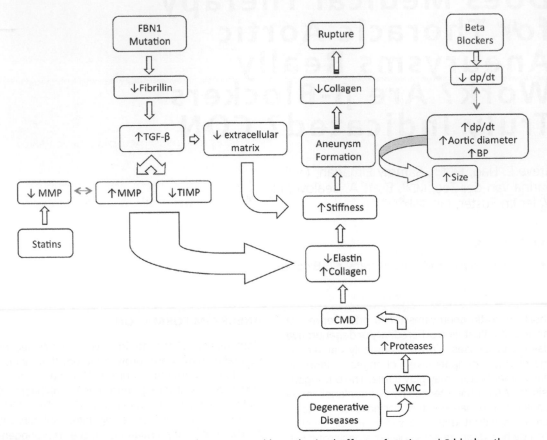

Fig. 1. Mechanisms of aortic aneurysm formation and hypothesized effects of statin and β-blocker therapy.

media that damages the elastin skeleton and leads to loss of VSMCs, and may disrupt the lamellar structure of the media (**Fig. 2**).[6]

An imbalance between MMP and TIMP activity leads to proteolysis and aortic wall weakening.[7–9] Elastin degradation fragments, in addition to inflammatory cytokines, chemokines, and prostaglandin derivates, promote leukocyte recruitment that perpetuates and amplifies the degradation cycle.[10,11] Together, the inflammatory milieu, elastic fiber fragmentation, medial attenuation, and decreased collagen reduce the structural integrity of the aorta and ultimately result in aneurysmal dilatation.[12–15]

Circumferential wall tension in the aorta is directly related to the transmural pressure (intravascular pressure minus the extravascular wall pressure) and the radius of the vessel (Laplace's law), and inversely proportional to wall thickness. Thus increases in aortic diameter or arterial pressure increase wall stress and the risk of aneurysm enlargement, rupture, or dissection. However, wall stress, as a predictor of adverse events, is more complex in aneurysmal tissue, because some of these physical assumptions may not relate to diseased aortic tissues (**Fig. 3**).[16]

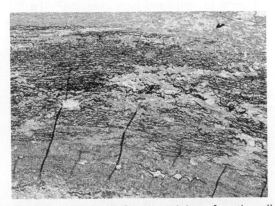

Fig. 2. Hematoxylin and eosin staining of aortic wall showing CMD. (*Courtesy of* John T. Fallon, MD, PhD, Department of Pathology, The Mount Sinai School of Medicine.)

PHARMACOLOGIC IMPLICATIONS

With increased understanding of the pathophysiologic processes that are involved in aneurysm

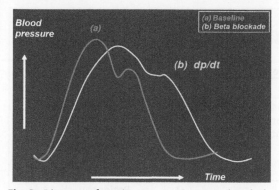

Fig. 3. Diagram of aortic pressure. Compared with the baseline state (*a*), β-blockade decreases aortic pressures and prolongs the cardiac cycle, thereby reducing dp/dt (*b*). (*Adapted from* Sanz J, Einstein AJ, Fuster V. Acute aortic dissection: anti-impulse therapy. New York: Taylor & Francis Inc; 2007:235; with permission.)

formation, greater attention is being given to evaluating pharmacologic interventions that may slow or arrest aneurysm formation. However, although promising results have been seen with the use of renin-angiotensin system blockade,[17–19] other medical therapies have not proved to be effective. In this section, pharmacologic agents other than those that affect the renin-angiotensin system that have been evaluated for the management of TAA are discussed.

β-Blockers

Medical therapy aimed at reducing wall tension through use of β-adrenergic blockade has its basis from a seminal work by Prokop and colleagues,[20] demonstrating that the pulsatile nature of the cardiac cycle places significant strain on the aorta, especially within the first 2 cm of the aorta. Pulsatile flow, characterized by a change in pressure over time (dp/dt), contributes to the progression of aortic dissections (see **Fig. 3**), whereas nonpulsatile flow does not. Because of their favorable effects on dp/dt,[20,21] β-blockers have become a cornerstone of the medical management of aortic dissection.

However, the benefit of β-adrenergic blockade is much better established in aortic dissection than in TAA. Although β-blockers provide the theoretical benefits of blood pressure and dp/dt reduction, no clinical trial has established a benefit of β-blocker therapy in TAA in the absence of Marfan syndrome.[22] Shores and colleagues[23] demonstrated that prophylactic β-blockade was effective in slowing the rate of aortic dilatation and reducing the development of aortic complications in Marfan syndrome; however, a subsequent meta-analysis failed to show any benefit. A recent

study is randomizing patients with Marfan syndrome to treatment with nebivolol, losartan, or a combination of both and is evaluating the progression of aortic root growth rate.[24]

β-Blockers have also been studied in abdominal aortic aneurysm (AAA) with mixed results. Initial animal studies[25–27] suggested that propranolol might have beneficial effects on aneursymal disease on the basis of its hemodynamic properties and biochemical effects on matrix proteins. However, the clinical data evaluating the effect of β-blockade on AAA growth rate have been conflicting. Three nonrandomized clinical studies showed that β-blocker use was associated with a decreased rate of AAA expansion,[28–30] whereas 2 other trials failed to show a statistically significant impact.[31,32] In the only 2 randomized controlled trials to evaluate the use of propranolol for AAA,[33,34] subjects did not tolerate the propranolol therapy well because of dyspnea and impaired quality of life, and neither study demonstrated a significant attenuation of AAA growth rate with propranolol. In the Propranolol Aneurysm Trial, the larger of the 2 studies (n = 548), a significant reduction in the rate of elective aneurysm resection was noted when the analysis was limited to those who could tolerate propranolol.[33] The second trial (n = 54) was stopped early after finding significantly increased mortality in the propranolol group (relative risk = 1.6; 95% confidence interval, 1.02–2.51) (**Table 1**).[34]

The theoretical benefits of β-blocker therapy for TAA have not been proven clinically. No data support their use in TAA with the possible exception of patients with Marfan syndrome. In fact, β-blockade may actually lead to increased mortality in patients with AAA.[34] In addition, there is evidence that β-blockers may decrease aortic wall elasticity, a serious concern given that reduced elasticity is a major pathologic component of aneursymal aortas.[35] Together, these data do not support the use of β-blocker therapy in patients with TAA.

Statins

Therapy with 3-hydroxy-3-methylglutaryl-coenzyme A reductase inhibitors (statins) disrupts many of the inflammatory pathways critical in the development of aortic aneurysms. Cerivastatin, simvastatin, and lovastatin inhibit secretion of MMP-1, -3, and -9 from rabbit and human VSMCs and from rabbit macrophages.[36] Collagenolytic and gelatinolytic activities are consequently reduced, but the statin effects are mediated via inhibition of isoprenoid rather than cholesterol biosynthesis.[36] Similarly, AAA tissue samples

Table 1
Clinical trials of β-blockers in management of aneurysms

Aneurysm Type	Author, Year Medication	Study Design		Results
TAA	No clinical trials available			
AAA	Lindholt, 1999 Propranolol	RCT of 54 asymptomatic patients with small AAA	(−)	Only 22% were treatable with propranolol for 2 years; increased mortality in β-blocker group
AAA	Propranolol Aneurysm Trial Investigators, CANADA, 2002 Propranolol	Three nonrandomized trials	(−)	Patients with AAAs did not tolerate propranolol well; no significant effect on the growth rate of small AAAs
AAA	Cronenwett; Gadowski; Leach, 1990, 1994, 2005 Propranolol	RCT of asymptomatic AAA (3.0–5.0 cm)	(+)	Decreased rate of AAA expansion in β-blocker group
Marfan syndrome	Shores, 1994 Propranolol	RCT of 70 patients	(+)	Decreased rate of aortic root dilatation and fewer aortic complications in β-blocker group
Marfan syndrome	Gersony, 2007 β-Blockers	Meta-analysis: 6 studies (5 nonrandomized; 1 was a prospective RCT with 802 patients)	(−)	No change in risk of aortic dissection or rupture, cardiovascular surgery, or death
Marfan syndrome	Gambarin, 2009 Losartan vs nebivolol	Open-label phase 3 study will include 291 patients	Ongoing	Primary end point: effect on the progression of aortic root growth

Abbreviations: AAA, abdominal aortic aneurysm; RCT, randomized controlled trial.

from patients receiving a statin preoperatively demonstrated less MMP-9 and -3 activity when compared with those from nonstatin users.[37–39] In a study specifically focusing on tissue samples from patients with TAA, increased reactive oxygen species were seen in aneurysmal tissue than in nonaneurysmal tissue, especially in areas of macrophage and monocyte infiltration.[40] The investigators also observed that expression of p22^{phox}, a component of the oxidase that is responsible for the generation of reactive oxygen species, was reduced in tissue samples from patients who received an angiotensin II receptor blocker or a statin, suggesting that both agents may have a role in inhibiting aneurysm formation.

Data from animal models of AAA suggest that statins inhibit MMP-9 activity, and reduce aneurysm development[41,42] and expansion.[43] Using gene microarray analysis, Kalyanasundaram and colleagues[43] demonstrated that statin therapy significantly changed the expression of 315 genes, most of which were related to inflammation, extracellular matrix remodeling, and oxidative stress. Shiraya and colleagues[41] suggest that the inhibitory effects of statins on aneurysm formation result from inhibition of macrophage infiltration. Atorvastatin inhibited the expression of intercellular adhesion molecule and monocyte chemotactic protein 1, which are involved in macrophage migration.[41]

However, there are no clinical data supporting the use of statins for TAA. Scant data from AAA are supportive. In a small study of 130 patients, those receiving a statin demonstrated no aneurysm expansion over 23 months of follow-up compared with an increase from 4.5 ± 0.6 cm to 5.3 ± 0.6 cm in nonstatin users.[44] Statin use was also associated with significantly reduced mortality (5% vs 16%, $P<.05$). A similar study of infrarenal AAA revealed slower aneurysm expansion in statin users over a 3-year follow-up period (2.0 mm/y vs 3.6 mm/y, $P = .001$).[45]

Macrolides and Tetracyclines

Theoretically, the use of antibiotic therapy for aortic aneurysms is justified by evidence of secondary infection with bacteria such as *Chlamydia pneumoniae* in both atherosclerotic plaques and AAA tissue[46,47] and by the effectiveness of specific antibiotic agents in attenuating metalloproteinase activity independent of their antibiotic activity.[48] Patients who were randomized to therapy with roxithromycin (300 mg) daily for 1 month demonstrated slower aneurysm expansion rate than placebo (1.56 vs 2.75 mm/y). However, there was no correlation between *C. pneumoniae* titers and inhibition of aneurysm expansion, suggesting that the mechanism of benefit is unrelated to specific antibiotic activity.[49]

Tetracyclines have been shown to antagonize a spectrum of MMPs in vitro and in animal models through mechanisms similar to those of endogenous TIMPs, which are independent of their antibiotic activity.[50–53] Doxycycline prevented the disruption of medial elastin in rodent models and attenuated the dilation of AAA by 33% to 66% compared with placebo.[54–56] Although the doses used in these studies (5–30 mg/kg/d) were substantially higher than the usual human dose (1–1.5 mg/kg/d or 200 mg/d), doxycycline (100 mg) administered twice daily in humans achieved

similar steady-state plasma concentrations to those required for aneurysm inhibition in rodents.[56] The safety of therapy with doxycycline (200 mg) daily for 6 months in patients with AAAs has been established in a phase 2 clinical trial, as has its efficacy in reducing MMP expression.[48,57] A randomized trial of 32 patients demonstrated attenuation of aneurysmal growth (from 3.0 mm/y to 1.5 mm/y) after 3 months of treatment with doxycycline (150 mg/d), again with no effect on *C. pneumoniae* titers.[58]

Results of macrolide and tetracycline therapy in animal and preliminary human studies are promising, but the studies have several important limitations in addition to their small size. First, most data were derived from AAA and may not be simply extrapolated to thoracic aorta disease. Second, even if the efficacy of attenuating thoracic aneursymal dilation is established, it must be confirmed that the inhibition of growth does not compromise the structural integrity of aneurysmal tissue such that it is prone to rupture at smaller diameters.

ANEURYSM PARITY

Much of the data regarding the use of pharmacologic agents in the management of aortic aneurysms has been generated from studies of patients with AAA or with Marfan syndrome. The question of whether the extrapolation of these data to TAA is appropriate remains. Several differences exist between TAA and AAA that encumber the ability to apply data from one disease process to another (**Table 2**). The epidemiology of each is distinct, with a 4-fold greater prevalence of AAA compared with TAA and a similar imbalance in the incidence of aneurysm rupture.[59] Several atherosclerotic risk factors, such as male gender, age, smoking, and hypertension, are strongly

Table 2
Differences between TAA, AAA, and Marfan syndrome

	TAA	AAA	Marfan Syndrome
Prevalence	1.25%	5%	1 in 10,000
Risk factors	Genetic predisposition Hypertension	Genetic predisposition Age Male gender Hypertension Smoking	Genetic predisposition
Histology	Cystic medial necrosis	Inflammatory infiltrate, VSMC apoptosis	Cystic medial necrosis
Rate of expansion and rupture	+	++	+++

associated with AAA, whereas genetic predisposition seems to play a larger role in TAA.[35,60–62] Although some similarities exist, several genetic loci are uniquely associated with aneurysm formation either in the thoracic or abdominal aorta.[63] These data suggest that different pathophysiologic processes are responsible for the development and progression of AAA and TAA. Nordon and colleagues[64] demonstrated that AAA are associated with a systemic propensity of the vasculature to dilate, whereas TAA are not. In addition, AAA are characterized by an active inflammatory process that results in smooth muscle cell apoptosis and fragmentation of the extracellular matrix.[65] On the other hand, medial necrosis, mucoid infiltration, and elastin degradation are characteristic of TAA.[63]

The pathophysiologic differences between Marfan syndrome and non-Marfan TAA are also significant (see **Table 2**). Marfan syndrome is an autosomal dominant disorder caused by mutations in the fibrillin-1 (FBN1) gene. Fibrillins form the structural framework of elastin fibers and are vital for normal aortic development and functioning. An important feature in the aortic pathology that is observed in Marfan syndrome is that fibrillin-1 inhibits TGF-β.[66–68] Consequently, elevated levels of TGF-β in patients with FBN1 mutations[2,68,69] correspond to increased MMP activity and extracellular matrix breakdown.[70–72] The result is progressive aortic root enlargement with possible aneurysm development, dissection, rupture, or aortic valve regurgitation. Conversely, reductions of TGF-β have been shown to suppress the characteristic histologic changes associated with Marfan syndrome.[69] The aortic pathology in Marfan syndrome is more aggressive than that seen in senile TAA, with rapid aneurysm enlargement and frequent rupture.[73] Although several aspects of Marfan syndrome are common to those with bicuspid aortic valves and familial TAA, these pathophysiologic features have not been demonstrated in senile TAA.

SUMMARY

The pathophysiology of aneurysm formation involves a complex interplay of genetic predisposition, cardiovascular risk factors, and hemodynamic forces. The medical community has resorted to the use of pharmacologic agents based on weak data transplanted from either AAA or Marfan syndrome. However, aneurysms differ significantly based on anatomic location and etiology. Epidemiologic and experimental data demonstrate that different genetic and nongenetic risk factors as well as diverse pathophysiologic processes are responsible for the development and progression of sporadic TAA, familial TAA (such as those found in Marfan syndrome), and AAA. Therefore, these disease processes need to be considered as distinct entities and not hastily grouped together. The extrapolation of data from one aneursymal disease process to another is ill founded and potentially harmful. Clinical trials in TAA are required before medical therapies, such as β-blockers, statins, and macrolide antibiotics, can be recommended.

REFERENCES

1. Agmon Y, Khandheria BK, Meissner I, et al. Is aortic dilatation an atherosclerosis-related process? Clinical, laboratory, and transesophageal echocardiographic correlates of thoracic aortic dimensions in the population with implications for thoracic aortic aneurysm formation. J Am Coll Cardiol 2003;42(6): 1076–83.
2. Nataatmadja M, West J, West M. Overexpression of transforming growth factor-beta is associated with increased hyaluronan content and impairment of repair in Marfan syndrome aortic aneurysm. Circulation 2006;114(Suppl 1):I371–7.
3. El-Hamamsy I, Yacoub MH. Cellular and molecular mechanisms of thoracic aortic aneurysms. Nat Rev Cardiol 2009;6(12):771–86.
4. Kadoglou NP, Liapis CD. Matrix metalloproteinases: contribution to pathogenesis, diagnosis, surveillance and treatment of abdominal aortic aneurysms. Curr Med Res Opin 2004;20(4):419–32.
5. O'Rourke MF, Hashimoto J. Mechanical factors in arterial aging: a clinical perspective. J Am Coll Cardiol 2007;50(1):1–13.
6. Elefteriades JA. Acute aortic diseases. 1st edition. New York: Taylor & Francis, Inc; 2007.
7. Knox JB, Sukhova GK, Whittemore AD, et al. Evidence for altered balance between matrix metalloproteinases and their inhibitors in human aortic diseases. Circulation 1997;95(1):205–12.
8. Pyo R, Lee JK, Shipley JM, et al. Targeted gene disruption of matrix metalloproteinase-9 (gelatinase B) suppresses development of experimental abdominal aortic aneurysms. J Clin Invest 2000; 105(11):1641–9.
9. Tamarina NA, McMillan WD, Shively VP, et al. Expression of matrix metalloproteinases and their inhibitors in aneurysms and normal aorta. Surgery 1997;122(2):264–71 [discussion: 271–2].
10. Shah PK. Inflammation, metalloproteinases, and increased proteolysis: an emerging pathophysiological paradigm in aortic aneurysm. Circulation 1997; 96(7):2115–7.
11. Herron GS, Unemori E, Wong M, et al. Connective tissue proteinases and inhibitors in abdominal aortic

aneurysms. Involvement of the vasa vasorum in the pathogenesis of aortic aneurysms. Arterioscler Thromb 1991;11(6):1667–77.

12. Baxter BT, McGee GS, Shively VP, et al. Elastin content, cross-links, and mRNA in normal and aneurysmal human aorta. J Vasc Surg 1992;16(2): 192–200.

13. Sakalihasan N, Heyeres A, Nusgens BV, et al. Modifications of the extracellular matrix of aneurysmal abdominal aortas as a function of their size. Eur J Vasc Surg 1993;7(6):633–7.

14. Dobrin PB, Mrkvicka R. Failure of elastin or collagen as possible critical connective tissue alterations underlying aneurysmal dilatation. Cardiovasc Surg 1994;2(4):484–8.

15. Satta J, Juvonen T, Haukipuro K, et al. Increased turnover of collagen in abdominal aortic aneurysms, demonstrated by measuring the concentration of the aminoterminal propeptide of type III procollagen in peripheral and aortal blood samples. J Vasc Surg 1995;22(2):155–60.

16. Elefteriades J. Acute aortic disease. New York: Informa Healthcare USA, Inc; 2007.

17. Lim DS, Lutucuta S, Bachireddy P, et al. Angiotensin II blockade reverses myocardial fibrosis in a transgenic mouse model of human hypertrophic cardiomyopathy. Circulation 2001;103(6):789–91.

18. Lavoie P, Robitaille G, Agharazii M, et al. Neutralization of transforming growth factor-beta attenuates hypertension and prevents renal injury in uremic rats. J Hypertens 2005;23(10):1895–903.

19. Brooke BS, Habashi JP, Judge DP, et al. Angiotensin II blockade and aortic-root dilation in Marfan's syndrome. N Engl J Med 2008;358(26):2787–95.

20. Prokop EK, Palmer RF, Wheat MW Jr. Hydrodynamic forces in dissecting aneurysms. In-vitro studies in a Tygon model and in dog aortas. Circ Res 1970; 27(1):121–7.

21. Sanz J, Einstein AJ, Fuster V. Acute aortic dissection: anti-impulse therapy. New York: Taylor & Francis, Inc; 2007.

22. Gersony DR, McClaughlin MA, Jin Z, et al. The effect of beta-blocker therapy on clinical outcome in patients with Marfan's syndrome: a meta-analysis. Int J Cardiol 2007;114(3):303–8.

23. Shores J, Berger KR, Murphy EA, et al. Progression of aortic dilatation and the benefit of long-term beta-adrenergic blockade in Marfan's syndrome. N Engl J Med 1994;330(19):1335–41.

24. Gambarin FI, Favalli V, Serio A, et al. Rationale and design of a trial evaluating the effects of losartan vs. nebivolol vs. the association of both on the progression of aortic root dilation in Marfan syndrome with FBN1 gene mutations. J Cardiovasc Med (Hagerstown) 2009;10(4):354–62.

25. Boucek RJ, Gunja-Smith Z, Noble NL, et al. Modulation by propranolol of the lysyl cross-links in aortic elastin and collagen of the aneurysm-prone turkey. Biochem Pharmacol 1983;32(2):275–80.

26. Brophy CM, Tilson JE, Tilson MD. Propranolol stimulates the crosslinking of matrix components in skin from the aneurysm-prone blotchy mouse. J Surg Res 1989;46(4):330–2.

27. Simpson CF, Kling JM, Palmer RF. Beta-aminopropionitrile-induced dissecting aneurysms of turkeys: treatment with propranolol. Toxicol Appl Pharmacol 1970;16(1):143–53.

28. Gadowski GR, Pilcher DB, Ricci MA. Abdominal aortic aneurysm expansion rate: effect of size and beta-adrenergic blockade. J Vasc Surg 1994;19(4): 727–31.

29. Leach SD, Toole AL, Stern H, et al. Effect of beta-adrenergic blockade on the growth rate of abdominal aortic aneurysms. Arch Surg 1988; 123(5):606–9.

30. Cronenwett JL, Sargent SK, Wall MH, et al. Variables that affect the expansion rate and outcome of small abdominal aortic aneurysms. J Vasc Surg 1990; 11(2):260–8 [discussion: 268–9].

31. Biancari F, Mosorin M, Anttila V, et al. Ten-year outcome of patients with very small abdominal aortic aneurysm. Am J Surg 2002;183(1):53–5.

32. Wilmink AB, Vardulaki KA, Hubbard CS, et al. Are antihypertensive drugs associated with abdominal aortic aneurysms? J Vasc Surg 2002;36(4):751–7.

33. Propranolol Aneurysm Trial Investigators. Propranolol for small abdominal aortic aneurysms: results of a randomized trial. J Vasc Surg 2002;35(1): 72–9.

34. Lindholt JS, Henneberg EW, Juul S, et al. Impaired results of a randomised double blinded clinical trial of propranolol versus placebo on the expansion rate of small abdominal aortic aneurysms. Int Angiol 1999;18(1):52–7.

35. Elefteriades JA. Thoracic aortic aneurysm: reading the enemy's playbook. Curr Probl Cardiol 2008; 33(5):203–77.

36. Luan Z, Chase AJ, Newby AC. Statins inhibit secretion of metalloproteinases-1, -2, -3, and -9 from vascular smooth muscle cells and macrophages. Arterioscler Thromb Vasc Biol 2003;23(5):769–75.

37. Wilson WR, Evans J, Bell PR, et al. HMG-CoA reductase inhibitors (statins) decrease MMP-3 and MMP-9 concentrations in abdominal aortic aneurysms. Eur J Vasc Endovasc Surg 2005;30(3):259–62.

38. Abisi S, Burnand KG, Humphries J, et al. Effect of statins on proteolytic activity in the wall of abdominal aortic aneurysms. Br J Surg 2008;95(3):333–7.

39. Evans J, Powell JT, Schwalbe E, et al. Simvastatin attenuates the activity of matrix metalloprotease-9 in aneurysmal aortic tissue. Eur J Vasc Endovasc Surg 2007;34(3):302–3.

40. Ejiri J, Inoue N, Tsukube T, et al. Oxidative stress in the pathogenesis of thoracic aortic aneurysm: protective

role of statin and angiotensin II type 1 receptor blocker. Cardiovasc Res 2003;59(4):988–96.

41. Shiraya S, Miyake T, Aoki M, et al. Inhibition of development of experimental aortic abdominal aneurysm in rat model by atorvastatin through inhibition of macrophage migration. Atherosclerosis 2009; 202(1):34–40.

42. Steinmetz EF, Buckley C, Shames ML, et al. Treatment with simvastatin suppresses the development of experimental abdominal aortic aneurysms in normal and hypercholesterolemic mice. Ann Surg 2005;241(1):92–101.

43. Kalyanasundaram A, Elmore JR, Manazer JR, et al. Simvastatin suppresses experimental aortic aneurysm expansion. J Vasc Surg 2006;43(1):117–24.

44. Sukhija R, Aronow WS, Sandhu R, et al. Mortality and size of abdominal aortic aneurysm at long-term follow-up of patients not treated surgically and treated with and without statins. Am J Cardiol 2006;97(2):279–80.

45. Schouten O, van Laanen JH, Boersma E, et al. Statins are associated with a reduced infrarenal abdominal aortic aneurysm growth. Eur J Vasc Endovasc Surg 2006;32(1):21–6.

46. Nieto FJ. Infective agents and cardiovascular disease. Semin Vasc Med 2002;2(4):401–15.

47. Lindholt JS, Ashton HA, Scott RA. Indicators of infection with Chlamydia pneumoniae are associated with expansion of abdominal aortic aneurysms. J Vasc Surg 2001;34(2):212–5.

48. Curci JA, Mao D, Bohner DG, et al. Preoperative treatment with doxycycline reduces aortic wall expression and activation of matrix metalloproteinases in patients with abdominal aortic aneurysm. J Vasc Surg 2000;31(2):325–42.

49. Vammen S, Lindholt JS, Ostergaard L, et al. Randomized double-blind controlled trial of roxithromycin for prevention of abdominal aortic aneurysm expansion. Br J Surg 2001;88(8):1066–72.

50. Golub LM, Lee HM, Lehrer G, et al. Minocycline reduces gingival collagenolytic activity during diabetes. Preliminary observations and a proposed new mechanism of action. J Periodont Res 1983; 18(5):516–26.

51. Golub LM, Lee HM, Ryan ME, et al. Tetracyclines inhibit connective tissue breakdown by multiple non-antimicrobial mechanisms. Adv Dent Res 1998;12(2):12–26.

52. Greenwald RA. Treatment of destructive arthritic disorders with MMP inhibitors. Potential role of tetracyclines. Ann N Y Acad Sci 1994;732:181–98.

53. Longo GM, Buda SJ, Fiotta N, et al. MMP-12 has a role in abdominal aortic aneurysms in mice. Surgery 2005;137(4):457–62.

54. Curci JA, Petrinec D, Liao S, et al. Pharmacologic suppression of experimental abdominal aortic aneurysms: a comparison of doxycycline and four chemically modified tetracyclines. J Vasc Surg 1998;28(6):1082–93.

55. Petrinec D, Liao S, Holmes DR, et al. Doxycycline inhibition of aneurysmal degeneration in an elastase-induced rat model of abdominal aortic aneurysm: preservation of aortic elastin associated with suppressed production of 92 kD gelatinase. J Vasc Surg 1996;23(2):336–46.

56. Prall AK, Longo GM, Mayhan WG, et al. Doxycycline in patients with abdominal aortic aneurysms and in mice: comparison of serum levels and effect on aneurysm growth in mice. J Vasc Surg 2002;35(5):923–9.

57. Baxter BT, Pearce WH, Waltke EA, et al. Prolonged administration of doxycycline in patients with small asymptomatic abdominal aortic aneurysms: report of a prospective (Phase II) multicenter study. J Vasc Surg 2002;36(1):1–12.

58. Mosorin M, Juvonen J, Biancari F, et al. Use of doxycycline to decrease the growth rate of abdominal aortic aneurysms: a randomized, double-blind, placebo-controlled pilot study. J Vasc Surg 2001; 34(4):606–10.

59. Dalsing MC, Lalka SG, Sawchuk AP, et al. Vascular medicine. In: Kelley WN, editor. Textbook of internal medicine. Philadelphia: Lippincott-Raven Publishers; 1997.

60. Bickerstaff LK, Pairolero PC, Hollier LH, et al. Thoracic aortic aneurysms: a population-based study. Surgery 1982;92(6):1103–8.

61. Bickerstaff LK, Hollier LH, Van Peenen HJ, et al. Abdominal aortic aneurysms: the changing natural history. J Vasc Surg 1984;1(1):6–12.

62. Golledge J, Muller J, Daugherty A, et al. Abdominal aortic aneurysm: pathogenesis and implications for management. Arterioscler Thromb Vasc Biol 2006; 26(12):2605–13.

63. Kuivaniemi H, Platsoucas CD, Tilson MD 3rd. Aortic aneurysms: an immune disease with a strong genetic component. Circulation 2008;117(2):242–52.

64. Nordon I, Brar R, Taylor J, et al. Evidence from cross-sectional imaging indicates abdominal but not thoracic aortic aneurysms are local manifestations of a systemic dilating diathesis. J Vasc Surg 2009;50(1):171–6, e171.

65. Thompson RW. Reflections on the pathogenesis of abdominal aortic aneurysms. Cardiovasc Surg 2002;10(4):389–94.

66. Kielty CM. Elastic fibres in health and disease. Expert Rev Mol Med 2006;8(19):1–23.

67. Isogai Z, Ono RN, Ushiro S, et al. Latent transforming growth factor beta-binding protein 1 interacts with fibrillin and is a microfibril-associated protein. J Biol Chem 2003;278(4):2750–7.

68. Neptune ER, Frischmeyer PA, Arking DE, et al. Dysregulation of TGF-beta activation contributes to pathogenesis in Marfan syndrome. Nat Genet 2003;33(3):407–11.

69. Habashi JP, Judge DP, Holm TM, et al. Losartan, an AT1 antagonist, prevents aortic aneurysm in a mouse model of Marfan syndrome. Science 2006;312(5770): 117–21.

70. Nataatmadja M, West M, West J, et al. Abnormal extracellular matrix protein transport associated with increased apoptosis of vascular smooth muscle cells in Marfan syndrome and bicuspid aortic valve thoracic aortic aneurysm. Circulation 2003; 108(Suppl 1):II329–34.

71. Ikonomidis JS, Jones JA, Barbour JR, et al. Expression of matrix metalloproteinases and endogenous inhibitors within ascending aortic aneurysms of patients with Marfan syndrome. Circulation 2006; 114(Suppl 1):I365–70.

72. Chung AW, Au Yeung K, Sandor GG, et al. Loss of elastic fiber integrity and reduction of vascular smooth muscle contraction resulting from the upregulated activities of matrix metalloproteinase-2 and -9 in the thoracic aortic aneurysm in Marfan syndrome. Circ Res 2007;101(5):512–22.

73. Davies RR, Goldstein LJ, Coady MA, et al. Yearly rupture or dissection rates for thoracic aortic aneurysms: simple prediction based on size. Ann Thorac Surg 2002;73(1):17–27 [discussion: 27–8].

Editorial Comment: Does Medical Therapy for Thoracic Aortic Aneurysms Really Work? Are β-Blockers Truly Indicated?

John A. Elefteriades, MD

The article by Dr Valentin Fuster and colleagues in this issue of *Cardiology Clinics* elegantly exposes the paucity of scientific and clinical evidence in favor of benefit from β-blockers in patients with thoracic aortic aneurysm (**Table 1**).

Dr John A. Elefteriades actually is a skeptic regarding the benefits of β-blockade. His article reviews the historical and modern evidence of benefit, but he does feel that, although theoretically reasonable, widespread use of β-blockers for protection of patients with thoracic aortic aneurysm is largely unproved (**Fig. 1**). He recommends that if a specific patient is intolerant of β-blockers, the drugs can reasonably be omitted.

Table 1
Does medical therapy for thoracic aortic aneurysms really work?

Pro: β-Blockers Are Indicated (Elefteriades)	Con: β-Blockers Are Not Indicated (Fuster)
Historical evidence in Tygon tubing and turkeys	No study has established the clinical benefit of β-blockers for chronic thoracic aortic aneurysm in patients without Marfan syndrome
Shores article showed slower rate of growth in patients with Marfan syndrome	One must not presume "aneurysm parity"—that is, data from Marfan patients cannot be extrapolated to patients with other types of aneurysms
Some clinical evidence of benefit in acute aortic dissection	Studies in abdominal aortic aneurysm are equivocal at best
Conflicting studies of impact on mechanical properties of aorta	Some evidence indicates that β-blockers impair aortic elasticity
New evidence implicating emotion/exertion in inciting acute dissection suggests that there may be benefit in blunting acute blood pressure spikes via β-blockage	Other drugs: • Very preliminary experimental and clinical evidence suggests there may be some benefit from statin drugs in aneurysm patients • Some evidence supports the use of tetracycline for its anti-MMP effects

Section of Cardiac Surgery, Department of Surgery, Yale University School of Medicine, Yale-New Haven Hospital, PO Box 208039, New Haven, CT 06520-8039, USA
E-mail address: john.elefteriades@yale.edu

Cardiol Clin 28 (2010) 271–272
doi:10.1016/j.ccl.2010.02.018

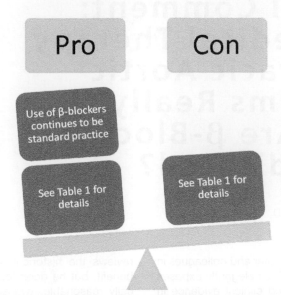

Fig. 1. Despite the lack of direct evidence, use of β-blockers continues to be standard practice on the basis of some positive evidence and strong theoretic merit. Randomized studies are under way.

Is Losartan the True Panacea for Aneurysm Disease? PRO

Michael J. Collins, MD[a], John A. Elefteriades, MD[b],*

KEYWORDS

- Aortic aneurysm • Marfan syndrome
- Angiotensin receptor blockers

Aneurysms of the aorta remain a significant and common medical problem in the twenty-first century. Despite advances in intensive care, aortic aneurysms remain the 13th most common cause of death in the United States,[1] with 150,000 hospital admissions for abdominal aortic aneurysms (AAAs) alone.[2] The mean age at onset ranges from 59 to 69 years, with a male to female ratio of between 2:1 and 4:1.[1] Aortic aneurysms are often associated with dissections of the aorta, the rupture of which represents a catastrophic event requiring emergency surgical intervention. There have been numerous recent advances in the treatment of aneurysms, especially with regard to the use of interventional procedures and new stent grafts; however, surgical repair remains the current standard of care.

Although most aneurysms occur spontaneously, there are a number of syndromes which predispose patients to aneurysm formation. Marfan syndrome is an autosomal dominant disorder of the connective tissue, with an incidence of 2 to 3 per 100,000 individuals. Aortic dilation and dissection is the main cause of morbidity and mortality in patients with Marfan syndrome. The mainstay of long-term management of the patients has focused on blood pressure control and beta blockade. Recent work examining the mechanisms of aneurysm formation has led to increased interest in medical therapy targeting factors involved in aneurysm formation and expansion.

In particular, inhibition of the renin-angiotensin system with angiotensin converting enzyme inhibitors (ACEis) and angiotensin receptor blockers (ARBs) has recently emerged as a potentially powerful treatment modality for the aortic aneurysms. In the present review, data from animal models, as well as early clinical results, are reviewed with particular attention to how these medications may target the mechanisms underlying aneurysm formation. These new data point to the use of ARBs as one of the new cornerstones in the management of aneurysmal disease.

PATHOGENESIS OF ANEURYSM FORMATION

Recent studies have begun to elucidate the molecular pathways responsible for aneurysm development and are reviewed elsewhere.[3] The mechanisms involved in aneurysm formation are complex and vary in different segments of the aorta. Although it is tempting to assume that aortic aneurysms proceed by a similar mechanisms regardless of their anatomic location, significant histologic differences have been observed. AAAs are frequently associated with severe complex atherosclerosis with heavy inflammatory infiltration of macrophages.[4] In contrast, high-grade inflammation is usually absent in thoracic aortic aneurysm tissue.[5] It is now accepted that nearly all aortic aneurysms result from a shift in the balance between extracellular matrix synthesis and

[a] Division of Cardiothoracic Surgery, Department of Surgery, Yale New Haven Hospital, Yale University School of Medicine, Post Office Box 208062, New Haven, CT 06520-8062, USA
[b] Section of Cardiac Surgery, Department of Surgery, Yale University School of Medicine, Yale-New Haven Hospital, PO Box 208039, New Haven, CT 06520-8039, USA
* Corresponding author.
E-mail address: john.elefteriades@yale.edu

Cardiol Clin 28 (2010) 273–277
doi:10.1016/j.ccl.2010.02.005
0733-8651/10/$ – see front matter © 2010 Published by Elsevier Inc.

degradation toward proteolysis. Numerous matrix degrading enzymes, particularly matrix metallo-proteinases (MMPs), especially MMP-2 and MMP-9, have been found in increased amounts in abdominal and ascending aortic aneurysms and are thought to play a central role in aneurysm pathogenesis.[6,7]

Regardless of the anatomic location, aortic aneurysms are associated with degenerative changes in the aortic media, including fragmentation and loss of the elastic laminae, loss of vascular smooth muscle cells (VSMCs), and deposition of mucopolysaccharides and/or collagen.[6] Pathology studies have shown that patients with Marfan syndrome show the most severe histologic changes with respect to elastin fragmentation and loss compared with other patients with aortic aneurysms, likely reflective of a disease process which has been ongoing since birth. Histologic changes were not only more severe but also showed a different pattern of changes from non-Marfan patients. Patients with Marfan syndrome tended to show transmural elastin loss with only very few strands of elastin remaining; however, smooth muscle cells were comparatively better preserved, which is consistent with a primary connective tissue defect.[8]

RENIN-ANGIOTENSIN BLOCKADE IN ANIMAL MODELS

Given that many features of aortic aneurysms include degradation of extracellular matrix components and an inflammatory response related to atherosclerosis, it is not surprising to discover the involvement of proinflammatory transcription factors in aneurysm pathogenesis. Expression of these proinflammatory proteases, as well as the production of other proinflammatory cytokines, is regulated by nuclear factor (NF) κB.[9] The renin-angiotensin system, particularly angiotensin II (AngII), is well known to be involved in atherosclerosis. Studies have shown that AngII exerts a proinflammatory effect through increased NF-κB-mediated expression of several mediators, including leukocyte adhesion molecules, heat shock proteins, growth factors, and endothelin-1. AngII is known to upregulate NF-κB, which provides a mechanistic link between the renin-angiotensin system and aneurysm pathogenesis.[10,11] Angiotensin converting enzyme is known to be increased in human AAA tissues.[12] In fact, AngII has been used to induce aneurysms in apolipoprotein E–deficient mice,[13] whereas ACEis have been shown to suppress aortic dilation in experimental AAA model.[14]

Two main AngII receptors have been identified. Most physiologic effects of AngII in adults are mediated by AngII type 1 receptor (AT1R), whereas AngII type 2 receptor (AT2R) signaling is generally inhibitory to AT1R signaling. AT2R levels are high in fetal tissues, but decrease rapidly after birth; however, multiple studies have shown that levels of AT2R are elevated in cardiovascular disease.[15,16] The role of AT2R signaling in aneurysm pathogenesis is unclear. AT2R messenger RNA expression is significantly increased in animal models of aortic aneurysms. In a study by Nagashima and colleagues,[17] rats were fed a diet containing β-aminopropionitrile, a chemical that inhibits collagen crosslinking and thus induces aneurysm dilation and dissection. Treatment of these rats with an ACEi over a 5-week period prevented dissection and VSMC apoptosis, and significantly preserved elastic fibers on histologic examination compared with controls. Interestingly, treatment with ACEis, which inhibits both AT1R and AT2R signaling but not AT1R-specific receptor blockers, prevented dissection in their animal model.

In contrast, Fujiwara and colleagues[18] used a rat model in which aortic aneurysm formation was induced by injection of elastase. Valsartan (an AT1R blocker) was administered daily through osmotic minipumps from the date of the operation to 4 weeks postoperation. The dose of valsartan was minimal and had no effect on blood pressure. Aneurysm progression was significantly decreased over the 4-week study period in valsartan-treated mice. Similarly, MMP-2, MMP-3, MMP-9, and MMP-12 levels were assessed using western blot and were found to be significantly decreased in valsartan-treated rats compared with controls. This effect was further confirmed by reverse transcription-polymerase chain reaction from isolated peritoneal macrophages, which showed that valsartan inhibited the expression of MMP-2 and MMP-9. NF-κB activation was also noted to be decreased in valsartan-treated rats. The reason for the discrepancy in these 2 studies likely relates to differences in animal models used to study aortic aneurysms. In most animal models, acute events (such as injection of elastase or chemical treatment) are necessary to induce aneurysm formation. These models, although easily reproducible, do not accurately mimic the complex multifactorial nature and time course through which aneurysms develop in human subjects.

To address these concerns, Habashi and colleagues[19] used a mouse model of Marfan syndrome with mice heterozygous for fibrillin-1 allele mutations that mimic those seen in human patients. Marfan syndrome results from mutations in fibrillin-1. Fibrillin-1 was initially thought to play primarily only a structural role in connective tissue. However, more recent data suggest an additional role as a regulatory player in cytokine transforming growth factor (TGF) β1 signaling. TGF-β1 is expressed by VSMCs in the artery wall, and its production is increased during wall repair in response to mechanical injury.[20] In aneurysmal, decellularized transplanted xenografts, TGF-β1 mRNA was increased mostly in the intima where VSMCs had been seeded. There were also increased levels of activated TGF-β1 in the entire thickness of the aneurysm wall, suggesting that TGF-β1 functions as an intimal paracrine factor. In vitro, TGF-β1 shifts MMP balance toward inhibition by downregulating various MMPs and upregulating tissue inhibitors of MMPs.[21]

Studies have shown that treatment with AT1R blockers antagonizes TGF signaling in animal models of chronic renal insufficiency and cardiomyopathy. In a mouse model of Marfan syndrome,[19] there was increased collagen deposition as well as phosphorylation and nuclear translocation of SMAD2, which are indicators of TGF-β1 signaling.

To assess the role of TGF-β1 signaling in aneurysm pathogenesis, these heterozygous mice were treated beginning at 7 weeks of age with intraperitoneal injections of TGF-neutralizing antibody. Treated mice showed markedly reduced elastic fiber fragmentation and reduced TGF-β1 signaling as evidenced by phosphorylation and nuclear translocation of SMAD2 compared with placebo-treated heterozygous mice. Furthermore, on echocardiographic examination at 8 weeks of life, there was no difference in TGF-neutralizing-antibody–treated heterozygous mice and wild-type controls. Combined, these data show that the disruption of TGF signaling in mouse models of Marfan syndrome help prevent aneurysm formation.

This mouse model was further used to evaluate the potential benefit of AT1R blockade. Heterozygous mice were treated with either oral losartan or propranolol and compared with wild-type mice. After 6 months of treatment, mice were killed. It was observed that losartan-treated mice showed improved preservation of the elastic media and reduced nuclear accumulation of SMAD2, indicative of reduced TGF-β1 signaling compared with propranolol-treated heterozygous mice. The aortic root growth rate, aortic wall thickness, and elastic fiber architecture were indistinguishable from those of wild-type mice during the study period for losartan-treated mice, suggesting that losartan may achieve full correction of phenotypic abnormalities of heterozygous Marfan mice.

The mechanism through which AT1R signaling antagonizes TGF-β1 signaling remains to be determined. AT1R signaling has been show to increase expression of TGF receptors as well as induce expression of thrombospondin-1, a potent activator of TGF-β1.[22]

ANGIOTENSIN BLOCKADE IN HUMAN PATIENTS

Nagashima and colleagues[23] reported evidence for the potential effectiveness of renin-angiotensin blockade in a series of 10 Marfan patients undergoing surgery for annuloaortic ectasia. These patients all had severe advanced aortic disease, with annuloaortic dimensions ranging from 6.7 to 9 cm. Tissue from these patients showed higher AngII concentration in tissues as measured with enzyme-linked immunosorbent assay and when calculated per wet weight, was significantly higher in Marfan aortas compared with non-Marfan control aortas.

Perhaps the most compelling data for the use of ARBs in the medical management of Marfan syndrome were reported by Brooke and colleagues.[24] This study was a retrospective review of all patients with Marfan syndrome undergoing care at the authors' institution. The study identified a cohort of 17 patients with Marfan syndrome aged 14 months to 16 years who had received ARB therapy for at least1 year. These patients had been prescribed ARB therapy as part of their medical care by their treating physicians based on their clinical discretion. This cohort was compared with 65 patients with Marfan syndrome who had undergone echocardiography during the study period and were not on ARB therapy. Patients on ARB therapy experienced a significant drop in the rate of change in aortic root diameter (3.54 mm/yr vs 0.46 mm/yr). A similar decrease in the rate of dilation of the sinotubular junction was also observed in ARB-treated patients. In contrast, more distal segments of the ascending aorta, which are generally not affected by the pathologic dilation in Marfan syndrome, showed no change after initiation of ARB therapy. There were no significant changes in mean systolic blood pressure with initiation of ARB therapy, suggesting that this observed reduction in the rate of root dilation is independent of blood pressure control. Although this review is retrospective, its findings provide powerful human data that support findings previously observed in animal models.

At present, clinical trials are underway to investigate the use of ARBs in the medical management of Marfan syndrome. The COMPARE (COzaar in Marfan Patients Reduces aortic Enlargement) trial,[25] which is currently enrolling patients, is an open-label randomized controlled trial with blinded end points. A total of 330 patients will be randomized to receive losartan and followed up for 3 years. The end points of the study include change in aortic diameter at any level as measured by magnetic resonance imaging.

SUMMARY

Aortic aneurysms remain a common medical condition in the twenty-first century. Although surgical repair remains the standard of care for patients with enlarging and advanced aneurysm disease, new insights into aortic aneurysm pathogenesis have resulted in an interest in targeting these pathways and reducing the rate of aneurysm expansion. The renin-angiotensin system has been shown to be involved in aneurysm pathogenesis, likely through the activation of the proinflammatory transcription factor NF-κB. Blockade of the rennin-angiotensin system has been shown to reduce the rate of aneurysm expansion and dissection and the expression of matrix degrading molecules. Data from mouse models of Marfan syndrome suggest that this effect may be related to disruption in TGF-β1 signaling. Most importantly, in a retrospective review of patients with Marfan syndrome, angiotensin receptor blockade resulted in significantly reduced rates of expansion of the aortic root and sinotubular junction.

These data have paved the way for new prospective randomized trials that are currently underway. Although additional study is clearly warranted to determine optimal dosing, duration of therapy, and timing of initiation of therapy, the use of angiotensin receptor blockade has the potential to revolutionize the medical management of aneurysmal disease.

REFERENCES

1. Coady MA, Rizzo JA, Goldstein LJ, et al. Natural history, pathogenesis, and etiology of thoracic aortic aneurysms and dissections. Cardiol Clin 1999;17: 615–35, vii.
2. Gillum RF. Epidemiology of aortic aneurysm in the United States. J Clin Epidemiol 1995;48: 1289–98.
3. Thompson RW. Basic science of abdominal aortic aneurysms: emerging therapeutic strategies for an unresolved clinical problem. Curr Opin Cardiol 1996;11:504–18.
4. Absi TS, Sundt TM 3rd, Tung WS, et al. Altered patterns of gene expression distinguishing ascending aortic aneurysms from abdominal aortic aneurysms: complementary DNA expression profiling in the molecular characterization of aortic disease. J Thorac Cardiovasc Surg 2003;126: 344–57 [discussion: 357].
5. Ikonomidis JS, Gibson WC, Butler JE, et al. Effects of deletion of the tissue inhibitor of matrix metalloproteinases-1 gene on the progression of murine thoracic aortic aneurysms. Circulation 2004;110: II268–73.
6. Annabi B, Shedid D, Ghosn P, et al. Differential regulation of matrix metalloproteinase activities in abdominal aortic aneurysms. J Vasc Surg 2002;35: 539–46.
7. Kadoglou NP, Liapis CD. Matrix metalloproteinases: contribution to pathogenesis, diagnosis, surveillance and treatment of abdominal aortic aneurysms. Curr Med Res Opin 2004;20:419–32.
8. Collins MJ, Dev V, Stauss BH, et al. Variation in histopathological features of patients with ascending aortic aneurysms: a study of 111 surgically excised cases. J Clin Pathol 2007;61:519–23.
9. Laundry DB, Couper LL, Bryant SR, et al. Activation of the NF-kB and 1-kB system in smooth muscle cells after rat arterial injury: induction of vascular cell adhesion molecules-1 and monocyte chemotactic protein-1. Am J Pathol 1997;151: 1085–95.
10. Suzuki J, Iwai M, Mogi M, et al. Eplerenone with valsartan effectively reduces atherosclerotic lesions by attenuation of oxidative stress and inflammation. Arterioscler Thromb Vasc Biol 2006; 26:917–21.
11. Manabe S, Okura T, Watanab S, et al. Effects of angiotensin II receptor blockade with valsartan on proinflammatory cytokines in patients with essential hypertension. J Cardiovasc Pharmacol 2005;46:735–9.
12. Nishimoto M, Takai S, Fukumoto H, et al. Increased local angiotensin II formation in aneurismal aortas. Life Sci 2002;71:2195–205.
13. Daugherty A, Manning MW, Cassis LA. Angiotensin II promotes atherosclerotic lesions and aneurysms in apolipoprotein E deficient mice. J Clin Invest 2000;105:1605–12.
14. Liao S, Miralles M, Kelley BJ, et al. Suppression of experimental abdominal aortic aneurysms in the rat by treatment with angiotensin-converting enzyme inhibitors. J Vasc Surg 2001;33:1057–64.
15. Lopez JJ, Lorell BH, Ingelfinger JR, et al. Distribution and function of cardiac angiotensin AT1 and AT2 receptor subtypes in hypertrophied rat hearts. Am J Phys 1994;267:H844–62.
16. Nio Y, Matsubara H, Murasawa S, et al. Regulation of gene transcription of angiotensin II receptor subtypes in myocardial infarction. J Clin Invest 1995;95:46–54.
17. Nagashima H, Uto K, Sakomura Y, et al. An angiotensin-converting enzyme inhibitor, not an angiotensin II type 1 receptor blocker prevents

B-aminopropionitrile monfumarate-induced aortic dissection in rats. J Vasc Surg 2002;36:818–23.

18. Fujiwara Y, Shiraya S, Miyake T, et al. Inhibition of experimental abdominal aortic aneurysm in a rat model by angiotensin receptor blocker valsartan. Int J Mol Med 2008;22:703–8.

19. Habashi JP, Judge DP, Holm TM, et al. Losartan, an AT1 anatagonist, prevents aortic aneurysm in a mouse model of marfan syndrome. Science 2007;312:117–21.

20. Losy F, Dai J, Pages C, et al. Paracrine secretion of transforming growth factor-beta1 in aneurysm healing and stabilization with endovascular smooth muscle cell therapy. J Vasc Surg 2003;37:1301–9.

21. Vaday GG, Schor H, Rahat MA, et al. Transforming growth factor-beta suppresses tumor necrosis factor alpha-induced matrix metalloproteinase-9 expression in monocytes. J Leukoc Biol 2001;69:613–21.

22. Zhou Y, Poczatek MH, Berecek KH, et al. Thrombospondin 1 mediates angiotensin II induction of TGF beta activation by cardiac and renal cells under both high and low glucose conditions. Biochem Biophys Res Commun 2006;339:633–41.

23. Nagashima H, Sakomura Y, Aoka Y, et al. Angiotensin II type 2 receptor mediates vascular smooth muscle cell apoptosis in cystic medial degeneration associated with Marfan's syndrome. Circulation 2001;104:I282–7.

24. Brooke BS, Habashi JP, Judge DP, et al. Angiotensin II blockade and aortic-root dilation in Marfan's syndrome. N Engl J Med 2008;358(26):2787–95.

25. Radonic T, de Witte P, Baars MJ, et al. Losartan therapy in adults with Marfan syndrome: study protocol of the multi center randomized controlled COMPARE trial. Trials 2010;11:3.

Is Losartan the True Panacea for Aneurysm Disease? CON

Peter Danyi, MD, MPH, MBA[a], Ion S. Jovin, MD, ScD[a,b,]*

KEYWORDS

- Aortic aneurysm • Angiotensin
- Angiotensin receptor blocker • Medical therapy

INCIDENCE, PREVALENCE, PATHOGENESIS, AND CLINICAL COURSE OF THORACIC AORTIC ANEURYSM

An aortic aneurysm is defined as a localized dilatation of the aorta, 50% more than the normal diameter, and it includes all 3 layers of the vessel (intima, media, adventitia).[1] Aortic aneurysms are the thirteenth leading cause of death in Western countries.[2] Thoracic aortic aneurysms (TAA) are less common than abdominal aortic aneurysms (AAA). The incidence of TAA is estimated to be between 4.5 and 5.9 per 100,000 person-years.[3,4] Overall, 5-year survival with TAA has been reported to be 64%,[4] with some studies reporting much lower rates.[3] This rate is significantly less than the survival with AAA (75%–80% over 8 years).[5] Risk factors include male gender, age, cigarette smoking, hypertension, chronic obstructive lung disease, and coronary artery disease.[6,7] Atherosclerotic disease, although associated with AAA, is not a well-established risk factor for TAA.[8] Genetic predisposition is another etiologic factor, and has a higher impact in TAA than in AAA. Approximately 20% of TAAs are attributed to a genetic syndrome.[4] The most common of these is Marfan syndrome (MFS), a connective tissue disorder affecting about 1 in 5000 persons.[9] Ehlers-Danlos syndrome type IV preferentially causes dilatation of the thoracic aorta.[4] Loeys-Dietz syndrome and the familial TAA and dissection syndrome are caused by mutations in growth factor receptors, which predispose patients to TAA.[10,11] The common congenital anomaly, bicuspid aortic valve, which affects 2% of the population, has also been associated with TAA. Much less common are certain inflammatory and infectious causes such as Takayasu arteritis, giant cell arteritis (temporal arteritis), and syphilis.

The pathogenesis of TAA is not well understood; however, it seems that aortic aneurysm is a chronic-inflammatory state of a focal portion of the aorta. All of these causes and risk factors exert their effects through localized-inflammatory changes culminating in cystic medial necrosis (degradation of extracellular matrix) and the apoptosis of vascular smooth muscle cells (VSMCs). Cystic medial necrosis is a nonspecific degenerative condition, which provides the anatomic background for dissection.[12] Numerous pathways have been proposed that can lead to these changes. One proposed mechanism is the development of reactive oxygen species (ROS) in response to the inflammatory state. ROS in turn can cause an imbalance between matrix metalloproteinases (MMPs) and their inhibitor proteins: tissue inhibitors of matrix metalloproteinases. MMPs (especially MMP2 and MMP9) are responsible for the degradation of extracellular matrix in aortic aneurysms.[13] The role of NADH/NADPH oxidase has also been shown in the development of ROS and its effect in the development of

There are no financial interests to declare.
[a] Department of Medicine, Virginia Commonwealth University, PO Box 980051, Richmond, VA 23298, USA
[b] Department of Medicine, McGuire VAMC, 1201 Broad Rock Boulevard 111J, Richmond, VA 23249, USA
* Corresponding author. Department of Medicine, McGuire VAMC, 1201 Broad Rock Boulevard 111J, Richmond, VA 23249.
E-mail address: isjovin@yahoo.com

TAA.[14] Elevated levels of transforming growth factor (TGF)-β have been found in certain aneurysmal segments, notably in MFS and other inherited diseases.[15] Two more possible pathways have been shown to participate in aneurysm formation: osteoprotegerin seems to be associated with VSMC proliferation and apoptosis in AAA, and its levels are associated with aneurysm size.[16] Satoh and colleagues[17] recently identified cyclophilin A as a key factor in the inflammatory response to angiotensin II through ROS in the development of aortic aneurysms.

The major cause of mortality from aortic aneurysms is dissection and rupture. The incidence of rupture increases with expanding aneurysm size.[4,18] The overall incidence of aortic dissection is 2.9 to 3.5 per 100,000 per year.[19,20] The rate of growth of aneurysm diameter is between 0.1 cm/y and 0.4 cm/y.[5,21] In the ascending aorta the complication rate steeply increases to about 30% once the diameter reaches 6 cm; in the descending aorta this increase occurs at 7 cm.[22]

PRINCIPLES AND GOALS OF THERAPY

The recommendation of therapy depends on the location and size of the aneurysm, its cause, and the patient's comorbidities. For aneurysms that are at high risk for rupture, surgical repair is recommended. Historically the risk of surgery has been associated with 5% to 10% surgical mortality for elective cases and at least 20% mortality for emergency procedures.[23] The consensus is that when the 1-year mortality risk from complications of aneurysm surpasses the surgical mortality risk, surgery is recommended. Medical therapy has traditionally been targeted to reduce the growth rate of aneurysm and delay surgery. The reduction of shear stress on the aneurysm along with the reduction of heart rate and blood pressure has been the one approach that has been shown to accomplish this.[24] More recently, the authors have gained better insight into the mechanisms of pathophysiologic changes that occur within aortic aneurysms. This has opened the door to possible therapies that would not only slow the expansion of aneurysm but also possibly affect the underlying disease process, from certain causes at least.[15,16]

Surgical Therapy

Open surgical repair became available in the early 1950s. Since then, the emphasis has been to determine the diameter that requires surgery.[25] Current recommendations are to perform surgical repair on an ascending TAA at 5.5 cm diameter (5.0 cm in case of patients with MFS) and 6.5 cm for descending TAA (6.0 cm for patients with MFS), or if the rate of growth is more than 1 cm per year. Other indications for surgery are aortic insufficiency and surgical emergencies from aneurysm complications.[26] In 2005 the Food and Drug Administration approved the Gore TAG thoracic endoprosthesis (W.L. Gore and Associates Inc, Flagstaff, AZ, USA), which opened the possibility for thoracic endovascular repair, with the aim of reducing perioperative mortality and spinal cord ischemia[27] as well as hospital length of stay. Major problems are graft endoleak and dealing with branch vessels of the aorta. Current recommendations for endovascular repair are for infrarenal aorta and descending TAA without abdominal extension.[28] New approaches have been investigated for treating aortic aneurysms in which branch vessels are involved.[29]

Medical Therapy

β-BLOCKERS, TETRACYCLINES, AND MACROLIDES; STATINS; ANGIOTENSIN-CONVERTING ENZYME INHIBITORS; OTHER AGENTS

The mainstay of medical therapy in patients with aortic aneurysm has been β-blocking drugs.[24] β-Blockers have been shown to reduce the rate of thoracic aortic dilatation, especially in patients with MFS.[30] For AAA the results are more controversial, with animal studies and retrospective data reports suggesting benefit, and prospective trials showing no significant benefit.[31–33] These trials also showed a significant negative effect on the quality of life among patients taking β-blockers and a high discontinuation rate.

Doxycycline can stop or slow elastin degradation and can decrease MMP levels in the aortic wall; it can also slow aneurysm development in animal models and in a small series of human subjects.[34–36] Roxithromycin, a macrolide, has also been shown to inhibit the rate of expansion of AAA.[37]

Statins reduce the progression of atherosclerosis through their lipid-lowering effects as well as through their so-called pleiotropic (eg, inflammatory and immunology response modulating) effects, and are one of the mainstays of therapy in cardiovascular diseases. Statins also reduce oxidative stress via the NADP/NADPH oxidase system.[14,38] Reduction of expansion rate of aneurysm by statins has been reported in AAA[39] but not in TAA.

Angiotensin-converting enzyme inhibitors (ACEIs) have been shown to stimulate and inhibit MMPs, as well as to stimulate and inhibit the degradation of extracellular matrix in aortic aneurysms.[40,41] TGF-β neutralizing antibodies have shown their efficacy by delaying or avoiding the development of TAA in MFS.[15]

Other agents that act on specifically proposed pathogenetic mechanisms have been tested in animal models of AAA, but not TAA; these include c-jun-N-terminal kinase inhibitor, glucocorticoids, leukocyte-depleting antibody (anti-CD18), and indomethacin. Lifestyle modifications, such as smoking cessation and other cardiovascular risk factor reduction, are also very important.

Angiotensin II receptor blockers in the treatment of TAA

Biology of angiotensin and mechanisms of action Angiotensin was discovered in the 1930s. An oligopeptide, it is a component of the renin-angiotensin system and increases aldosterone levels. Angiotensin is derived from its precursor, angiotensinogen, which is produced in the liver. Angiotensinogen levels are increased by cortico-steroids, estrogen, thyroid hormone, and angiotensin II itself. Angiotensin occurs in 4 forms. Angiotensin I, formed by the action of renin on angiotensinogen, is a precursor of angiotensin II and appears to have no biologic effect. In addition to increasing blood pressure, angiotensin II promotes vascular hypertrophy, cell proliferation, production of extracellular matrix, activation of macrophages, and activation of NADH/NADPH oxidase of VSMCs. Angiotensin II is derived from angiotensin I via angiotensin-converting enzyme (ACE), mainly in the lung capillaries. Angiotensin II is degraded to angiotensin III and IV; both have some pressor and aldosterone-producing activities. There are 4 angiotensin (AT) receptors. AT1 mediates vasoconstriction, aldosterone production, vasopressin secretion, cardiac hypertrophy, VSMC proliferation, renin inhibition, and extracellular matrix formation. AT2 modulates cell growth (inhibition), fetal tissue development, extracellular matrix, apoptosis, and cellular differentiation. Although AT2-receptor density is highest in fetal tissue and decreases significantly after birth, enhanced expression has been reported in adults in the settings of atherosclerosis, hypertension,[42] and MFS.[43] AT2 has been shown to mediate VSMC apoptosis in tissue culture experiments with cells obtained from patients with MFS.[43] AT3 and AT4 are as yet poorly characterized subtypes.

ACEIs were first discovered in 1975. ACEIs not only inhibit the RAS pathway but also inhibit the breakdown of bradykinin and in turn activate nitric oxide synthetase. There are alternative pathways of angiotensin II production; through serine proteases, such as kallikrein, cathepsin, and chymase,

which are not blocked by ACEIs. Angiotensin II receptor blockers (ARBs) block angiotensin's effect on the AT1 receptor. ARBs have a 1000- to 20,000-fold affinity for AT1 versus AT2. In MFS, a mutation occurs in the gene encoding fibrillin-1 (Fbn1), a component of the extracellular matrix microfibril,[44] which in turn leads to various Marfanoid manifestations including TAA. In mouse models low levels of Fbn1 produces an MFS-like syndrome. Fbn1 not only has important structural function but also regulates TGF-β. TGF-β has been associated with thickening of the aortic wall and the fragmentation and disarray of elastic fibers.[15] TGF-β influences cellular proliferation, differentiation, and survival of different cell types. ARBs are known to inhibit the effects of TGF-β. Angiotensin II has also been shown to activate the NADH/NADPH oxidative system in VSMC cultures[45] that produce ROS and induce oxidative stress. Angiotensin II plays a role in aneurysm development possibly by activating MMPs and cyclophilin A (**Fig. 1**).

Preclinical evidence ARBs, and specifically losartan, have been studied for TGF-β antagonizing effects in human and animal models of cardiomyopathy and renal insufficiency.[46,47] Ejiri and colleagues[14] demonstrated that ARBs suppressed the expression of NADH/NADPH oxidase in human thoracic aneurysmal segments and ACEI did not, suggesting an AT1-mediated pathway. Habashi and colleagues[15] found that in a mouse model of MFS losartan inhibited elastic-fiber fragmentation, but propranolol did not (**Table 1**). This group provided evidence that losartan achieved its effect through AT1 receptor blockade, mediated via downstream TGF-β signaling inhibition. The effect of losartan was comparable to TGF-β neutralizing antibody. Daugherty and colleagues[48] found that signaling through AT2 receptors antagonizes any effects of AT1. In theory this would mean that while AT1 blockade should produce a beneficial effect on TAAs, ACE blockade, which blocks AT1 as well as AT2 effects, should at least have a smaller effect or no effect at all. The effects of angiotensin II on aneurysm formation were observed in the apolipoprotein (Apo) E-deficient mouse model.[49] Nagashima and colleagues[50] found that β-amino-propionitrile monofumarate (BAPN)-induced aortic dissection is not prevented by ARBs, but by ACEIs. These findings suggested that instead of AT1 receptor participation, AT2 receptor expression is upregulated in organ culture of aortic aneurysm, and also indicate that ACEIs and not ARBs block VSMC apoptosis.[43] In the case of elastase-induced AAA in the rat model, Liao and colleagues[51] also found that ACE inhibition but

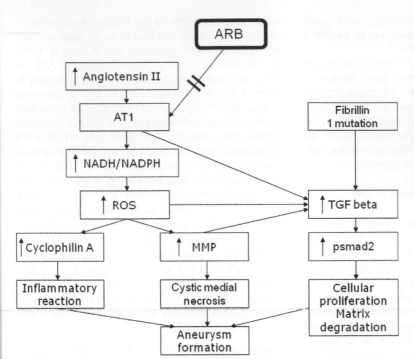

Fig. 1. Angiotensin II and ARB in aneurysm formation. Angiotensin promotes aneurysm formation through AT1 receptors. Increased angiotensin II causes an increase of ROS through the NADH/NADPH system, which in turn increases cyclophilin A and MMP levels. This promotes inflammatory reaction and subsequent cystic medial necrosis, leading to aneurysm formation. Fibrillin gene mutation causes elevated signaling of TGF-β, resulting in cellular proliferation and matrix degradation probably through signaling via the psmad2 system. ARBs are believed to inhibit the above pathways via inhibition of the AT1 receptors.

not AT1 blockade suppressed aneurysm formation.

Clinical evidence To date there has been one retrospective study on 18 subjects with MFS who were followed for at least 1 year after ARB therapy initiation. The patients were followed for a median length of 26.1 months. The mean rate of aortic root enlargement before ARB therapy was 3.54 ± 2.87 cm/y and after ARB therapy, 0.46 ± 0.62 cm/y.[52] Other clinical data pertain to AAA. Hackam and colleagues[53] analyzed a database in Ontario, Canada and found that use of ACEI but not the use of ARBs had a beneficial effect in preventing rupture of AAA (see **Table 1**). Another report from this dataset suggested that the

Table 1
Preclinical and clinical studies of angiotensin receptor blockers in aortic aneurysms

First Author[Ref]	Model/Population	Subject Number	Findings
Habashi[15]	Mouse, Marfan	10	ARB prevented aneurysm formation
Daugherty[49]	Mouse, apoE deficient, AAA	15	AT1 blockade (losartan) prevented aneurysm formation, AT2 blockade promoted it
Nagashima[50]	Rat, β-aminopropionitrile monofumarate-induced cystic medial degeneration and aortic dissection	15	ACEI but not ARB prevented cystic medial degeneration and aortic dissection
Liao[51]	Rat, elastase-induced, AAA	9	ACEIs but not ARB suppressed AAA formation
Brooke[52]	Human, Marfan (retrospective)	18	ARB significantly slowed aortic root dilatation
Hackam[53]	Human, AAA (retrospective)	15326	ACEIs were, but ARBs not protective against aortic aneurysm rupture

discontinuation of ACE inhibitor prior to admission had a deleterious effect on aneurysm rupture.[54]

Potential benefits of ARB therapy in TAA The use of ARB in TAA has the theoretical benefit of blood pressure lowering and subsequent shear force reduction. In animal models of MFS and ApoB deficiency, ARBs preferentially blocked extracellular-matrix degradation and VSMC apoptosis, and slowed or arrested aneurysm expansion and formation. This was thought to be achieved by blocking TGF-β signaling by preferentially blocking AT1 receptors. Other potential benefits could be exerted through blocking the NADH/NADPH oxidase system and reducing ROS production.

Potential risks of ARB therapy in TAA Some of the preclinical studies of the effects of ARB on aortic aneurysms have produced conflicting results. Some animal models (elastase and BAPN) suggested that AT2 receptor signaling was more important in the development of aneurysms than AT1 receptor signaling. In these models ARBs did not produce any beneficial results, whereas ACEIs (dual AT1 and AT2 blockade) did. This result suggests that whereas ARBs could be beneficial in some cases of TAAs, in other cases they could have little or no effect.

There are also contraindications to ARB use in the general population (eg, pregnancy, allergy), and without more knowledge of ARB action in TAA from different causes, it is impossible to know if there are more specific contraindications in these patients. Also, it is impossible to know if any ARB effect would be sustained over a longer period of time or if their long-term effects are equal, worse, or better than β-blockers.

SUMMARY

TAA is a significant health problem with potentially devastating consequences. More is known about the genetics and molecular genesis of the disease than ever before, and potential treatments are on the horizon. The results of AT1-receptor blocker treatments in MFS are exciting. However, only retrospective data from a small number of individuals with only one subtype of aneurysm is available. The underlying biochemical and molecular mechanisms of aneurysm formation are varied, and a full understanding of the different mechanisms that contribute to the different causes is needed. Although it is tempting to generalize, caution should be used. The tendency to extrapolate the scant available data should be avoided to prevent any harm that can be caused to patients. There are many unknowns, and the answers will come from ongoing or future studies; but for now losartan (and ARBs in general) cannot be regarded as a panacea for all patients with thoracic aortic disease.

REFERENCES

1. Johnston KW, Rutherford RB, Tilson MD, et al. Suggested standards for reporting on arterial aneurysms. Subcommittee on Reporting Standards for Arterial Aneurysms, Ad Hoc Committee on Reporting Standards, Society for Vascular Surgery and North American Chapter, International Society for Cardiovascular Surgery. J Vasc Surg 1991;13(3): 452–8.
2. Isselbacher EM. Thoracic and abdominal aortic aneurysms. Circulation 2005;111(6):816–28.
3. Bickerstaff LK, Pairolero PC, Hollier LH, et al. Thoracic aortic aneurysms: a population-based study. Surgery 1982;92(6):1103–8.
4. Coady MA, Rizzo JA, Goldstein LJ, et al. Natural history, pathogenesis, and etiology of thoracic aortic aneurysms and dissections. Cardiol Clin 1999;17(4): 615–35, vii.
5. Lederle FA, Wilson SE, Johnson GR, et al. Immediate repair compared with surveillance of small abdominal aortic aneurysms. N Engl J Med 2002; 346(19):1437–44.
6. Davies RR, Gallo A, Coady MA, et al. Novel measurement of relative aortic size predicts rupture of thoracic aortic aneurysms. Ann Thorac Surg 2006;81(1):169–77.
7. Lederle FA, Johnson GR, Wilson SE, et al. Prevalence and associations of abdominal aortic aneurysm detected through screening. Aneurysm Detection and Management (ADAM) Veterans Affairs Cooperative Study Group. Ann Intern Med 1997;126(6):441–9.
8. Ito S, Akutsu K, Tamori Y, et al. Differences in atherosclerotic profiles between patients with thoracic and abdominal aortic aneurysms. Am J Cardiol 2008; 101(5):696–9.
9. Judge DP, Dietz HC. Marfan's syndrome. Lancet 2005;366(9501):1965–76.
10. Loeys BL, Chen J, Neptune ER, et al. A syndrome of altered cardiovascular, craniofacial, neurocognitive and skeletal development caused by mutations in TGFBR1 or TGFBR2. Nat Genet 2005;37(3):275–81.
11. Pannu H, Fadulu VT, Chang J, et al. Mutations in transforming growth factor-beta receptor type II cause familial thoracic aortic aneurysms and dissections. Circulation 2005;112(4):513–20.
12. Elefteriades JA. Thoracic aortic aneurysm: reading the enemy's playbook. Yale J Biol Med 2008;81(4): 175–86.
13. Palombo D, Maione M, Cifiello BI, et al. Matrix metalloproteinases. Their role in degenerative chronic

diseases of abdominal aorta. J Cardiovasc Surg (Torino) 1999;40(2):257–60.

14. Ejiri J, Inoue N, Tsukube T, et al. Oxidative stress in the pathogenesis of thoracic aortic aneurysm: protective role of statin and angiotensin II type 1 receptor blocker. Cardiovasc Res 2003;59(4): 988–96.

15. Habashi JP, Judge DP, Holm TM, et al. Losartan, an AT1 antagonist, prevents aortic aneurysm in a mouse model of Marfan syndrome. Science 2006; 312(5770):117–21.

16. Moran CS, McCann M, Karan M, et al. Association of osteoprotegerin with human abdominal aortic aneurysm progression. Circulation 2005;111(23): 3119–25.

17. Satoh K, Nigro P, Matoba T, et al. Cyclophilin A enhances vascular oxidative stress and the development of angiotensin II-induced aortic aneurysms. Nat Med 2009;15(6):649–56.

18. Davies RR, Goldstein LJ, Coady MA, et al. Yearly rupture or dissection rates for thoracic aortic aneurysms: simple prediction based on size. Ann Thorac Surg 2002;73(1):17–27 [discussion: 27–8].

19. Meszaros I, Morocz J, Szlavi J, et al. Epidemiology and clinicopathology of aortic dissection. Chest 2000;117(5):1271–8.

20. Clouse WD, Hallett JW Jr, Schaff HV, et al. Acute aortic dissection: population-based incidence compared with degenerative aortic aneurysm rupture. Mayo Clin Proc 2004;79(2):176–80.

21. United Kingdom Small Aneurysm Trial Participants. Long-term outcomes of immediate repair compared with surveillance of small abdominal aortic aneurysms. N Engl J Med 2002;346(19):1445–52.

22. Coady MA, Rizzo JA, Hammond GL, et al. What is the appropriate size criterion for resection of thoracic aortic aneurysms? J Thorac Cardiovasc Surg 1997;113(3):476–91 [discussion: 89–91].

23. Conrad MF, Cambria RP. Contemporary management of descending thoracic and thoracoabdominal aortic aneurysms: endovascular versus open. Circulation 2008;117(6):841–52.

24. Fuster V, Andrews P. Medical treatment of the aorta. I. Cardiol Clin 1999;17(4):697–715, viii.

25. Crawford ES. Thoraco-abdominal and abdominal aortic aneurysms involving renal, superior mesenteric, celiac arteries. Ann Surg 1974;179(5):763–72.

26. Bonow RO, Carabello B, de Leon AC Jr, et al. Guidelines for the management of patients with valvular heart disease: executive summary. A report of the American College of Cardiology/American Heart Association Task Force on Practice Guidelines (Committee on Management of Patients with Valvular Heart Disease). Circulation 1998;98(18):1949–84.

27. Bavaria JE, Appoo JJ, Makaroun MS, et al. Endovascular stent grafting versus open surgical repair of descending thoracic aortic aneurysms in low-risk patients: a multicenter comparative trial. J Thorac Cardiovasc Surg 2007;133(2):369–77.

28. Svensson LG, Kouchoukos NT, Miller DC, et al. Expert consensus document on the treatment of descending thoracic aortic disease using endovascular stent-grafts. Ann Thorac Surg 2008;85(1 Suppl): S1–41.

29. Inoue K, Hosokawa H, Iwase T, et al. Aortic arch reconstruction by transluminally placed endovascular branched stent graft. Circulation 1999;100(19 Suppl):II316–21.

30. Shores J, Berger KR, Murphy EA, et al. Progression of aortic dilatation and the benefit of long-term beta-adrenergic blockade in Marfan's syndrome. N Engl J Med 1994;330(19):1335–41.

31. Gadowski GR, Pilcher DB, Ricci MA. Abdominal aortic aneurysm expansion rate: effect of size and beta-adrenergic blockade. J Vasc Surg 1994;19(4): 727–31.

32. Propanolol Aneurysm Trial Investigators. Propanolol for small abdominal aortic aneurysms: results of a randomized trial. J Vasc Surg 2002;35(1):72–9.

33. Lindholt JS, Vammen S, Juul S, et al. The validity of ultrasonographic scanning as screening method for abdominal aortic aneurysm. Eur J Vasc Endovasc Surg 1999;17(6):472–5.

34. Xiong W, Knispel RA, Dietz HC, et al. Doxycycline delays aneurysm rupture in a mouse model of Marfan syndrome. J Vasc Surg 2008;47(1):166–72 [discussion: 72].

35. Baxter BT, Pearce WH, Waltke EA, et al. Prolonged administration of doxycycline in patients with small asymptomatic abdominal aortic aneurysms: report of a prospective (Phase II) multicenter study. J Vasc Surg 2002;36(1):1–12.

36. Mosorin M, Juvonen J, Biancari F, et al. Use of doxycycline to decrease the growth rate of abdominal aortic aneurysms: a randomized, double-blind, placebo-controlled pilot study. J Vasc Surg 2001; 34(4):606–10.

37. Vammen S, Lindholt JS, Ostergaard L, et al. Randomized double-blind controlled trial of roxithromycin for prevention of abdominal aortic aneurysm expansion. Br J Surg 2001;88(8):1066–72.

38. Wassmann S, Laufs U, Muller K, et al. Cellular antioxidant effects of atorvastatin in vitro and in vivo. Arterioscler Thromb Vasc Biol 2002;22(2):300–5.

39. Guessous I, Periard D, Lorenzetti D, et al. The efficacy of pharmacotherapy for decreasing the expansion rate of abdominal aortic aneurysms: a systematic review and meta-analysis. PLoS One 2008;3(3):e1895.

40. Yamamoto D, Takai S, Jin D, et al. Molecular mechanism of imidapril for cardiovascular protection via inhibition of MMP-9. J Mol Cell Cardiol 2007;43(6): 670–6.

41. Rizzoni D, Rodella L, Porteri E, et al. Effects of losartan and enalapril at different doses on cardiac and

renal interstitial matrix in spontaneously hypertensive rats. Clin Exp Hypertens 2003;25(7):427–41.

42. Otsuka S, Sugano M, Makino N, et al. Interaction of
mRNAs for angiotensin II type 1 and type 2 receptors to vascular remodeling in spontaneously hypertensive rats. Hypertension 1998;32(3):467–72.

43. Nagashima H, Sakomura Y, Aoka Y, et al. Angiotensin II type 2 receptor mediates vascular smooth
muscle cell apoptosis in cystic medial degeneration
associated with Marfan's syndrome. Circulation
2001;104(12 Suppl 1):I282–7.

44. Dietz HC, Cutting GR, Pyeritz RE, et al. Marfan
syndrome caused by a recurrent de novo missense
mutation in the fibrillin gene. Nature 1991;352(6333):
337–9.

45. Griendling KK, Minieri CA, Ollerenshaw JD, et al.
Angiotensin II stimulates NADH and NADPH oxidase
activity in cultured vascular smooth muscle cells.
Circ Res 1994;74(6):1141–8.

46. Lavoie P, Robitaille G, Agharazii M, et al. Neutralization of transforming growth factor-beta attenuates
hypertension and prevents renal injury in uremic
rats. J Hypertens 2005;23(10):1895–903.

47. Lim DS, Lutucuta S, Bachireddy P, et al. Angiotensin
II blockade reverses myocardial fibrosis in a transgenic mouse model of human hypertrophic cardiomyopathy. Circulation 2001;103(6):789–91.

48. Daugherty A, Manning MW, Cassis LA. Antagonism
of AT2 receptors augments angiotensin II-induced
abdominal aortic aneurysms and atherosclerosis.
Br J Pharmacol 2001;134(4):865–70.

49. Daugherty A, Manning MW, Cassis LA. Angiotensin
II promotes atherosclerotic lesions and aneurysms
in apolipoprotein E-deficient mice. J Clin Invest
2000;105(11):1605–12.

50. Nagashima H, Uto K, Sakomura Y, et al. An angiotensin-converting enzyme inhibitor, not an angiotensin
II type-1 receptor blocker, prevents beta-aminopropio-
nitrile monofumarate-induced aortic dissection in rats.
J Vasc Surg 2002;36(4):818–23.

51. Liao S, Miralles M, Kelley BJ, et al. Suppression of
experimental abdominal aortic aneurysms in the rat
by treatment with angiotensin-converting enzyme
inhibitors. J Vasc Surg 2001;33(5):1057–64.

52. Brooke BS, Habashi JP, Judge DP, et al. Angiotensin II blockade and aortic-root dilation in Marfan's syndrome. N Engl J Med 2008;358(26):
2787–95.

53. Hackam DG, Thiruchelvam D, Redelmeier DA.
Angiotensin-converting enzyme inhibitors and aortic
rupture: a population-based case-control study.
Lancet 2006;368(9536):659–65.

54. Lederle FA, Taylor BC. ACE inhibitors and aortic
rupture. Lancet 2006;368(9547):1571 [author reply: 2].

Editorial Comment: Losartan-Based Medical Therapy for Aneurysm Disease

John A. Elefteriades, MD

The situation with angiotensin receptor blockers (ARBs) is currently one of great anticipation, justified by animal trials but as yet with unproved efficacy in the clinical arena. Even if or when efficacy is shown in Marfan disease, this raises the question of efficacy in other aneurysm diseases, which are mediated by different pathophysiologic pathways (**Fig. 1, Table 1**). The article by Drs Michael Collins and John A. Elefteriades in this issue of *Cardiology Clinics* argues the pro side of the question, while Drs Peter Danyi and Ion S. Jovin argue the con side.

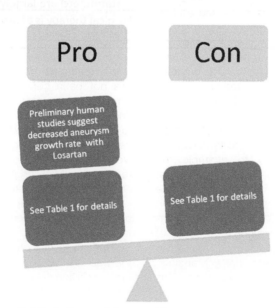

Fig. 1. The argument inclines slightly in favor of the pro side.

Section of Cardiac Surgery, Department of Surgery, Yale University School of Medicine, Yale-New Haven Hospital, PO Box 208039, New Haven, CT 06520-8039, USA
E-mail address: john.elefteriades@yale.edu

Cardiol Clin 28 (2010) 287–288
doi:10.1016/j.ccl.2010.02.015
0733-8651/10/$ – see front matter © 2010 Elsevier Inc. All rights reserved.

Table 1
Medical therapy for aneurysm disease

Losartan is a Panacea: Pro (Collins)	Losartan is a Panacea: Con (Jovin)
Animal investigations suggest a role for the rennin-angiotensin system in the pathophysiology of aneurysm disease (via nuclear factor κB, proteolytic enzymes, and transforming growth factor β1 signaling)	Only some animal models of thoracic aortic aneurysm (TAA) showed benefit of ARBs, whereas other models showed no benefit, suggesting that patients with TAAs of different etiologies may react differently to ARB therapy
Preliminary human studies suggest decreased aneurysm growth rate with losartan (in Marfan disease)	In humans, only 1 retrospective study (n = 18) showed benefits (in patients with Marfan disease); findings not yet reproduced
The COMPARE trial will yield prospective information on the effectiveness of losartan in ameliorating the aortic course in Marfan disease	Because the benefits of ARB therapy in all patients have not been established and because there are risks associated with ARB therapy, the risk/benefit ratio is unknown
	The long-term effects of ARBs, even in TAA patients who had short-term beneficial results, are not known
	Even other therapies (β-blockers, antibiotics, statins, etc) are largely unproved
	Surgical therapy is of proved benefit and durable as well

Should Aortas in Patients with Bicuspid Aortic Valve Really be Resected at an Earlier Stage than Tricuspid? PRO

Ori Wald, MD, PhD, Amit Korach, MD, Oz M. Shapira, MD*

KEYWORDS

- Aorta • Bicuspid aortic valve • Aneurysm

DEFINITION AND EXTENT OF DISEASE

Bicuspid aortic valve (BAV) disease is increasingly recognized as a disease of the entire proximal aorta up to the level of the ligamentum arteriosum.[1] The anatomic structures involved in BAV disease include the aortic annulus, sinuses of Valsalva, coronary ostia, sinotubular junction, ascending aorta, aortic arch up to the ligamentum arteriosum, and the pulmonary trunk.[2] This is likely explained by the semilunar valves and the conotruncal-derived vessels (proximal aorta and pulmonary artery) sharing a common embryonic origin: the neural crest.[3,4]

Patients with BAV develop valvular and vascular complications. The clinical scope of BAV disease includes severe valvular aortic stenosis or insufficiency, aortic valve endocarditis, and aortic aneurysm or dissection.[5] BAV is formed due to fusion of 2 of the 3 valve cusps. Classification of BAV according to the cusps fused was described recently. Fusion of the left coronary and right coronary cusps (type A) is the most common form of BAV, occurring in 74% of cases; the next most common form is fusion of the right coronary and the noncoronary cusps (type B) occurring in 24% of the cases, and least common form of BAV is the fusion of left coronary and the noncoronary cusps (type C), occurring in 2% of the cases. The anatomy of type A BAV is associated with a more severe degree of aortic wall degeneration and earlier dilatation of the aortic root.[6,7]

EPIDEMIOLOGY OF BAV AND ASSOCIATED DISORDERS
BAV Epidemiology

BAV is the most frequent congenital cardiac anomaly, affecting 1% to 2% of the population.[8] Between 2.8 million and 5.6 million Americans are affected by BAV disease, and the majority eventually develops valvular or aortic complications by the age of 70 years.[9,10] Only 15% to 28% of BAV are reported as normal in necropsy series.[9,11] The incidence of BAV among patients operated for aortic valve disease ranges from 27% to 32%.[12,13] Between 10% and 30% of patients with BAV develop infective endocarditis, and 25% of patients with BAV develop native-valve infective endocarditis.[14,15]

Department of Cardiothoracic Surgery, Hadassah Medical Center, Hebrew University, Ein-Kerem, PO Box 12000, Jerusalem 91120, Israel
* Corresponding author.
E-mail address: ozshapira@hadassah.org.il

Cardiol Clin 28 (2010) 289–298
doi:10.1016/j.ccl.2010.01.005
0733-8651/10/$ – see front matter © 2010 Elsevier Inc. All rights reserved.

BAV-Associated Aortic Dilatation

Aortic root dilatation occurs in up to 50% to 60% of patients with a normally functioning BAV. Several reports examined the prevalence of aortic disease according to age in patients with BAV. In these studies aortic dilatation was found to begin early in life, affecting 56% of patients younger than 30 years. The disease was progressive and affected up to 88% of patients older than 80 years.[9,16–18]

Aortic Dissection in BAV Patients

Patients with BAV tend to develop aortic dilatation at an early age; this is associated with increased risk of acute dissection or rupture. In the International Registry of Acute Aortic Dissection database, younger aortic dissection patients (<40 years) were more likely to have a BAV than older patients (>40 years) (9% vs 1%, respectively; *P*<.001).[17] Furthermore, aortic dissection occurs at a younger age in patients with BAV relative to trileaflet aortic valve (TAV). Several reports indicate that the median age of patients with BAV presenting with dissection is about a decade younger than patients with TAV. It is estimated that aortic dissection occurs 5 to 10 times more frequently in patients with BAV than in those with TAV. BAV is present in 4% to 15% of unselected cases of aortic dissection.[17,19–22]

INHERITANCE AND GENETICS

The genetics of BAV is not fully elucidated. It seems that the mode of inheritance is autosomal dominant with varied penetration and male predominance (male-to-female ratio 3:1).[23,24] BAV is associated with familial clustering in 17% to 34% of cases.[25] Biner and colleagues[26] showed that the aortic root is functionally abnormal and that dilation is common (32%) in first-degree relatives (FDR) of patients with BAV (**Fig. 1**).

Several genetic syndromes have been associated with BAV, including Williams syndrome, Anderson syndrome, DiGeorge syndrome, Loeys-Dietz syndrome, and Turner syndrome.[27–31] Thirteen percent to 34% of patients with Turner syndrome have BAV, and 3% to 42% develop aortic aneurysm.[32,33]

The specific genes and metabolic pathways involved in BAV and associated disorders are subjects for intense investigations. Single gene mutations have been linked to BAV disease and to aortic dilatation. Two such examples include the NOTCH1 and ACTA2 genes. Mutations in the NOTCH1 gene (chromosome 9q) lead to signaling abnormalities responsible not only for development of a bicuspid aortic valve but also accelerated valvular calcium deposition.[34,35] Mutations in the ACTA2 gene (chromosome 10q), which encodes vascular smooth muscle cell (VSMC) β-actin, are associated with BAV and familial thoracic aortic aneurysms.[36]

The biologic processes leading to BAV-associated aortic dilatation have been extensively studied. The aortic wall normally undergoes a continuous process of extracellular matrix deposition and degradation. Imbalance in this process results in weakening of the aortic wall and subsequent formation of aneurysm.[13,37,38] **Fig. 2** shows the importance of the extracellular matrix component fibrillin-1 in the preservation of normal aortic wall structure. Fibrillin-1 deficiency leads to VSMC detachment, matrix metalloproteinase (MMP) release, matrix disruption, and apoptosis of VSMCs.[39] These processes result in the loss of structural support and elasticity (see **Fig. 2**). Several additional molecular pathways have been investigated. One mechanism considered to be important is lower expression level of endothelium-derived nitric oxide synthase.[40] Another metabolic disorder identified in association with BAV aortic disease is increased activity of MMPs 2 and 9.[41–45] Finally, the expression of metallothioneins, proteins that play a pivotal role in the response of ascending aortic smooth muscle cells to oxidative stress signals by regulation of MMP expression, was found to be reduced in cases of ascending aortic aneurysms of BAV patients.[46]

HISTOPATHOLOGY OF BAV DISEASE
Aortic Valve Pathology

Compared with TAV, histologic assessment of BAVs typically shows cusp calcification (involving either the base or the body of the cusp), areas of frank ossification, cartilaginous metaplasia, and ulceration. In some patients the dominant valve pathology is myxomatous degeneration.[13] These degenerative processes lead to accelerated deterioration of BAV function in the form of stenosis or insufficiency, and predispose patients with BAV to infective endocarditis.[13,15] The hemodynamic changes observed in patients with BAV may subsequently enhance the development of ascending aortic aneurysm.[47]

Pathology of the Ascending Aorta

Normal aortic wall consists of collagen, elastin, and smooth muscle cells. With age, degenerative changes lead to breakdown of the collagen and elastin, and to the loss of smooth muscle cells; these changes are termed cystic medial necrosis.[38,48] This process is characterized by

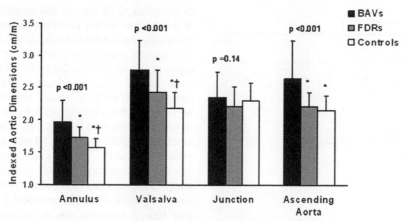

Fig. 1. Indexed (cm²/m) aortic root dimensions in patients with BAV, FDRs of BAVs, and control healthy individuals (Controls), at aortic root, annulus, sinuses of Valsalva, sinotubular junction, and proximal ascending aorta. Variance results are shown as *P* values on the top of each group of black bars. *P lesser than .05 versus BAV patients. †P lesser than .05 versus FDRs. (*From* Biner S, Rafique A, Ray I, et al. Aortopathy is prevalent in relatives of bicuspid aortic valve patients. J Am Coll Cardiol 2009;53(24):2291; with permission.)

loss of cells, the accumulation of basophilic ground substance in the media, and formation of cystlike pools.[49] As a result of the metabolic abnormalities described earlier, the aortas of BAV patients undergo accelerated degeneration characterized by early cystic medial necrosis, elastic fragmentation, and abnormal smooth muscle cell orientation (**Fig. 3**).[6] Similar changes are found in the main pulmonary arteries. Bauer and colleagues[37] studied the aortic pathology in patients with BAV. These investigators found that BAV aortas have thinner elastic lamellae in the aortic media and greater distance between the elastic lamellae than TAV aortas (see **Fig. 3**).[5] de Sa and colleagues[2] found that 75% of patients with BAV had advanced degenerative changes, compared with 14% of patients with TAV. These histologic changes result in weakening of the aortic wall and predispose the aorta to an ongoing process of dilatation, and subsequently to dissection or rupture.[50]

Gross inspection of dilated aortas reveals 2 types of aortic dilatation. In type 1 the diameter of the aorta at the sinuses of Valsalva exceeds that of the ascending aorta above the sinotubular junction, and in type 2 the reverse is true, as the ascending aorta is larger than the sinuses of Valsalva. Type 1 is more common in BAV patients (72%).[51,52]

PATHOPHYSIOLOGY AND MECHANICS OF AORTIC DILATATION

The inherent morphologic and histologic characteristics of the BAV and ascending aorta predispose these structures to early structural and mechanical deterioration. Biner and colleagues[26] recently evaluated the mechanical properties of the aortas of patients with BAV. The evaluation showed that BAV is associated with lower aortic distensibility and greater stiffness.

An abnormal flow pattern across the BAV results in turbulence and promotes inflammatory changes, fibrosis, and calcification, leading to accelerated valvular stenosis, insufficiency, or both.[12,13] Abnormal blood flow pattern across the valve exposes the already weakened aortic wall to increased shear forces, which enhance aortic dilatation. Aortic annular and root dilation results in impaired aortic valve cusp coaptation, leading directly to aortic insufficiency. Thus, a vicious cycle of increasing volume load and aortic dilatation is generated.[53] This entire process is aggravated in the presence of systemic hypertension and active smoking.[54]

NATURAL HISTORY OF BAV

Most patients with BAV disease develop serious complications (severe aortic stenosis, insufficiency, endocarditis, or aortic dissection) by the age of 70 years.[55] Pediatric patients usually present with aortic stenosis or endocarditis. Aortic insufficiency is typically observed in young adults.[56] Aortic stenosis and dissection occur at an earlier age in patients with BAV than in those with TAVs.[55] Only 20% of bicuspid valves are reported as normal in autopsy studies.[13]

Aortic stenosis progresses more rapidly in BAV. In one study, the aortic valve gradient increased at a rate of approximately 20 mm Hg per decade in BAV patients, which is much faster than TAV stenosis.[57]

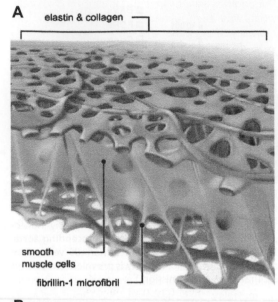

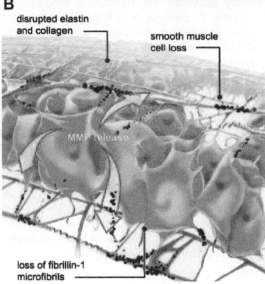

Fig. 2. The elastic laminae of the aortic media provide structural support and elasticity to the aorta. In normal patients with tricuspid valve (*A*), fibrillin-1 microfibrils tether smooth muscle cells to adjacent elastin and collagen matrix components. In patients with BAV (*B*), deficient microfibrillar elements result in smooth muscle cell detachment, MMP release, matrix disruption, cell death, and a loss of structural support and elasticity. (*From* Fedak PW, Verma S, David TE, et al. Clinical and pathophysiological implications of a bicuspid aortic valve. Circulation 2002;106:903; with permission.)

The progression rate of aortic dilatation in patients with BAV is substantially faster compared with TAV.[5,48] Thanassoulis and colleagues[7] reported a mean annual rate of progression of 0.18 mm at the aortic annulus, 0.17 mm at the sinus

of Valsalva, 0.18 mm at the sinotubular junction, and 0.37 mm at the proximal ascending aorta. In this study, type A BAV, fusion of left and right coronary cusps, was associated with increased risk of rapid aortic dilatation. Other studies documented even faster rates of annual aortic dilatation in patients with BAV up to 0.7 mm at the annulus, and ranging from 0.5 mm to 0.9 mm at the sinuses of Valsalva, 0.5 mm to 1.06 mm at the sinotubular junction, and 0.9 mm to 1.18 mm at the proximal ascending aorta.[16,58–60] According to Laplace's law (and not unique to BAV disease) the rate of aortic dilatation is exponential, thus larger aortas expand faster. Poorly controlled blood pressure and heavy smoking are additional risk factors, accelerating the process of aortic dilatation.[54]

About 50% of BAV patients present with no evidence of aortic dilatation.[9] The incidence of newly diagnosed aortic dilatation in patients with BAV is 4 cases per 100 patient-years.[5,61] FDR of patients with BAV are prone to develop aortic aneurysms and dissection even if they have TAV morphology.[25,26,62]

Several reports evaluated the link between the extent of aortic dilatation, expansion rate, and aneurysm-related complications to the type and severity of valvular disease.[47,62,63] Two studies showed an association between severe aortic regurgitation and larger aortic root measurements and accelerated rate of aortic dilatation.[47,64] In another study, patients with BAV and valvular aortic stenosis had a higher risk of rupture, dissection, or death compared with those who had normally functioning aortic valves.[62]

Although abnormal function of the BAV may adversely affect aortic pathology, it seems that replacing the valve, by itself, does not modify the natural history of the ascending aortic pathology and related complications. Yasuda and colleagues[64] found that aortic valve replacement (AVR) did not prevent progressive aortic dilatation in BAV, suggesting that aortic dilatation in BAV is mainly due to the inherent fragility of the aortic wall rather than hemodynamic factors. Russo and colleagues[65] reported that 10% of BAV patients undergoing AVR suffered late acute aortic dissection compared with none with TAV. In this study, sudden death occurred in 14% of BAV patients and in none of the TAV group. Borger and colleagues[55] reported a 10-year follow-up of 201 patients who underwent AVR for BAV without ascending aortic replacement. At the time of the primary operation ascending aortic size was 4.0 cm in 57%, 4.0 to 4.4 cm in 32%, and 4.5 to 4.9 cm in 11% of patients. Aortas greater than 5.0 cm in diameter (representing 17% of BAV patients) were replaced at the primary operation. During

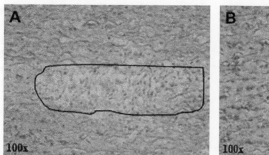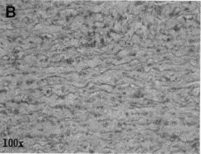

Fig. 3. (*A*) Histologic section from the ascending aorta in a patient with type A valve anatomy shows severe cystic medial necrosis, grade 3 (*circled area*), and fragmentation of elastic fibers. (*B*) Histologic section from the ascending aorta in a patient with type B valve anatomy shows fibrosis, fragmentation of elastic fibers, and misalignment of smooth muscle cells (5-μm sections, Masson trichrome elastic stain, original magnification ×100). (*From* Russo CF, Cannata A, Lanfranconi M, et al. Is aortic wall degeneration related to bicuspid aortic valve anatomy in patients with valvular disease? J Thorac Cardiovasc Surg 2008;136(4):940; with permission.)

follow-up, 9% of the patients required late ascending aortic replacement because of progressive aortic dilatation. Freedom from ascending aortic complications was 78%, 81%, and 43% in the 3 described size groups, respectively. In this study, major aortic complications became clinically evident starting from the sixth postoperative year, and were more common in patients with aortic diameter equal to or greater than 45 mm (**Fig. 4**).

Studies evaluating the association of acute aortic dissection with BAV reveal that aortic dissection occurs in approximately 5% of BAV patients, whereas BAV are found in 15% of patients with type A aortic dissections.[14,66] BAV disease carries an approximately 6% lifetime risk of aortic dissection, which is ninefold higher than the age- and gender-matched general population.[10]

In summary, a large body of evidence suggests that due to inherent aortic wall weakness and, perhaps, hemodynamic alterations, BAV is associated with accelerated development aortic

aneurysms at an earlier age. These aneurysms enlarge at a faster rate and have a tendency to dissect early in life. It seems that replacing the aortic valve, by itself, does not modify the natural history of the aortic disease in patients with BAV.

PREDICTING THE RISK OF AORTIC DISSECTION AND THE RATIONALE FOR ELECTIVE OPERATION

Up to 40% of patients with acute type A aortic dissection die in hospital. Thirty-day mortality after emergency surgical repair is in the range of 14% to 32%. Long-term survival after acute aortic dissection is also compromised, ranging between 45% and 55% at 10 years.[67–70] Many patients remain with persistent false lumen and are prone to late aortic complications.[71–73] In contrast, operative mortality after elective repair of ascending aortic aneurysm in the current era is in the range of 2.5% to 5.0%.[74] In experienced

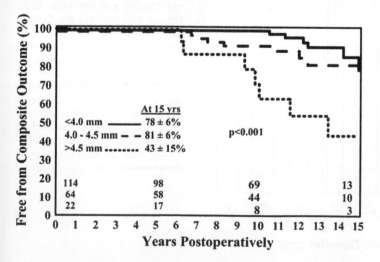

Fig. 4. Freedom from ascending aortic complications for patients with BAV disease versus number of postoperative years is shown. Patients with moderate dilation of the ascending aorta (4.5–4.9 cm) had a significantly increased risk of future aortic complications (aneurysm, dissection, or sudden death). (*From* Borger MA, Preston M, Ivanov J, et al. Should the ascending aorta be replaced more frequently in patients with bicuspid aortic valve disease? J Thorac Cardiovasc Surg 2004;128(5):680; with permission.)

centers operative mortality is reported to be as low as 1% to 2%.[75–77] Thus, elective surgical repair should be offered to the patient whenever the risk of dissection is estimated to be higher than the operative mortality and major morbidity of elective repair.

The key and very difficult point is the ability to precisely predict the risk of a dissection or rupture in each individual case. A tool that can predict the risk is currently unavailable. Current guidelines for treatment of non-BAV associated idiopathic ascending aortic aneurysms are based mostly on size.[78] Elective surgical repair is recommended when the aortic root diameter reaches 55 mm. This recommendation is based on observational studies examining the natural history of ascending aortic aneurysms.[79–81] Several long-term follow-up studies showed that aortic aneurysm diameter equal to or greater than 6.0 cm is associated with a dramatically increased risk of dissection or rupture.[79,02,83] However, 2 large series have shown that acute dissection frequently occurs in small-diameter aortas.[17,84] Nearly 60% of aortic dissections occur in patients with an aortic diameter of less than 55 mm, 40% percent occur at a diameter of less than 50 mm, and nearly 20% at a diameter of less than 45 mm (**Fig. 5**).[17,84] Thus, it is clear that absolute size alone is a crude and imprecise criterion. Novel and, perhaps, more accurate predictors of aortic dissection or rupture are currently being evaluated; these include indexed-size measurements and morphologic criteria.

A common method used to better predict the risk of dissection is to index aortic diameter to body height or surface area. In one study, a ratio of aortic diameter in centimeters to body surface area in square meters of 4.25 cm/m^2 was found to be a reliable predictor of dissection, rupture, or death.[85] Another metric found to be useful is the ratio of aortic area in square centimeters to body height in meters, using a ratio of 10 as an indicator of increased risk.[86]

Poullis and colleagues[87] suggested that the aortic curvature is a more sensitive predictor of the force acting on the aortic wall, and speculated that this finding may explain the occurrence of acute dissection in patients with normal-diameter aortas. Other investigators used echocardiography to measure aortic distensibility and elasticity, and related these parameters to aortic dissection or rupture.[88–90] Large studies with long-term follow-up are necessary to validate these newer criteria. At present, the various size criteria remain the accepted indicators determining the timing of elective surgical repair.

INDICATIONS FOR ELECTIVE SURGICAL REPAIR OF DILATED ASCENDING AORTA IN PATIENTS WITH BAV

The authors believe that the data presented in this review regarding the epidemiology, genetics, histopathology, pathophysiology, and natural history of BAV-associated aortic disease strongly support the use of more liberal criteria for

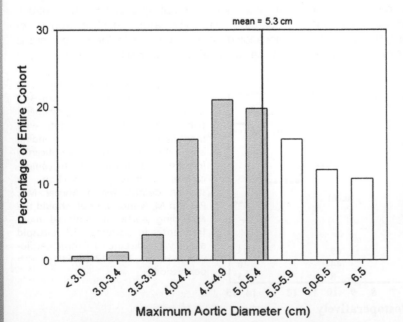

Fig. 5. Distribution of maximum aortic size at the time of presentation with acute type A aortic dissection (cm) in a cohort of 177 non-Marfan patients with TAVs. Shaded bars indicate the 62% of patients with maximum diameters lesser than 5.5 cm. More than 20% of the cohort had a maximum aortic diameter lesser than 4.5 cm. (*From* Parish LM, Gorman JH 3rd, Kahn S, et al. Aortic size in acute type A dissection: implications for preventive ascending aortic replacement. Eur J Cardiothorac Surg 2009;35(6):943; with permission.)

recommending early repair of the dilated ascending aortas of BAV patients as compared with TAV.

The authors suggest the following criteria for elective replacement of the ascending aorta in patients with BAV:

1. Aortic diameter larger than 5.0 cm
2. Aortic diameter larger than 4.5 cm associated with any of the following:
   - Expansion rate larger than 0.5 cm/y in an adult
   - Aortic coarctation, corrected or uncorrected
   - FDR with ascending aortic dissection or rupture
   - Long smoking history, especially with chronic obstructive pulmonary disease
   - Uncontrolled or partially controlled hypertension
   - Small adult body size, indicated by either of the following:
     - Ratio of aortic area to body height larger than 10 cm^2/m
     - Ratio of aortic diameter to body surface area larger than 4.25 cm/m^2
3. Aortic diameter larger than 4.0 cm in patients undergoing concomitant AVR or other cardiac operation if operative risk is low and expected postoperative survival is a decade or longer.

REFERENCES

1. Matthias Bechtel JF, Noack F, Sayk F, et al. Histopathological grading of ascending aortic aneurysm: comparison of patients with bicuspid versus tricuspid aortic valve. J Heart Valve Dis 2003; 12(1):54–9 [discussion: 59–61].
2. de Sa M, Moshkovitz Y, Butany J, et al. Histologic abnormalities of the ascending aorta and pulmonary trunk in patients with bicuspid aortic valve disease: clinical relevance to the Ross procedure. J Thorac Cardiovasc Surg 1999;118(4):588–94.
3. Kirby ML, Waldo KL. Neural crest and cardiovascular patterning. Circ Res 1995;77(2):211–5.
4. Stoller JZ, Epstein JA. Cardiac neural crest. Semin Cell Dev Biol 2005;16(6):704–15.
5. Cannata A, Russo CF, Vitali E. Bicuspid aortic valve: about natural history of ascending aorta aneurysms. Ann Thorac Surg 2008;85(1):362–3.
6. Russo CF, Cannata A, Lanfranconi M, et al. Is aortic wall degeneration related to bicuspid aortic valve anatomy in patients with valvular disease? J Thorac Cardiovasc Surg 2008;136(4):937–42.
7. Thanassoulis G, Yip JW, Filion K, et al. Retrospective study to identify predictors of the presence and rapid progression of aortic dilatation in patients

with bicuspid aortic valves. Nat Clin Pract Cardiovasc Med 2008;5(12):821–8.
8. Fedak PW, David TE, Borger M, et al. Bicuspid aortic valve disease: recent insights in pathophysiology and treatment. Expert Rev Cardiovasc Ther 2005; 3(2):295–308.
9. Borger MA, David TE. Management of the valve and ascending aorta in adults with bicuspid aortic valve disease. Semin Thorac Cardiovasc Surg 2005;17(2): 143–7.
10. Sabet HY, Edwards WD, Tazelaar HD, et al. Congenitally bicuspid aortic valves: a surgical pathology study of 542 cases (1991 through 1996) and a literature review of 2,715 additional cases. Mayo Clin Proc 1999;74(1):14–26.
11. Roberts WC. The congenitally bicuspid aortic valve. A study of 85 autopsy cases. Am J Cardiol 1970; 26(1):72–83.
12. Butany J, Collins MJ, Demellawy DE, et al. Morphological and clinical findings in 247 surgically excised native aortic valves. Can J Cardiol 2005;21(9):747–55.
13. Collins MJ, Butany J, Borger MA, et al. Implications of a congenitally abnormal valve: a study of 1025 consecutively excised aortic valves. J Clin Pathol 2008;61(4):530–6.
14. Ward C. Clinical significance of the bicuspid aortic valve. Heart 2000;83(1):81–5.
15. Kahveci G, Bayrak F, Pala S, et al. Impact of bicuspid aortic valve on complications and death in infective endocarditis of native aortic valves. Tex Heart Inst J 2009;36(2):111–6.
16. Ferencik M, Pape LA. Changes in size of ascending aorta and aortic valve function with time in patients with congenitally bicuspid aortic valves. Am J Cardiol 2003;92(1):43–6.
17. Pape LA, Tsai TT, Isselbacher EM, et al. Aortic diameter > or = 5.5 cm is not a good predictor of type A aortic dissection: observations from the International Registry of Acute Aortic Dissection (IRAD). Circulation 2007;116(10):1120–7.
18. Cecconi M, Manfrin M, Moraca A, et al. Aortic dimensions in patients with bicuspid aortic valve without significant valve dysfunction. Am J Cardiol 2005;95(2):292–4.
19. Larson EW, Edwards WD. Risk factors for aortic dissection: a necropsy study of 161 cases. Am J Cardiol 1984;53(6):849–55.
20. Ando M, Okita Y, Matsukawa R, et al. Surgery for aortic dissection associated with congenital bicuspid aortic valve. Jpn J Thorac Cardiovasc Surg 1998;46(11):1069–73.
21. Ando M, Okita Y, Morota T, et al. Thoracic aortic aneurysm associated with congenital bicuspid aortic valve. Cardiovasc Surg 1998;6(6):629–34.
22. Tsai TT, Trimarchi S, Nienaber CA. Acute aortic dissection: perspectives from the International

Registry of Acute Aortic Dissection (IRAD). Eur J Vasc Endovasc Surg 2009;37(2):149–59.

23. Tutar E, Ekici F, Atalay S, et al. The prevalence of bicuspid aortic valve in newborns by echocardiographic screening. Am Heart J 2005;150(3):513–5.

24. Basso C, Boschello M, Perrone C, et al. An echocardiographic survey of primary school children for bicuspid aortic valve. Am J Cardiol 2004;93(5):661–3.

25. Cripe L, Andelfinger G, Martin LJ, et al. Bicuspid aortic valve is heritable. J Am Coll Cardiol 2004;44(1):138–43.

26. Biner S, Rafique AM, Ray I, et al. Aortopathy is prevalent in relatives of bicuspid aortic valve patients. J Am Coll Cardiol 2009;53(24):2288–95.

27. De Rubens Figueroa J, Rodriguez LM, Hach JL, et al. Cardiovascular spectrum in Williams-Beuren syndrome: the Mexican experience in 40 patients. Tex Heart Inst J 2008;35(3):279–85.

28. Andelfinger G, Tapper AR, Welch RC, et al. KCNJ2 mutation results in Andersen syndrome with sex-specific cardiac and skeletal muscle phenotypes. Am J Hum Genet 2002;71(3):663–8.

29. John AS, McDonald-McGinn DM, Zackai EH, et al. Aortic root dilation in patients with 22q11.2 deletion syndrome. Am J Med Genet A 2009;149A(5):939–42.

30. Arrington CB, Sower CT, Chuckwuk N, et al. Absence of TGFBR1 and TGFBR2 mutations in patients with bicuspid aortic valve and aortic dilation. Am J Cardiol 2008;102(5):629–31.

31. Matura LA, Ho VB, Rosing DR, et al. Aortic dilatation and dissection in Turner syndrome. Circulation 2007;116(15):1663–70.

32. Bondy CA. Aortic dissection in Turner syndrome. Curr Opin Cardiol 2008;23(6):519–26.

33. Sachdev V, Matura LA, Sidenko S, et al. Aortic valve disease in Turner syndrome. J Am Coll Cardiol 2008;51(19):1904–9.

34. Garg V, Muth AN, Ransom JF, et al. Mutations in NOTCH1 cause aortic valve disease. Nature 2005;437(7056):270–4.

35. Mohamed SA, Aherrahrou Z, Liptau H, et al. Novel missense mutations (p.T596M and p.P1797H) in NOTCH1 in patients with bicuspid aortic valve. Biochem Biophys Res Commun 2006;345(4):1460–5.

36. Guo DC, Pannu H, Tran-Fadulu V, et al. Mutations in smooth muscle alpha-actin (ACTA2) lead to thoracic aortic aneurysms and dissections. Nat Genet 2007;39(12):1488–93.

37. Bauer M, Pasic M, Meyer R, et al. Morphometric analysis of aortic media in patients with bicuspid and tricuspid aortic valve. Ann Thorac Surg 2002;74(1):58–62.

38. Collins MJ, Dev V, Strauss BH, et al. Variation in the histopathological features of patients with ascending aortic aneurysms: a study of 111 surgically excised cases. J Clin Pathol 2008;61(4):519–23.

39. Fedak PW, Verma S, David TE, et al. Clinical and pathophysiological implications of a bicuspid aortic valve. Circulation 2002;106(8):900–4.

40. Aicher D, Urbich C, Zeiher A, et al. Endothelial nitric oxide synthase in bicuspid aortic valve disease. Ann Thorac Surg 2007;83(4):1290–4.

41. Boyum J, Fellinger EK, Schmoker JD, et al. Matrix metalloproteinase activity in thoracic aortic aneurysms associated with bicuspid and tricuspid aortic valves. J Thorac Cardiovasc Surg 2004;127(3):686–91.

42. Fedak PW, de Sa MP, Verma S, et al. Vascular matrix remodeling in patients with bicuspid aortic valve malformations: implications for aortic dilatation. J Thorac Cardiovasc Surg 2003;126(3):797–806.

43. Ikonomidis JS, Jones JA, Barbour JR, et al. Expression of matrix metalloproteinases and endogenous inhibitors within ascending aortic aneurysms of patients with bicuspid or tricuspid aortic valves. J Thorac Cardiovasc Surg 2007;133(4):1028–36.

44. Wilton E, Bland M, Thompson M, et al. Matrix metalloproteinase expression in the ascending aorta and aortic valve. Interact Cardiovasc Thorac Surg 2008;7(1):37–40.

45. Koullias GJ, Korkolis DP, Ravichandran P, et al. Tissue microarray detection of matrix metalloproteinases, in diseased tricuspid and bicuspid aortic valves with or without pathology of the ascending aorta. Eur J Cardiothorac Surg 2004;26(6):1098–103.

46. Phillippi JA, Klyachko EA, Kenny JP 4th, et al. Basal and oxidative stress-induced expression of metallothionein is decreased in ascending aortic aneurysms of bicuspid aortic valve patients. Circulation 2009;119(18):2498–506.

47. Keane MG, Wiegers SE, Plappert T, et al. Bicuspid aortic valves are associated with aortic dilatation out of proportion to coexistent valvular lesions. Circulation 2000;102(19 Suppl 3):III35–9.

48. Tadros TM, Klein MD, Shapira OM. Ascending aortic dilatation associated with bicuspid aortic valve: pathophysiology, molecular biology, and clinical implications. Circulation 2009;119(6):880–90.

49. Braverman AC, Guven H, Beardslee MA, et al. The bicuspid aortic valve. Curr Probl Cardiol 2005;30(9):470–522.

50. El-Hamamsy I, Yacoub MH. A measured approach to managing the aortic root in patients with bicuspid aortic valve disease. Curr Cardiol Rep 2009;11(2):94–100.

51. Schaefer BM, Lewin MB, Stout KK, et al. The bicuspid aortic valve: an integrated phenotypic classification of leaflet morphology and aortic root shape. Heart 2008;94(12):1634–8.

52. Della Corte A, Bancone C, Quarto C, et al. Predictors of ascending aortic dilatation with bicuspid

aortic valve: a wide spectrum of disease expression. Eur J Cardiothorac Surg 2007;31(3):397–404 [discussion: 404–5].

53. Koullias G, Modak R, Tranquilli M, et al. Mechanical deterioration underlies malignant behavior of aneurysmal human ascending aorta. J Thorac Cardiovasc Surg 2005;130(3):677–83.

54. Golledge J, Eagle KA. Acute aortic dissection. Lancet 2008;372(9632):55–66.

55. Borger MA, Preston M, Ivanov J, et al. Should the ascending aorta be replaced more frequently in patients with bicuspid aortic valve disease? J Thorac Cardiovasc Surg 2004;128(5):677–83.

56. Tzemos N, Therrien J, Yip J, et al. Outcomes in adults with bicuspid aortic valves. JAMA 2008; 300(11):1317–25.

57. Beppu S, Suzuki S, Matsuda H, et al. Rapidity of progression of aortic stenosis in patients with congenital bicuspid aortic valves. Am J Cardiol 1993;71(4):322–7.

58. La Canna G, Ficarra E, Tsagalau E, et al. Progression rate of ascending aortic dilation in patients with normally functioning bicuspid and tricuspid aortic valves. Am J Cardiol 2006;98(2):249–53.

59. Beroukhim RS, Kruzick TL, Taylor AL, et al. Progression of aortic dilation in children with a functionally normal bicuspid aortic valve. Am J Cardiol 2006; 98(6):828–30.

60. Novaro GM, Griffin BP. Congenital bicuspid aortic valve and rate of ascending aortic dilatation. Am J Cardiol 2004;93(4):525–6.

61. Cecconi M, Nistri S, Quarti A, et al. Aortic dilatation in patients with bicuspid aortic valve. J Cardiovasc Med (Hagerstown) 2006;7(1):11–20.

62. Davies RR, Kaple RK, Mandapati D, et al. Natural history of ascending aortic aneurysms in the setting of an unreplaced bicuspid aortic valve. Ann Thorac Surg 2007;83(4):1338–44.

63. Novaro GM, Tiong IY, Pearce GL, et al. Features and predictors of ascending aortic dilatation in association with a congenital bicuspid aortic valve. Am J Cardiol 2003;92(1):99–101.

64. Yasuda H, Nakatani S, Stugaard M, et al. Failure to prevent progressive dilation of ascending aorta by aortic valve replacement in patients with bicuspid aortic valve: comparison with tricuspid aortic valve. Circulation 2003;108(Suppl 1):II291–4.

65. Russo CF, Mazzetti S, Garatti A, et al. Aortic complications after bicuspid aortic valve replacement: long-term results. Ann Thorac Surg 2002;74(5): S1773–6 [discussion: S1792–9].

66. Edwards WD, Leaf DS, Edwards JE. Dissecting aortic aneurysm associated with congenital bicuspid aortic valve. Circulation 1978;57(5): 1022–5.

67. Olsson C, Eriksson N, Stahle E, et al. Surgical and long-term mortality in 2634 consecutive patients operated on the proximal thoracic aorta. Eur J Cardiothorac Surg 2007;31(6):963–9 [discussion: 969].

68. Olsson C, Thelin S, Stahle E, et al. Thoracic aortic aneurysm and dissection: increasing prevalence and improved outcomes reported in a nationwide population-based study of more than 14,000 cases from 1987 to 2002. Circulation 2006;114(24):2611–8.

69. Clouse WD, Hallett JW Jr, Schaff HV, et al. Acute aortic dissection: population-based incidence compared with degenerative aortic aneurysm rupture. Mayo Clin Proc 2004;79(2):176–80.

70. Ehrlich MP, Ergin MA, McCullough JN, et al. Results of immediate surgical treatment of all acute type A dissections. Circulation 2000;102(19 Suppl 3): III248–52.

71. Geirsson A, Bavaria JE, Swarr D, et al. Fate of the residual distal and proximal aorta after acute type a dissection repair using a contemporary surgical reconstruction algorithm. Ann Thorac Surg 2007; 84(6):1955–64 [discussion: 1955–64].

72. Olsson C, Thelin S. Quality of life in survivors of thoracic aortic surgery. Ann Thorac Surg 1999; 67(5):1262–7.

73. Trimarchi S, Nienaber CA, Rampoldi V, et al. Contemporary results of surgery in acute type A aortic dissection: the International Registry of Acute Aortic Dissection experience. J Thorac Cardiovasc Surg 2005;129(1):112–22.

74. Achneck HE, Rizzo JA, Tranquilli M, et al. Safety of thoracic aortic surgery in the present era. Ann Thorac Surg 2007;84(4):1180–5 [discussion: 1185].

75. Elefteriades JA. Natural history of thoracic aortic aneurysms: indications for surgery, and surgical versus nonsurgical risks. Ann Thorac Surg 2002; 74(5):S1877–80 [discussion: S1892–8].

76. Isselbacher EM. Thoracic and abdominal aortic aneurysms. Circulation 2005;111(6):816–28.

77. Narayan P, Caputo M, Rogers CA, et al. Early and mid-term outcomes of surgery of the ascending aorta/arch: is there a relationship with caseload? Eur J Cardiothorac Surg 2004;25(5):676–82.

78. Coady MA, Rizzo JA, Elefteriades JA. Developing surgical intervention criteria for thoracic aortic aneurysms. Cardiol Clin 1999;17(4):827–39.

79. Coady MA, Rizzo JA, Goldstein LJ, et al. Natural history, pathogenesis, and etiology of thoracic aortic aneurysms and dissections. Cardiol Clin 1999;17(4): 615–35, vii.

80. Bonow RO, Carabello BA, Chatterjee K, et al. 2008 Focused update incorporated into the ACC/AHA 2006 guidelines for the management of patients with valvular heart disease: a report of the American College of Cardiology/American Heart Association Task Force on Practice Guidelines (Writing Committee to Revise the 1998 Guidelines for the Management of Patients With Valvular Heart Disease): endorsed by the Society of

Cardiovascular Anesthesiologists, Society for Cardiovascular Angiography and Interventions, and Society of Thoracic Surgeons. Circulation 2008;118(15):e523–661.

81. Bonow RO, Carabello BA, Kanu C, et al. ACC/AHA 2006 guidelines for the management of patients with valvular heart disease: a report of the American College of Cardiology/American Heart Association Task Force on Practice Guidelines (writing committee to revise the 1998 Guidelines for the Management of Patients With Valvular Heart Disease): developed in collaboration with the Society of Cardiovascular Anesthesiologists: endorsed by the Society for Cardiovascular Angiography and Interventions and the Society of Thoracic Surgeons. Circulation 2006;114(5):e84–231.

82. Davies RR, Coe MP, Mandapati D, et al. Thoracic surgery directors association award. What is the optimal management of late-presenting survivors of acute type A aortic dissection? Ann Thorac Surg 2007;83(5):1593–601 [discussion: 1601–2].

83. Davies RR, Goldstein LJ, Coady MA, et al. Yearly rupture or dissection rates for thoracic aortic aneurysms: simple prediction based on size. Ann Thorac Surg 2002;73(1):17–27 [discussion: 27–8].

84. Parish LM, Gorman JH 3rd, Kahn S, et al. Aortic size in acute type A dissection: implications for preventive ascending aortic replacement. Eur J Cardiothorac Surg 2009;35(6):941–5 [discussion: 945–6].

85. Davies RR, Gallo A, Coady MA, et al. Novel measurement of relative aortic size predicts rupture of thoracic aortic aneurysms. Ann Thorac Surg 2006;81(1):169–77.

86. Svensson LG, Kim KH, Lytle BW, et al. Relationship of aortic cross-sectional area to height ratio and the risk of aortic dissection in patients with bicuspid aortic valves. J Thorac Cardiovasc Surg 2003; 126(3):892–3.

87. Poullis MP, Warwick R, Oo A, et al. Ascending aortic curvature as an independent risk factor for type A dissection, and ascending aortic aneurysm formation: a mathematical model. Eur J Cardiothorac Surg 2008;33(6):995–1001.

88. Nistri S, Sorbo MD, Basso C, et al. Bicuspid aortic valve: abnormal aortic elastic properties. J Heart Valve Dis 2002;11(3):369–73 [discussion: 373–4].

89. Nemes A, Soliman OI, Csanady M, et al. Aortic distensibility in patients with bicuspid aortic valves. Am J Cardiol 2008;102(3):370.

90. Nistri S, Grande-Allen J, Noale M, et al. Aortic elasticity and size in bicuspid aortic valve syndrome. Eur Heart J 2008;29(4):472–9.

Should Aortas in Patients with Bicuspid Aortic Valve Really Be Resected at an Earlier Stage than Tricuspid? CON

Michael A. Coady, MD, MPH[a],*, Philip H. Stockwell, MD[b],
Michael P. Robich, MD[a], Athena Poppas, MD[b],
Frank W. Sellke, MD[a]

KEYWORDS

• Aorta • Bicuspid • Tricuspid • Aortic resection

Bicuspid aortic valve (BAV) is the most common congenital heart malformation, affecting 1% to 2% of the population, and constitutes an important risk factor for the development of aortic valve disease. Unlike patients with normal tricuspid aortic valves (TAVs), only 20% of patients with congenitally BAV will maintain a normally functioning valve, and most will develop BAV-related complications.[1] BAV results in early valvular calcification and stenosis in three-quarters of patients, valvular insufficiency in 15%, and a mixed lesion in 10%.[2] Thirty percent of patients with BAV will also develop infective endocarditis. In addition, BAV is intimately associated with abnormalities of the aortic wall, such as ascending aortic dilatations and aneurysm formation.[3] The prevalence of aneurysmal dilatation in the literature ranges from 33% to 80%. This variation is based on aortic size cutoffs for definitions of aortic aneurysms and normative values for age and body surface area.[4]

Given the high incidence of sequelae, BAV accounts for considerable morbidity and mortality compared with other congenital cardiac abnormalities. The aortic dilatation that occurs with BAV arises more frequently and at a younger age than it does in patients with TAV, and the clinical significance of the correlation between BAV and ascending aortic dilatation is based on the potential for aortic dissection and rupture.[5] Indeed, the associated aortic pathology has significantly complicated the surgical treatment regimens in patients with BAV, because clinicians have realized that the disease process between the valve and aortic wall is intimately associated, yet the underlying etiologic link, whether physiologic or genetic, is still not completely understood. Defining the physiologic or potential molecular biologic basis for aneurysm formation in BAV is critical for understanding disease progression and designing appropriate evidence-based strategies for intervention.

This review explores the pathologic process in the development of BAV, examines the relationship between ascending aortic dilatation and aneurysm formation in the setting of valvular stenosis, explores the relevant genetic basis for aneurysm formation in BAV, and evaluates the current recommended treatment guidelines for

a Division of Cardiothoracic Surgery, Alpert School of Medicine at Brown University, Rhode Island Hospital, Two Dudley Street, Suite 500, Providence, RI 02905, USA
b Divisions of Cardiology, Alpert School of Medicine at Brown University, Rhode Island Hospital, 2 Dudley Street, Suite 360, Providence, RI 02905, USA
* Corresponding author.
E-mail address: mcoady@lifespan.org

Cardiol Clin 28 (2010) 299–314
doi:10.1016/j.ccl.2010.02.003

concomitant aneurysms in patients with BAV. Based on the available evidence, the authors extend a strong argument for a more conservative approach to treatment of concomitant ascending aortic dilatation in BAV disease.

THE BAV

Normal development of the semilunar valves occurs with the advent of valve swellings of subendocardial tissue located near the luminal surface of the aorticopulmonary trunk. Morphologic changes occur during valvulogenesis, which include tissue resorbtion and remodeling, ultimately leading to formation of the thin-walled trileaflet semilunar cusps of the TAV. In BAV development, there is a disruption of this developmental process.

The normal aortic valve is a TAV, with 3 equal-sized leaflets or cusps and 3 clear lines of coaptation. Congenital BAVs are a genetic variant in 1% to 2% of the population, with 2 functional cusps, unequal in size due to fusion during valvulogenesis. This variant is the result of a complex developmental process, not simply the fusion of 2 normal cusps. The larger leaflet in BAV is referred to as the conjoined leaflet. This fused leaflet contains a central raphe, or fibrous ridge, representing the site of congenital fusion. The central raphe is identifiable in most patients with BAV, and has been shown not to contain valve tissue on pathologic examination.[6] In contrast, the TAV is characterized by 3 distinct cusps without a raphe (**Fig. 1**).

In congenital BAV, the cusps are conjoined. Two commissures are present, and neither is partially fused. The shallow, upper aspect of the raphe is usually distinctly below the sinotubular junction, terminating well below the cuspid line of closure.[7,8] The circumferential distances between each of the 3 commissures are approximately equal in the normal TAV, and in congenital BAV the distances between the 2 commissures are also similar.

In a minority of cases, BAV occurs as an acquired pathologic process related to rheumatic heart disease or a degenerative, nonrheumatic inflammatory process. In these cases, the true commissure is fused.[8] This commonly originates at the level of the sinotubular junction, and is maintained at a level similar to the closing edge of the remainder of the valve.

In congenitally bicuspid valves, fusion of the raphe is typically observed between the right and left cusps in 86% of BAV cases.[2] The coronary arteries also tend to arise from the front of the cusps in which the raphe is present. In congenital BAV, the left main coronary artery is frequently up to 50% shorter and the coronary circulation tends to be a left-dominant pattern, more than in normal TAV hearts.[6,8]

BAV in the General Population

Prevalence of BAV in the population is 1% to 2%. The numbers are surprising when the potential clinical consequences are considered in light of a current population of the United States of approximately 305 million. Thus, there are 3 million to 6.1 million United States citizens with BAVs.

Most of the information available regarding prevalence of BAV in the population originated from pathology centers with a wide range of variation. BAV has not been considered rare since 1886, when Osler reported that 1.2% of 800 routine autopsies revealed this congenital malformation, excluding infective endocarditis (**Table 1**).[1,9] In 1970, Roberts[9] found 13 BAVs in 1440 routine post mortems on adults (0.9%), but he argued that this could reach 2% by including patients with cardiac disease. The most reliable

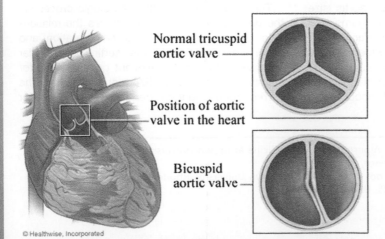

Normal tricuspid aortic valve

Position of aortic valve in the heart

Bicuspid aortic valve

© Healthwise, Incorporated

Fig. 1. The 3 distinct cusps, equal in size in the normal TAV. In BAV, 2 functional cusps are present with the conjoined leaflet containing a central raphe or fibrous ridge (Bicuspid aortic valve image provided courtesy of Healthwise, Incorporated. All rights reserved.).

Table 1
Prevalence of BAV in reported necropsy studies

Author	Year	Study Population (n)	Male/Female	BAV Prevalence (%)	BAV (%)	Prevalence in Men
Osler	1886	800	NA	1.2	NA	
Lewis and Grant	1923	215	NA	1.39	NA	
Wauchope	1928	9.966	NA	0.5	NA	
Grant et al	1928	1.350	NA	0.89	NA	
Gross	1937	5.000	NA	0.56	NA	
Roberts	1970	1.440	NA	0.9	NA	
Larson and Edwards	1984	21.417	NA	1.37	NA	
Datta et al	1988	8.800	NA	0.59	NA	
Pauperio et al	1999	2.000	3/1	0.65	0.87	

Reproduced from Basso C, Boschello M, Perrone C, et al. An echocardiographic survey of primary school children for bicuspid aortic valve. Am J Cardiol 2004;93:663; with permission.

rate of BAV prevalence has been considered to be the 1.37% reported by Larson and Edwards,[10] because of the large number of autopsies (293 BAVs out of 21,417 consecutive autopsies) and their expertise in aortic valve disease.[1,10] Certain groups have been shown to have a higher prevalence of associated BAV, including those with aortic coarctation, Turner syndrome, patent ductus arteriosus, supravalvular aortic stenosis (AS), Williams syndrome, ventricular septal defects, Shone syndrome, and congenital coronary anatomic variants.[6]

Disease Process in BAV

BAV may be identified in patients of any age. It may also be an incidental finding at autopsy. Most patients with BAV are asymptomatic. The BAV may be completely competent, producing no regurgitant flow. If symptoms develop, they are typically related to AS, aortic insufficiency, or both, and the presentation may be variable. Pediatric patients typically present with AS or endocarditis. Young adults often present with aortic regurgitation (AR), with or without associated endocarditis. Middle-aged adults may present with aortic dilatation, aortic dissection, or AS. The elderly patient typically presents with AS.[11]

Early sources of morbidity for patients with BAV include critical AS and infective endocarditis. Stenosis is caused by calcification and sclerosis, and can occur if the aortic cusps are asymmetric or in the anteroposterior position. AR may be caused by fibrosis and retraction of the commissural margins, cusp prolapse, aneurysmal enlargement of the aortic root and valvular annulus, or

valvular destruction secondary to endocarditis. Some degree of prolapse occurs in approximately 85% of patients with BAV, and the degree of prolapse is greater in those with regurgitation than in those without.

Associated Aortic Dilatation with BAV

The precise mechanisms underlying the development and progression of thoracic aortic disease in BAV patients have not been clearly delineated. Two logical considerations are most frequently believed to play a major role in this context[1]: similar to that seen in TAV-associated AS, increased hemodynamic load on the proximal aorta results in progressive aortic dilatation; and[2] that an as-yet unidentified genetic or developmental abnormality in the proximal aortic tissue clinically results in altered integrity of the extracellular matrix with consequent weakness of the aortic wall.

Although the first hypothesis of poststenotic dilatation has the advantage of relative simplicity, some studies suggest that hemodynamic alterations alone cannot be solely responsible for aortic dilatation in these patients because aortic dilatation can occur in the presence of normally functioning BAV.[11,12] In addition, Yasuda and colleagues[11] have shown that aortic valve replacement (AVR) alone does not prevent aortic dilatation in patients with BAV. However, postvalvular flow alterations may be underestimated in BAV by common diagnostic methods.[13,14] This has been interpreted as possibly supporting the hemodynamic hypothesis for aortic dilatation.

The presence of aortic valve dysfunction has consequences for the proximal aorta. In patients with BAV, concomitant AS increases the growth rate of the proximal ascending aorta and significantly increases the risk of rupture or dissection.[12] Although the mechanism for this effect is unknown, the altered hemodynamics resulting from a high-pressure aortic ejection jet may place a greater burden on the proximal aorta.

The other hypothesis for the high incidence of aortic disease in BAV patients is that it is an inborn congenital defect in aortic structure, and this may seem more compelling. The aortic valve and ascending aorta share a common embryologic origin in that both develop from neural crest cells. The pulmonary trunk has also been shown to undergo histopathologic changes similar to those of the ascending aorta in BAV patients.[15] The association between BAV and coarctation of the aorta with and without Turner syndrome may point toward BAV disease involving the ascending aorta and aortic arch.[16] However, despite extensive investigation, no clear genetic substrate and no specific pathogenic sequence has been identified for BAV-related aortic dilatation.

As mentioned earlier, the prevalence of aortic dilatation in BAV has been estimated at between 33% and 80%, depending on the different study populations and settings but also on the criteria used for definition of dilatation.[4] In a study of the features and predictors of ascending aortic dilatation in patients with congenital BAV, Della Corte and colleagues[4] used echocardiography to examine 280 adult patients with isolated BAV. In contrast with previous studies on this topic, root dilatation was distinguished from midascending dilatation. Aortic ectasia or dilatation was found to be present in 83.3% of patients. Dilatation prevailed at the midascending tract (dilatation at the tubular ascending portion alone), with normal sinuses and an unaffected root in 83.7% of these patients.[4] The investigators discovered BAV to represent a heterogeneous population in terms of risk and features of aortic disease. Midascending dilatation in this study was also proportional to the severity of stenosis, suggesting a poststenotic causative mechanism. This is in contrast with other echo studies showing absence of a statistical relationship between the severity of valvular stenosis and the degree of poststenotic aortic dilatation.[17–19]

Root dilatation was rarer in the Della Corte[4] study, and mostly observed in younger men. When the root was involved, it was unrelated to the presence and severity of stenosis. The investigators concluded that the 2 different aortic dilatation phenotypes (midascending and root) may be subtended by a different pathogenesis.

La Canna and colleagues[20] prospectively evaluated the rate of changes in ascending aortic dimensions and outcomes in patients with ascending aortic aneurysms in patients with BAV compared with ascending aortic aneurysms and TAV. Serial transesophageal echocardiograms were performed in 113 consecutive patients with ascending aortic diameters of 40 mm or more, and 60 mm or less, without significant aortic valve stenosis or regurgitation. During an average 3-year follow-up, the rate of ascending aortic diameter progression was similar for BAV and TAV groups. Patients with BAV did not have increased rates of aortic-related complications compared with patients with TAV.[20,21] Because the valve function was normal in this study, the rate of progression of ascending aortic diameters was not influenced by the hemodynamic conditions present in cases of valvular dysfunction. The investigators concluded that, although a general consensus favors the aggressive treatment of ascending aortic dilatation in patients with BAV, using the same size criteria recommended for Marfan syndrome, strong evidence supporting this treatment option still does not exist.[20]

The Yale group[12] recently reported on the natural history of 514 unrepaired ascending aortic aneurysms (>35 mm); TAV were found in 445, and BAV in 70. Patients with BAV had a higher rate of aortic growth (0.19 cm/y) than patients with TAV (0.13 cm/y), (P = .0102). However, despite somewhat faster rates of growth, patients with BAV had similar rates of aortic rupture, dissection, and death, and higher long-term survival. Among patients with BAV, those with AS had a higher risk of rupture, dissection, or death before operative repair than patients with normally functioning valves. The presence of aortic valve dysfunction was found to have consequences for the proximal aorta. In all patients, AS increased the growth rate of the proximal ascending aorta. Although the mechanism for this effect was not addressed in the Yale study,[12] it is possible that the altered hemodynamics resulting from a high-pressure aortic ejection jet places a greater burden on an already dilated proximal aorta.

Despite aneurysmal formation in BAV disease, aortic dissection is a rare event. In a pooled series of studies, the likelihood of BAV in a population of patients with aortic dissections is 59 of 1431 patients, or 4%. Among all aortic dissections in the International Registry of Acute Aortic Dissection (IRAD) database, only 3% had BAVs, and 5% had Marfan syndrome.[20] Thus, aortic dissection should not be directly attributed to aortic dilatation alone in BAV if the patient had hypertension, because that risk factor is much more prevalent in the IRAD database than BAV (73% vs 3%).[20] Roberts[1] found no aortic dissections in 85 autopsies in patients with BAV. Borger and colleagues,[22] in a series of 201 patients with BAV who had valve replacements without aortic replacement, found that only 1 had subsequent aortic dissection (0.5%).

Poststenotic Dilatation Revisited

A complex, long-standing puzzle in hemodynamics of the circulation is the dilatation of a blood vessel immediately downstream of a stenosed aortic valve (bicuspid or tricuspid) or vascular stenosis. Poststenotic dilatation has been studied theoretically and experimentally for the last century. In the early 1900s several investigators explored the concept of poststenotic dilatation, and demonstrated it in the laboratory. Halsted,[23] in 1916, intrigued by the phenomenon of poststentotic dilatation, turned to the animal laboratory, and was the first to investigate the phenomenon experimentally. After a decade of work, he succeeded in producing poststenotic dilatation in 7 dogs by constricting the lumen of the aorta to one-third of its original size. Halsted[23] was the first to observe the whirlpool eddies of blood in the backwaters of the poststenotic segment. He also noted that, when the constriction was slight or complete, dilation was not observed.

Campbell and Kauntze[24] later postulated that poststenotic dilatation in AS could be explained by the Bernoulli principle; that is, that dilatation arises from a relative elevation in lateral pressure in an area downstream from the level of stenosis. They believed that the presence of turbulence may also be a contributing factor in poststentotic dilatation.

Holman[25] was the first to submit the concept of poststenotic dilatation to exhaustive physical analysis. He theorized that physical stress over time led to a state of high kinetic energy in the poststenotic jet stream. Similar to the Bernoulli equation, kinetic energy was converted to lateral pressure by the swirling of blood, causing structural fatigue of the vessel wall. Holman[25] hypothesized that, as a high-velocity jet from the stenosis was suddenly retarded by a slow-moving stream distal to the stenosis, this caused a local conversion of kinetic energy into lateral pressure. This process leads to eddies of turbulent flow and reversed flow that strike the vessel and lead to vibration.

Holman[25] turned to an artificial circulatory system that included a pump and conduits of rigid plastic tubing with segments of elastic rubber in which he could regulate velocity of flow by altering the stroke output, and could record the effect on the elastic segment by varying the pressure and velocity of the flow system. Striking dilatations developed after 21 to 96 hours. These results presented strong evidence indicating that poststenotic dilatation is caused by a dynamic interaction between the blood flow and vessel wall. Three factors are paramount to Holman's[25] analysis: pressure increase secondary to the Bernoulli effect, irregular impact against an elastic wall by turbulent motion, and pulsation of the main flow.

Although Holman gained a deeper insight into the phenomenon than did Halsted,[23] he overlooked the viscous dissipation in the poststenotic region, where the Bernoulli principle ceased to be valid.[26] Fluid dynamics reveal that the pressure downstream of an obstacle is, in general, lower than that upstream under conditions of moderate or large turbulence (high Reynolds numbers). Therefore Holman's first and second factors are disputed.[26]

Following this lead, Robicsek and colleagues[27] refined this concept of fluid dynamics by finding increased turbulence but no experimental or clinical evidence of an increase in lateral pressure in the poststenotic region. They injected dye into a glass model of stenosis with a poststenotic dilatation, and found a maximum turbulence in the distal end of the dilated region. Robicsek and colleagues[27] believed that turbulence was an explanation for vessel weakening, by destroying elastic fibers of the vessel wall secondary to irregular variation of pressure distribution. Many investigators believe that turbulence is the sine qua non for aneurysm development and that the arterial wall undergoes histologic change by turbulence-related vibration.[26]

In 1959, Bruns and colleagues[28] radically challenged the classic concept that poststenotic dilatation was due to turbulence within the blood stream, attributing dilatation to vibrations of the vessel wall, akin to acoustic vibrations, sufficient to produce structural fatigue in the poststenotic vascular segment (**Fig. 2**). Bruns explored physical forces that may play a part in the development of poststentotic dilatation using thin-walled rubber tubes. It had been shown that murmurs of coarctation, recorded directly from the aorta, are maximal in intensity in the region of greatest poststenotic dilatation. Bruns and colleagues[28] hypothesized that vibration of the vessel wall, causing a thrill, produces sufficient energy to cause structural fatigue and eventual dilatation. Using distended elastic tubes, vibration of discrete segments of these tubes led to dilatation in that area. The energy of the pressure fluctuations is of the order of acoustic intensities and, if strong enough, will be transmitted to the vessel wall, causing it to vibrate. With time, this leads to structural fatigue of the elastic tissue with dilatation.

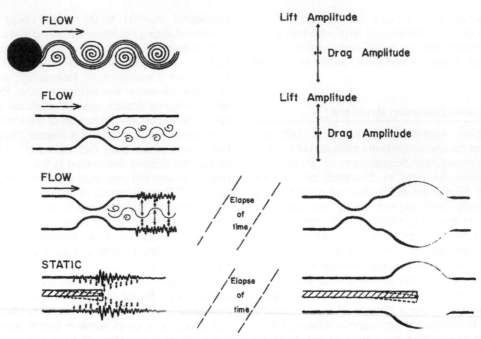

Fig. 2. The theoretical basis of the production of murmurs, thrills, and poststenotic dilatation. With flow past a wire or cylinder, vortices that cause periodic pressure fluctuations in the wake are shed. The bulk of the energy is radiated in a direction perpendicular to the flow (the lift amplitude) rather than parallel to the flow (the drag amplitude). Flow through a stenosis is a modification of this basic pattern. The energy of the pressure fluctuations is of the order of acoustical intensities and, if strong enough, will be transmitted to the vessel wall, causing it to vibrate. With time, this could lead to structural fatigue of the elastic tissue, resulting in dilatation. A vibrating blade can reproduce these physical forces experimentally. By using a static tube, physical forces resulting from fluid flow can be eliminated and the effectiveness of vibrational fatigue more clearly tested. In practice, the point of maximal vibration of the tubing wall was usually found to be 0.5 cm proximal to the blade tip. (*Reproduced from* Bruns DL, Connolly JE, Holman E, et al. Experimental observations on poststenotic dilatation. J Thorac Cardiovasc Surg 1959;38(5):664; with permission.)

In 1962, Kline and colleagues[29] used high-speed cinefluorography in conjunction with droplets of iodized oil to show in vivo the flow pattern within poststenotic segments of the great vessels in a weanling pig. They showed significant aneurysmal growth in the poststenotic segment, with a whirlpool pattern of maximum turbulence, confirming theories postulated by Holman[25] and Robicsek and colleagues.[27] The speed of the central jet stream reached a high velocity before shattering on the vessel wall.

The phenomenon was explored more broadly by Rodbard and colleagues,[30] who noted that an increase in the caliber of the lumen of a vessel may be considered to result from 3 general categories of effects: mechanical distension as a result of increased pressure, functional dilatation, and anatomic reorganization.

Mechanical distension

Mechanical distension is produced acutely as increased pressure stretches the vessel without changing its anatomic organization. In experimental animals, some of the poststenotic dilatations seen grossly at exploratory thoracotomy before sacrifice were not apparent after the aortic pressure decreased at the death of the animal. Thus, the arterial pressure could account for distension and enlargement of the vessels in these instances.

Functional dilatation

Functional dilatation of a vessel refers to a reduction in the tone of the vascular smooth muscle. Such reduction in tone reduces the modulus of elasticity of the vessel wall, resulting in enlargement of the vessel lumen. Vibrations of an arterial segment can produce a reduction in the modulus of elasticity of the arterial wall.

Anatomic reorganization

Anatomic reorganization is observed as changes from the normal pattern of the lines of elastic tissue and the amount of muscle in the wall. Such examples include congenital anomalies, atrophy, trauma after injury, or mechanical forces. Mechanical forces include chronically heightened intravascular

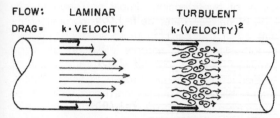

Fig. 3. Laminarity, turbulence, and drag. The sketch indicates a cross section of a vessel. At left, a laminar flow pattern is indicated by the arrows, the length of which show a parabolic distribution of the velocities of the stream line. The drag forces (proportional to the mean velocity) are indicated as the thick arrows in the boundary layers adjacent to the walls. In nonlaminar (turbulent) flow, the parabolic distribution of velocities is lost. Drag (*heavy lines adjacent to the wall*) increases with the square of the mean velocity of the stream. (*Reproduced from* Rodbard S, Ikeda K, Montes M. An analysis of mechanisms of post-stenotic dilatation. Angiology 1967;18(6):364; with permission.)

pressure, vibrations, turbulence, cavitation, structural fatigue of the wall, and drag (**Figs. 3** and **4**).[27,31]

In the 1980s, Kawaguti and Hamano[32] numerically studied steady and pulsatile flows of viscous fluid through a channel with a rectangular hump as a two-dimensional model of blood flow in a constricted artery to elucidate poststenotic dilatation from a hydrodynamic point of view. From numerical calculations, the investigators found that there are hydrodynamic forces causing endothelial injury and contributing to subsequent poststenotic dilatation; these can be found in the large temporal variation of shear stress (**Fig. 5**) behind a constructed portion of the artery.

In 2004, Robicsek and colleagues[13] made observations on cryopreserved, and later thawed, human aortic roots containing congenitally BAV. Valvular function, as studied in the left heart simulator using conventional and 500-frames/s cinematography, by intravascular ultrasound, by preparation of silicone molds, and by computerized digital modeling. The group showed that the clinically normal BAV is characterized by excessive folding and creasing, which (unlike the TAV) persist throughout the cardiac cycle; extended areas of leaflet contact; significant morphologic stenosis; and asymmetrical flow patterns and turbulence. These features subject the congenital BAV to abnormally high stresses that lead to early thickening and eventually calcification and stenosis. The abnormal flow patterns also predict dilatation and dissection of the ascending aorta (**Fig. 6**).[13]

Genetics of BAV

Despite extensive investigation, no clear genetic substrate, and no specific pathogenic sequence, has been identified for BAV-related aortic dilatation. This lack is in distinct contrast with the disease process in Marfan syndrome, in which the culprit gene defect has been isolated.

The ascending aorta and the pulmonary trunk originate from the truncus arteriosus during embryologic development. In patients with Marfan syndrome, the pulmonary artery is always dilated, whereas the pulmonary artery associated with BAV has never been reported to be dilated in situ.[20] Rare families with repeated occurrences of BAV have suggested a Mendelian inheritance, but, again, this has been infrequent compared with 1% to 2% of the general population with BAV.[20]

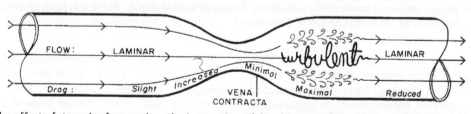

Fig. 4. The effect of stenosis of a vessel on the interaction of the elements of the stream with the wall. The stream lines are shown passing through a tube that is constricted in its mid portion. At the left, the central lamina passes directly through the narrowing without interaction with the wall; this lamina produces no direct effect on the wall. The stream lines near the walls interact with, and exert a drag force on, the vessel lining. Drag and interaction increase in the nozzle leading to the constriction. Immediately downstream from the point of maximal narrowing, the higher velocity of the stream lines deviates them from the wall so that interaction of stream and wall is minimal in the vena contracta; drag is also minimal in this site. Immediately beyond the vena contracta the high stream velocity disturbs laminarity, and turbulence occurs. In such a region of nonlaminar flow, drag and interaction of stream and wall are maximal. The tendency for reestablishment of laminarity becomes dominant further downstream, and drag and the interaction of the elements of the stream with wall are reduced. (*Reproduced from* Rodbard S, Ikeda K, and Montes M. An analysis of mechanisms of post-stenotic dilatation. Angiology 1967;18(6);364; with permission.)

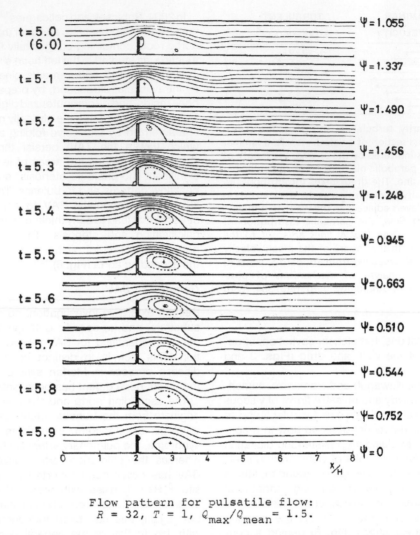

Flow pattern for pulsatile flow:
$R = 32$, $T = 1$, $Q_{max}/Q_{mean} = 1.5$.

Fig. 5. This model assumes that, for a constricted vessel, both ends can be approximated by pulsatile (Womersley) flow. Fluid in the standing vortex mixes with the main flow, and stasis of the blood does not occur even when the flow is laminar. Temporal change of shear stress induces cyclic pulling of the wall in the flow direction and may give rise to fatigue and breakdown of the wall. (*From* Kawaguti M, Hamano A. Numerical study on post-stenotic dilatation. Biorheology 1983;20(5):513; with permission.)

In familial clusters, the primary mode of inheritance seems to be autosomal dominant, similar to that seen in thoracic aortic aneurysms.[33,34] However, genetic heterogeneity is apparent, in that X-linked dominant and recessive modes also are evident. Mutations in the *NOTCH1* gene have recently been identified that lead to signaling abnormalities that may be related to the development of a bileaflet aortic valve and possibly accelerated calcium deposition.[35] In addition, missense mutations in the *ACTA2* gene, which encodes vascular smooth muscle [α]-actin, has been identified as being associated with familial thoracic aortic aneurysms and dissections in BAV.[36]

From a histopathologic perspective, BAV aortic disease shares some similarities with other collagen vascular disorders like Marfan syndrome, with cystic medial degeneration, an increase in matrix metalloproteinase (MMP) expression, and decreased fibrillin-1 content in the aortic wall in some cases. Although the fibrillin-1 content has been shown to be significantly decreased in BAV compared with TAV aortas, mutations in the *FBN1* have not been found to be associated with BAV disease.[37] However, it is likely that a heterogeneity of pathology of the aortic wall is present in association with BAV, and that several genetic factors may come into play.

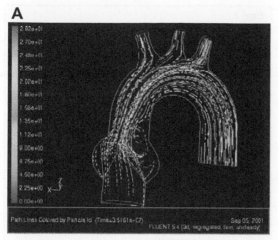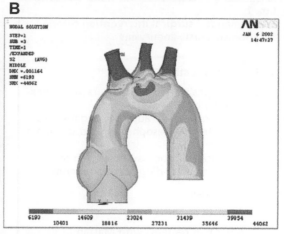

Fig. 6. (*A*) Flow and (*B*) stress patterns of an eccentric bicuspid valve. The valve opening is tilted to the left. The commissure attachment is 5 mm from the center of the valve. Valve dimensions: annulus, 20 mm; sinotubular junction, 20 mm; leaflet height, 16 mm; leaflet free-edge length, 26 mm. The area of the orifice is approximately 50% of that in the nonstenotic valve. For the stenotic valve, the left ventricle needs to contract harder and, as a result, the blood may carry a higher momentum (energy, velocity) into the aorta. Consequently, the aortic arch needs to provide a larger force to turn the flow path into the descending aorta. This force causes a higher and uneven stress distribution in the ascending aorta. (*From* Robicsek F, Thubrikar MJ, Cook JW, et al. The congenital bicuspid aortic valve: how does it function? Why does it fail? Ann Thorac Surg 2004;77:183; with permission.)

Whatever the underlying cause, ascending aortic aneurysms associated with BAV have increased expression of different and distinct MMPs and tissue inhibitors of MMPs (TIMPs) compared with patients with TAVs. Levels of MMP-2 (gelatinase A) and MMP-9 (gelatinase B) are commonly implicated as being increased in aneurysms associated with BAV.[38,39] However, this has not uniformly been the case, with some researchers finding MMP-2 expression in BAV and MMP-9 in trileaflet aortic valves.[40] Marfan syndrome features increased expression of MMP-12 (elastase) and TIMP-2, with decreased MMP-2 and TIMP-3.[41] These distinct patterns of MMP and TIMP expression may reflect different pathophysiological mechanisms, which are in turn dependent on the origin of the aortic disease and subsequent environmental and hemodynamic stressors.

Ascending Aortic Dilatation in TAV patients

The natural history of aortic rupture or dissection is clearly related to the size of the aorta. In the setting of a TAV, ascending aortic dilatation can occur alone, or in the setting of concomitant AS or insufficiency. Dilatation may be a poststenotic phenomenon in the case of AS, or can be part of the process of a dilating root in patients with aortic insufficiency. Aneurysm formation can also be a familial process in some instances or can be sporadic.

In most cases, unlike in BAV disease, treatment of an aneurysm (in isolation or concomitantly) is straightforward in patients with TAV. The Yale group[42] previously reported that the natural history of patients with Marfan syndrome argues for earlier repair of aortic aneurysms in these patients. Size criteria (**Box 1**) have been proposed for an enlarging aorta, based on the risk of rupture or dissection.[42] As noted, the recommended size criterion threshold for patients with Marfan syndrome (5 cm) is lower than in patients without Marfan syndrome (5.5 cm) because of the propensity for these individuals to rupture or dissect at smaller aortic sizes.[42]

Ascending Aortic Dilatation in BAV

The American College of Cardiology (ACC) and American Heart Association (AHA) Committee on Management of Patients With Valvular Heart Disease 2008 update report represents the most current and comprehensive consensus opinions of experts in cardiology and cardiac surgery; this monograph is designed to assist health care providers in the management of cardiovascular disorders.

The ACC/AHA uses a standard classification of conditions and proposed treatment rationales (divided into class I, II or III) and a report of the weight of evidence in support of recommendations for each listed indication (level of evidence A, B, or C) (**Box 2**).[43] **Fig. 7** shows the schema

---

Box 1
Recommended surgical intervention criteria for thoracic aortic aneurysms

1. Rupture
2. Symptomatic states
   a. Pain consistent with rupture and unexplained by other causes
   b. Compression of adjacent organs, especially trachea, esophagus, and left main stem bronchus
   c. Significant aortic insufficiency in conjunction with ascending aortic aneurysm
3. Absolute size
   a. Ascending aorta

   5.0 cm in patients with Marfan syndromea[a]
   5.5 cm in patients without Marfan syndrome

   b. Descending aorta

   6.0 cm in patients with Marfan syndrome
   6.5 cm in patients without Marfan syndrome

4. Documented enlargement

   a. Growth greater than or equal to 1 cm/y or substantial growth, and aneurysm is rapidly approaching criteria in number 3

5. Acute aortic dissection

   a. Ascending requires urgent operation
   b. Descending requires complication-specific approach

[a] The Marfan intervention criteria should also apply if there exists a family history of aortic disease other than Marfan syndrome.

Reprinted from Coady MA, et al. What is the appropriate size criterion for resection of thoracic aortic aneurysms? J Thorac Cardiovasc Surg 1997;113(3):488; with permission.

Box 2
ACC/AHA classification for practice guidelines

Class I

Conditions for which there is evidence for and/or general agreement that the procedure or treatment is beneficial, useful, and effective

Class II

Conditions for which there is conflicting evidence and/or a divergence of opinion about the usefulness/efficacy of a procedure or treatment

Class IIa

Weight of evidence/opinion is in favor of usefulness/efficacy

Class IIb

Usefulness/efficacy is less well established by evidence/opinion

Class III

Conditions for which there is evidence and/or general agreement that the procedure/treatment is not useful/effective, and in some cases may be harmful

Level of evidence A

Data derived from multiple randomized clinical trials

Level of evidence B

Data derived from a single randomized trial or nonrandomized studies

Level of evidence C

Only consensus opinion of experts, case studies, or standard of care

From Bonow RO, Carabello BA, Chatterjee K, et al. 2008 focused update incorporated into the ACC/AHA 2006 guidelines for the management of patients with valvular heart disease: a report of the American College of Cardiology/American Heart Association Task Force on Practice Guidelines (Writing Committee to revise the 1998 guidelines for the management of patients with valvular heart disease). Endorsed by the Society of Cardiovascular Anesthesiologists, Society for Cardiovascular Angiography and Interventions, and Society of Thoracic Surgeons. J Am Coll Cardiol 2008;52(13):e6; with permission.

---

for classification of recommendations and level of evidence summarized in **Box 2**, and also illustrates how the grading system provides estimates of the size of the treatment effect and the certainty of the treatment effect.[43] The ACC/AHA recommendations for bicupid aortic valve with dilated ascending aorta are described in **Box 3**.[43]

As seen in **Box 3**, the current guidelines supported by the ACC/AHA are largely backed only by being level of evidence C, or simply a consensus opinion of experts. These recommendations are not based on objective evidence such as data derived from multiple randomized controlled clinical trials or nonrandomized studies. These types of studies have not been done for BAV-related aortic dilatation.

Although specific size criteria are proposed in the recommendations, no data are presented on the actual risk of surgery for aortic replacement or the risk for dissection in a population of subjects with BAV, adjusted for age and, importantly, hypertension.[20,43]

The implications of the ACC/AHA guidelines are profound. Of an estimated 305 million Americans,

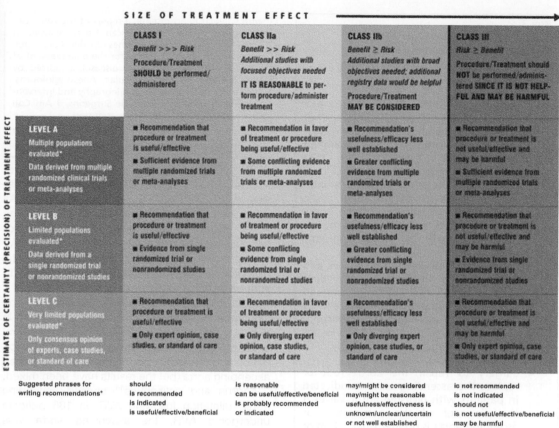

Fig. 7. Applying classification of recommendations and level of evidence. (*From* Bonow RO, Carabello BA, Chatterjee K, et al. 2008 focused update incorporated into the ACC/AHA 2006 guidelines for the management of patients with valvular heart disease: a report of the American College of Cardiology/American Heart Association Task Force on Practice Guidelines (Writing Committee to revise the 1998 guidelines for the management of patients with valvular heart disease). Endorsed by the Society of Cardiovascular Anesthesiologists, Society for Cardiovascular Angiography and Interventions, and Society of Thoracic Surgeons. J Am Coll Cardiol 2008; 52(13):e7; with permission.)

3 million to 6.1 million will, statistically, have BAVs. These guidelines recommend prophylactic aortic replacement for even an asymptomatic patient with a BAV when the aortic dimensions are smaller than arbitrary ranges based on Marfan syndrome, without comparing risk estimates of aortic dissection with operative risks (see **Box 3**).[42]

The suggestion that this large population lives under the threat of sudden death from aortic dissection, with a risk similar to that of patients with Marfan syndrome, is not firmly backed by data.[20] In addition, as discussed earlier, dissection in BAV disease is a rare event.

Special Considerations

Like TAV disease, several aspects need to be considered when evaluating the most appropriate surgical treatment in patients with BAV. Determining the morphology of the BAV, the size of the ascending aorta, and the extent and rate of progression of aortic dilatation are important to determine an individualized surgical approach. Of paramount importance in the decision making is an adequate risk assessment of the difficulty of the surgical procedure and the patient's associated comorbidities.

The risk of long-term aortic complications must be balanced against the increased perioperative risk associated with more complex procedures. The mortality for aortic root replacement is not trivial, considering the published statistics from centers of excellence. Early mortality has been reported as approximately 4%, and total mortality approximates 10%.[20] The early mortality from surgery is the same as the prevalence of BAV in a population of more than 1000 patients with aortic dissections from the IRAD database.[20] There is no prospective, large series of patients with BAV who have been followed without surgery.

with valvular heart disease: a report of the American College of Cardiology/American Heart Association Task Force on Practice Guidelines (Writing Committee to revise the 1998 guidelines for the management of patients with valvular heart disease). Endorsed by the Society of Cardiovascular Anesthesiologists, Society for Cardiovascular Angiography and Interventions, and Society of Thoracic Surgeons. J Am Coll Cardiol 2008;52(13):e38; with permission.

Box 3
Current ACC/AHA recommendations for bicuspid aortic valve with dilated ascending aorta

Class I

1. Patients with known bicuspid aortic valves should undergo an initial transthoracic echocardiogram to assess the diameters of the aortic root and ascending aorta (level of evidence: B)
2. Cardiac magnetic resonance imaging or cardiac computed tomography is indicated in patients with bicuspid aortic valves when morphology of the aortic root or ascending aorta cannot be assessed accurately by echocardiography (level of evidence: C)
3. Patients with bicuspid aortic valves and dilatation of the aortic root or ascending aorta (diameter >4.0 cm) should undergo serial evaluation of aortic root/ascending aorta size and morphology by echocardiography, cardiac magnetic resonance, or computed tomography on a yearly basis (level of evidence: C)
4. Surgery to repair the aortic root or replace the ascending aorta is indicated in patients with bicuspid aortic valves if the diameter of the aortic root or ascending aorta is greater than 5.0 cm or if the rate of increase in diameter is 0.5 cm/y or more (level of evidence: C)
5. In patients with bicuspid valves undergoing AVR because of severe AS or AR, repair of the aortic root or replacement of the ascending aorta is indicated if the diameter of the aortic root or ascending aorta is greater than 4.5 cm (level of evidence: C)

Class IIa

1. It is reasonable to give β-adrenergic blocking agents to patients with bicuspid valves and dilated aortic roots (diameter >4.0 cm) who are not candidates for surgical correction and who do not have moderate to severe AR. (level of evidence: C)
2. Cardiac magnetic resonance imaging or cardiac computed tomography is reasonable in patients with bicuspid aortic valves when aortic root dilatation is detected by echocardiography to further quantify severity of dilatation and involvement of the ascending aorta (level of evidence: B)

From Bonow RO, Carabello BA, Chatterjee K, et al. 2008 focused update incorporated into the ACC/AHA 2006 guidelines for the management of patients

---

Ascending Aortic Dilatation After AVR

Replacement of the ascending aorta at the time of AVR is controversial because the risk of progressive dilatation following AVR is uncertain. As mentioned earlier, the natural history of ascending aortic dilatation and risk factors for aortic dissection and rupture in the setting of a replaced BAV are unknown. The clinical effect of poststenotic dilatation is also unknown, making it difficult to support specific treatment regimens.

Little information is currently available on the incidence of aortic complications after AVR in patients with a dilated ascending aorta. Several small studies have attempted to clarify the incidence and risk factors for progression of a dilated ascending aorta, but the results have been mixed.

Andrus and colleagues[44] studied ascending aortic dilatation following AVR. In 185 patients undergoing AVR, the ascending aorta was measured 2 cm above the sinotubular ridge, using transesophageal echocardiography before surgery and during follow-up. Progressive aortic dilatation was defined as an increase in diameter of more than 0.3 cm from the preoperative measurement. This condition was only found in 15% of the study population. No patients with baseline aortic dilatation (3.5–5.3 cm) dilated to more than 5.5 cm during the follow-up period (n = 107, mean 33.6 months). There were no clinical or valvular characteristics that predicted progressive aortic dilatation. Their conclusion was therefore against routine replacement of the ascending aorta at the time of AVR.

Matsuyama and colleagues[45] studied 34 patients with a preoperative dilated ascending aorta of more than 4 cm and followed them after AVR. The baseline aortic diameter in the study population ranged from 4.0 to 5.5 cm and the mean follow-up period was 8.1 ($\pm$ 3.5) years. There was a high frequency of bicuspid valve disease in patients with a dilated ascending aorta (57%). Aortic events occurred in 5 patients (1 aortic dissection, 2 aortic rupture, and 2 reoperations). One aortic dissection developed at a baseline aortic size of 42 mm, whereas 2 aortic ruptures occurred at baseline aortic sizes of 47 mm and 50 mm. There was no statistically significant

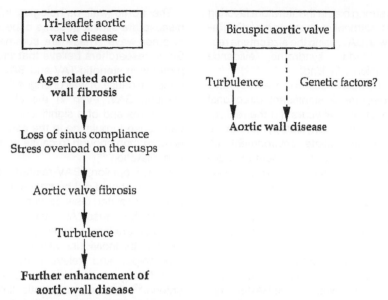

Fig. 8. Summary of hypothesized aortic wall pathophysiology in TAV and BAV disease. (*From* Robicsek F. Bicuspid versus tricuspid aortic valves. J Heart Valve Dis 2003;12:52–3; with permission.)

univariate association between any of the patient clinical characteristics and late aortic events or ascending aortic progression. The investigators concluded that the clinical course of patients with dilated ascending aorta is unpredictable, and complications may occur even in patients with a baseline aortic diameter less than 5.0 cm. They concluded that preventative aortic surgery at the time of AVR should be considered, to prevent aortic rupture and dissection, in patients with ascending aorta of 4.0 to 5.0 cm.

Aortic Dilatation in the Setting of Aortic Valvular Disease

Replacement of the ascending aorta at the time of an AVR in patients with mild to moderate aortic dilatation is controversial, especially for BAV.

This is partly because of the lack of evidence for progressive dilatation following AVR, and partly because of the increased risk associated with aortic root replacement. The perioperative risk is twice as high for root replacement as for isolated valve replacement.[22] Current ACC/AHA guidelines are presented in **Box 3**. In patients with bicuspid valves undergoing AVR because of severe AS or AR, repair of the aortic root or replacement of the ascending aorta is recommended if the diameter of the aortic root or ascending aorta is greater than 4.5 cm.

Borger and colleagues[22] reviewed all 201 patients with BAVs undergoing AVR at their institution from 1979 to 1993. The mean follow-up was 10.3 (±3.8) years and the average patient age was 56 (±15) years. The ascending aorta was normal (<4.0 cm) in 115 (57%) patients, mildly dilated (4.0–4.4 cm) in 64 (32%) patients, and moderately dilated (4.5–4.9 cm) in 22 (11%) patients. All patients with BAV with marked dilation (>5.0 cm) underwent replacement of the ascending aorta and were therefore excluded. Fifteen-year survival was 67%. During follow-up, 44 patients required reoperation, predominantly for aortic valve prosthesis failure. Twenty-two patients had long-term complications related to the ascending aorta: 18 required an operative procedure to replace the ascending aorta (for aortic aneurysm), 1 had aortic dissection, and 3 experienced sudden cardiac death. Fifteen-year freedom from ascending aorta–related complications was 86%, 81%, and 43% in patients with an aortic diameter of less than 4.0 cm, 4.0 to 4.4 cm, and 4.5 to 4.9 cm, respectively (*P*<.001). The investigators concluded that patients undergoing operations for BAV disease should be considered for concomitant replacement of the ascending aorta if the diameter is 4.5 cm or greater.

SUMMARY

The most serious weakness in making sound recommendations for earlier surgical intervention in BAV-related aortic disease is the absence of prospective randomized trials and uncertainty about its etiology. BAV-associated aortopathy is a complex phenomenon, and the current lack of univocal interpretation of its causes and treatment can be ascribed to the multiform nature of its clinical presentation.[4]

Although there is strong bias in the literature favoring more aggressive treatment of ascending aortic dilatation in patients with BAV, using the size criteria recommended for Marfan syndrome, evidence supporting this opinion is lacking.

The focus of medical research in aortic valve disease has undergone 2 significant directional changes in the past several years: (1) the realization that aortic valve pathophysiology cannot be separated from its immediate environment; (2) a shift of interest from surgical treatment to unanswered questions of causation.[46] This review discusses some of the relevant issues relating to causation: why the ascending aorta dilates in BAV. This discussion is an effort to better analyze the current recommendations used to guide surgical management.

Two prominent theories, poststenotic dilatation and genetic factors, may, independently or synergistically, lead to the development of BAV-related aortic pathology. The concept of poststenotic dilatation has been overshadowed in recent years by a quest for a genetic basis for aortic dilatation in BAV. However, despite significant effort, no pathogenic sequence or genetic substrate has been identified, and it is possible that the genetic predisposition is dependent on more than 1 genetic locus.

The current management advocated by many experts, including the ACC/AHA, combines BAV-associated aortic dilatation in the same category as Marfan-related disease, supporting more aggressive treatment of aortic dilatation at smaller aortic sizes than those currently recommended for ascending aortic aneurysms in the setting of TAVs.[1,12] These recommendations are at a level of evidence C: simply a consensus opinion of experts. The AHA/ACC guidelines do not present data on the actual risk of surgery for aortic replacement, or the risk for dissection in a population of subjects with BAV adjusted for age and hypertension.[47]

Although this change has occurred because of the fear that BAV has a genetic basis, the original hypothesis regarding poststenotic dilatation, initially proposed a century ago, has never been discounted as a plausible causal, or strong contributing, factor. Indeed, rare families with repeated occurrences of BAV have suggested the possibility of Mendelian inheritance, but this has been infrequent compared with the large population of patients with BAVs. In addition, no gene been identified in these patients.[47] The current level of genetic evidence is simply not as strong as it is for Marfan syndrome. There is also evidence that there may be more than 1 aortic dilatation phenotype in BAV disease: midascending and root, subtended by different pathogeneses.[4]

The aortic wall pathologies in TAV and BAV disease are similar in some aspects, but different in other ways. These are summarized in **Fig. 8**. Some researchers believe that the abnormal flow patterns in stenotic TAV and BAV disease are the principal cause of wall changes.[46] Morphologically stenotic BAV, even in the absence of clinical symptoms and of a significant pressure gradient, can cause turbulence in the ascending aorta that is more than enough to cause aortic wall changes and dilatation.[46]

In our opinion, BAV-related ascending aortic dilatation should not be treated more aggressively than TAV-related disease without further confirmation of the cause. At least, the data to support doing so are largely lacking. Treatment should be tailored by individual valvular pathology, clinical phenotype, and relevant comorbidities, using well-documented evidence-based clinical size criteria.[42] Because a genetic link has not been clearly identified, solid recommendations similar to or exceeding current Marfan recommendations are controversial. The risk in the current ACC/AHA guidelines for BAV-related aortopathy is that documents such as these often become the standard of care and, as such, reduce the legitimate choices available to practicing cardiologists and cardiac surgeons.[20,43]

REFERENCES

1. Roberts WC. The congenitally bicuspid aortic valve. A study of 85 autopsy cases. Am J Cardiol 1970; 26(1):72–83.
2. Sabet HY, Edwards WD, Tazelaar HD, et al. Congenitally bicuspid aortic valves: a surgical pathology study of 542 cases (1991 through 1996) and a literature review of 2,715 additional cases. Mayo Clin Proc 1999;74:14–26.
3. Vallely MP, Semsarian C, Bannon PG. Management of the ascending aorta in patients with bicuspid aortic valve disease. Heart Lung Circ 2008;17:357–63.
4. Della Corte A, Bancone C, Quarto C, et al. Predictors of ascending aortic dilatation with bicuspid aortic valve: a wide spectrum of disease expression. Eur J Cardiothorac Surg 2007;37:397–405.
5. Tadros TM, Klein MD, Shapira OM. Ascending aortic dilatation associated with bicuspid aortic valve: pathophysiology, molecular biology, and clinical implications. Circulation 2009;119:880–90.
6. Braerman AC, Guven H, Beardslee MA, et al. The bicuspid aortic valve. Curr Probl Cardiol 2005; 30(9):470–522.
7. Cardella JF, Kan VI, Edwards JE. Association of the acquired bicuspid aortic valve with rheumatic disease of atrioventricular valves. Am J Cardiol 1989;63(12):876–7.

8. Lerer PK, Edwards WD. Coronary arterial anatomy in bicuspid aortic valve. Necropsy study of 100 hearts. Br Heart J 1981;45:142–7.

9. Basso C, Boschello M, Perrone C, et al. An echocardiographic survey of primary school children for bicuspid aortic valve. Am J Cardiol 2004; 93(5):661–3.

10. Larson EW, Edwards WD. Risk factors for aortic dissection: a necropsy study of 161 cases. Am J Cardiol 1984;53:849–55.

11. Yasuda H, Nakatani S, Stugaard M, et al. Failure to prevent progressive dilation of ascending aorta by aortic valve replacement in patients with bicuspid aortic valve: comparison with tricuspid aortic valve. Circulation 2003;108(Suppl 1):II291–4.

12. Davies RR, Kaple RK, Mandapati D, et al. Natural history of ascending aortic aneurysms in the setting of an unreplaced bicuspid aortic valve. Ann Thorac Surg 2007;83:1338–44.

13. Robicsek F, Thubrikar MJ, Cook JW, et al. The congenital bicuspid aortic valve: how does it function? Why does it fail? Ann Thorac Surg 2004;77: 177–85.

14. Richards KE, Deserranno D, Donal E, et al. Influence of structural geometry on the severity of bicuspid aortic stenosis. Am J Physiol Heart Circ Physiol 2004;287:1410–6.

15. Niwa K, Perloff JK, Bhuta SM, et al. Structural abnormalities of great arterial walls in congenital heart disease: light and electron microscopic analyses. Circulation 2001;103:393–400.

16. Becker AE, Becker MJ, Edwards JE. Anomalies associated with coarctation of aorta particular reference to infancy. Circulation 1970;41:1067–75.

17. Nistri S, Sorbo MD, Marin M, et al. Aortic root dilatation in young men with normally functioning bicuspid aortic valves. Heart 1999;82:19–22.

18. Keane MG, Wiegers SE, Plappert T, et al. Bicuspid aortic valves are associated with aortic dilatation out of proportion to coexistent valvular lesions. Circulation 2000;102:III35–9.

19. Cecconi M, Manfrin M, Moraca A, et al. Aortic dimensions in patients with bicuspid aortic valve without significant valve dysfunction. Am J Cardiol 2005;95:292–4.

20. La Canna G, Ficarra E, Tsagalau E, et al. Progression rate of ascending aortic dilatation in patients with normally functioning bicuspid and tricuspid aortic valves. Am J Cardiol 2006;98:249–53.

21. Titus JL, Edwards JE. The aortic root and valve: anatomy and congenital anomalies. In: Emery RW, Arom KV, editors. The aortic valve. Philadelphia: Hanley & Belfus, Inc; 1991. p. 1–8.

22. Borger MA, Preston M, Ivanov J, et al. Should the ascending aorta be replaced more frequently in patients with bicuspid aortic valve disease? J Thorac Cardiovasc Surg 2004;128:677–83.

23. Halsted WS. An experimental study of the circumscribed dilation of an artery immediately distal to a partially occluding band and its bearing on the dilation of the subclavian artery observed in certain cases of cervical rib. J Exp Med 1916;24:271–6.

24. Campbell M, Kauntze R. Congenital aortic valvular stenosis. Br Heart J 1953;15(2):179–94.

25. Holman E. The obscure physiology and poststenotic dilatation: its relation to the development of aneurysms. J Thorac Surg 1954;28:109.

26. Matunobu Y, Arakawa A. Model experiment of the post-stenotic dilatation in blood vessels. Biorheology 1974;11:456–64.

27. Robicsek F, Sanger PW, Taylor FH, et al. Pathogenesis and significance of post-stenotic dilatation in great vessels. Ann Surg 1958;147:835.

28. Bruns DL, Connolly JE, Holman E, et al. Experimental observations on post-stenotic dilatation. J Thorac Cardiovasc Surg 1959;38(5):662–9.

29. Kline JL, Gimenez JL, Maloney RJ. Post-stenotic vascular dilatation: confirmation of an old hypothesis by a new method. J Thorac Cardiovasc Surg 1962; 44(6):738–48.

30. Rodbard S, Ikeda K, Montes M. An analysis of mechanisms of post-stenotic dilatation. Angiology 1967;18(6):349–67.

31. Talbot SA, Boyer SH. Does cavitation contribute to cardiovascular sound? IRE Trans Med Electron 1957;PGME-9:8–10.

32. Kawaguti M, Hamano A. Numerical study on post-stenotic dilatation. Biorheology 1983;20:507–18.

33. Coady MA, Davies RR, Roberts M, et al. Familial patterns of thoracic aortic aneurysms. Arch Surg 1999;134:361–7.

34. Huntington K, Hunter AG, Chan KL. A prospective study to assess the frequency of familial clustering of congenital bicuspid aortic valve. J Am Coll Cardiol 1997;30:1809–12.

35. Garg V, Muth AN, Ransom JF, et al. Mutations in NOTCH1 cause aortic valve disease. Nature 2005; 437:270–4.

36. Guo DC, Pannu H, Tran-Fadulu V, et al. Mutations in smooth muscle alpha-actin (ACTA2) lead to thoracic aortic aneurysms and dissections. Nat Genet 2007; 39:1488–93.

37. Lee TC, Zhao YD, Courtman DW, et al. Abnormal aortic valve development in mice lacking endothelial nitric oxide synthase. Circulation 2000;101: 2345–8.

38. Ikonomidis JS, Jones JA, Barbour JR, et al. Expression of matrix metalloproteinases and endogenous inhibitors within ascending aortic aneurysms of patients with bicuspid or tricuspid aortic valves. J Thorac Cardiovasc Surg 2007;133:1028–36.

39. Koullias GJ, Korkolis DP, Ravichandran P, et al. Tissue microarray detection of matrix metalloproteinases, in diseased tricuspid and bicuspid aortic

valves with or without pathology of the ascending aorta. Eur J Cardiothorac Surg 2004;26:1098–103.

40. LeMaire S, Wang X, Wilks J, et al. Matrix metalloproteinases in ascending aortic aneurysms: bicuspid versus trileaflet aortic valves. J Surg Res 2005;123: 40–8.

41. Ikonomidis JS, Jones JA, Barbour JR, et al. Expression of matrix metalloproteinases and endogenous inhibitors within ascending aortic aneurysms of patients with Marfan syndrome. Circulation 2006; 114(Suppl):I365–70.

42. Coady MA, Rizzo JA, Hammond GL, et al. What is the appropriate size criterion for resection of thoracic aortic aneurysms? J Thorac Cardiovasc Surg 1997;113:476–91.

43. Bonow RO, Carabello BA, Chatterjee K, et al. 2008 focused update incorporated into the ACC/AHA 2006 guidelines for the management of patients with valvular heart disease: a report of the American College of Cardiology/American Heart Association Task Force on Practice Guidelines (Writing Committee to revise the 1998 guidelines for the management of patients with valvular heart disease). Endorsed by the Society of Cardiovascular Anesthesiologists, Society for Cardiovascular Angiography and Interventions, and Society of Thoracic Surgeons. J Am Coll Cardiol 2008;13:e1–142.

44. Andrus BW, O'Rourke DJ, Dacey LJ, et al. Stability of ascending aortic dilatation following aortic valve replacement. Circulation 2003;108(Suppl):II295–9.

45. Matsuyama KA, Akita T, Yoshikawa M, et al. Natural history of a dilated ascending aorta after aortic valve replacement. Circ J 2005;69:392–6.

46. Robicsek F. Bicuspid versus tricuspid aortic valves. J Heart Valve Dis 2003;12:52–3.

47. Guntheroth WG. A critical review of the American College of Cardiology/American Heart Association practice guidelines on bicuspid aortic valve with dilated ascending aorta. Am J Cardiol 2008;102: 107–10.

Editorial Comment: Should Aortas in Patients with Bicuspid Aortic Valve Really Be Resected at an Earlier Stage Than Those in Patients with Tricuspid Valve?

John A. Elefteriades, MD

In their article in this issue of *Cardiology Clinics*, Dr Oz M. Shapira and colleagues do a masterful job at guiding us through the epidemiologic, genetic, molecular, and clinical aberrations consequent on having a bicuspid aortic valve (**Table 1**). They make a strong case that the entire segment from aortic valve and annulus to ligamentum arteriosum is inherently abnormal in bicuspid

Table 1
Should aortas in patients with bicuspid aortic valve be resected at an earlier stage than those in patients with tricuspid valve?

Pro (Shapira)	Con (Coady)
Bicuspid valve disease encompasses all tissues from aortic valve to ligamentum arteriosum (including ascending aorta): • Common embryologic origin from neural crest • Genetic basis • Aorta continues to grow even after AVR	No clear genetic substrate yet established for bicuspid aortic valve and aortopathy
Complex pathophysiology in aortic wall	No clear pathophysiologic pathway yet established for bicuspid aortopathy
Abnormal mechanical properties in aortic wall	Study by LaCanna found no increased growth rate or complication rate compared to trileaflet valves
Excess hemodynamic stress in aortic wall (due to turbulence across valve)	Yale study found similar rates of rupture, dissection, and death compared to trileaflet valves (and better long-term survival)
Bicuspid aortas grow more quickly	Aortic dissection is actually rare in bicuspid patients, according to several studies
Dissections tend to occur early in life	ACC/AHA recommendations for early intervention are based only on class C evidence
Elective aortic resection is safe, in contrast to emergent resection during acute dissection	Aortic dissection is unlikely in patients with moderately dilated aortas at the time of AVR

Abbreviations: ACC, American College of Cardiology; AHA, American Heart Association; AVR, aortic valve replacement.

Section of Cardiac Surgery, Department of Surgery, Yale University School of Medicine, Yale-New Haven Hospital, PO Box 208039, New Haven, CT 06520-8039, USA
E-mail address: john.elefteriades@yale.edu

Cardiol Clin 28 (2010) 315–316
doi:10.1016/j.ccl.2010.02.020

aortic valve disease. They take a leap of faith, however, in making their specific recommendations. There is no proved scientific basis for applying the earlier criteria that they enumerate at the end of their installment. The editor agrees fully, however, with those criteria as enumerated, sharing the clinical judgment of the authors.

The article by Dr Michael A. Coady and colleagues deftly pinpoints the weaknesses in the arguments for early intervention. They emphasize areas where supporting data are sparse or inconsistent.

It is very hard to make a decision on this controversy (**Fig. 1**). The editor tends to agree clinically with the early interventionists, all the while recognizing the paucity and variability of supporting data.

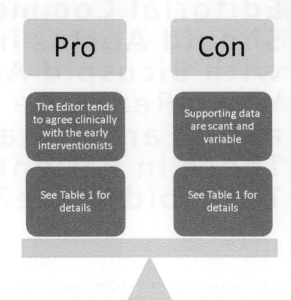

Fig. 1. The weight of evidence is not clearly on either side in this controversy.

Acute Type A Aortic Dissection: Surgical Intervention for All: PRO

Anthony L. Estrera, MD*, Hazim J. Safi, MD

KEYWORDS

- Type A aortic dissection • Aortic surgery
- Tamponade • Malperfusion

Acute aortic dissection remains the most common of all aortic catastrophes and is associated with significant morbidity and mortality. The mortality for acute type A aortic dissection has been suggested to be 1% per hour in the first 48 hours, but in reality, as reported by Hirst, was 21% at 1 day, 37% at 2 days, 62% at 1 week, 74% at 2 weeks, and 93% at 1 year.[1] Without surgical intervention, early death occurs as a result of malperfusion syndromes (cerebrovascular, visceral, renal, or peripheral ischemia), cardiac complications (acute aortic insufficiency, coronary ischemia, cardiac tamponade), or free rupture.

Thus for most patients, expeditious surgical intervention for this devastating condition should be undertaken.[2,3] Certain conditions or situations such as acute stroke, previous cardiac surgery (PCS), and older age have been associated with poor outcomes and have led some to recommend nonoperative or medical management for acute type A aortic dissection. Every patient should be individualized, and there are certain cases such as neurologic devastation that should not undergo surgical intervention, but in general, most patients with acute type A aortic dissection should undergo expeditious repair. The authors describe a relatively uniform approach to acute type A aortic dissection and provide recommendations and details on how they deal with these less-favorable situations.

INITIAL PRESENTATION

Because most patients with acute aortic dissection (either type A or type B) initially present with hypertension, the immediate aim is to control blood pressure, alleviate pain, and halt the progression of dissection. Less frequent (<10%) are those that present with refractory hypotension; these patients should be considered for emergent transfer to the operating room even if the diagnosis has not been confirmed. In these cases, the use of transesophageal echocardiography becomes pivotal in differentiating proximal aortic involvement (type A) from distal aortic involvement (type B). But for most, admission to the cardiovascular intensive care unit (CVICU) for administration of anti-impulse therapy can be undertaken. Even if urgent surgery is decided on, transfer to CVICU is still performed because monitoring and administration of antihypertensive agents can be performed more expeditiously in an intensive care setting than in the emergency center.

Rupture remains the primary concern at initial presentation with acute type A aortic dissection, but, interestingly, few data exist regarding the effect of adequate anti-impulse therapy (mean arterial pressure <80 mm Hg, heart rate <60) on the risk of rupture in this setting. Although rare, cases of early rupture and death have occurred in the authors' experience only when anti-impulse

Department of Cardiothoracic and Vascular Surgery, University of Texas Medical School, Memorial Hermann Heart and Vascular Institute, 6400 Fannin Street Suite 2850, Houston, TX 77030, USA
* Corresponding author.
E-mail address: Anthony.l.estrera@uth.tmc.edu

Cardiol Clin 28 (2010) 317–323
doi:10.1016/j.ccl.2010.01.012
0733-8651/10/$ – see front matter © 2010 Elsevier Inc. All rights reserved.

therapy could not achieve the optimal hemodynamics. Thus, for the framework of the following discussion, when surgical intervention is discussed, it is assumed that optimal medical management (adequate anti-impulse therapy) has already been applied. The authors believe that medical management should be applied to all patients regardless of comorbidities; persons not candidates for surgical repair (very rare) are thus considered nonoperative.

SURGICAL APPROACH

In principle, like others, the authors[4] prefer a simplistic approach to repair that addresses the primary problems: prevention of rupture/tamponade with replacement of the ascending aorta, correction of aortic valvular insufficiency with resuspension and aortic root reconstruction, and avoidance of further malperfusion with excision of the tear and obliteration of the false lumen if possible. At present, it is rare that the aortic valve (<5%), aortic root (<5%), or transverse aortic arch (<5%) is replaced.

In patients managed surgically, repair is via a median sternotomy, using full heparinization, cardiopulmonary bypass, and profound hypothermic circulatory arrest with retrograde cerebral perfusion. Arterial cannulation is accessed most often via the femoral artery, with few occasions requiring axillary or aortic access. Open distal anastomosis is performed under circulatory arrest. The authors[4] agree that open distal reconstruction allows for complete excision of the ascending aorta and prevents anastomotic leaks. Cerebral oximetry, transcranial Doppler ultrasound, and systemic and nasopharyngeal temperatures aid in cerebral monitoring. Electroencephalograms are used to monitor cerebral function and determine the time to initiate circulatory arrest. For typical dissection, obliteration of the false channel is performed with resection of the tear if feasible. All patients are supplemented with retrograde cerebral perfusion. After completion of the distal anastomosis, antegrade systemic flow is reestablished via a commercially available side-armed branched graft. Abnormal aorta is resected to the sinotubular junction. The aortic valve is resuspended, and the aortic root is reconstructed with complete obliteration of the false lumen. This watertight root reconstruction prevents retrograde dissection, maintains valve competency, and prevents late root enlargement.[5]

CEREBRAL MALPERFUSION

Cerebral malperfusion can occur at any point in the operative period during repairs of acute type A aortic dissection, leading to neurologic complications. The incidence of stroke and temporary neurologic dysfunction can be as high as 40%, with devastating long-term consequences.[6,7]

It was previously hypothesized that identifying and correcting cerebral malperfusion would improve neurologic outcome during these repairs, and the authors demonstrated that during the course of operative repair, significant cerebral malperfusion occurred in 29% of patients.[8] Thus, the high incidence of cerebral malperfusion during repairs of acute type A aortic dissection remains a problem and may go undetected without any neurologic monitoring.

CEREBRAL MONITORING EQUALS CEREBRAL PROTECTION

The results of the study using power motion mode transcranial Doppler ultrasound (PM-TCD) to guide retrograde cerebral perfusion during repairs of the ascending and transverse aortic arch was previously reported.[9] In this study, it was identified that an "opening" retrograde cerebral perfusion (RCP) pressure was required to identify reversal of blood flow in the middle cerebral arteries. In addition, when using standard RCP flow and pressure (0.5 L/min and <25 mm Hg), reversal of middle cerebral artery (MCA) blood flow was identified in only 20% of cases, and 80% of cases required some modification of RCP flow. More recently, the use of PM-TCD during repairs of acute type A aortic dissection was examined. About 78.5% of patients required modification of RCP flow to identify reversal of MCA blood flow. In addition, the RCP pressures in this study were significantly higher than in the control group, 33.3 ± 7.1 versus 26.7 ± 10.6, $P = .008$. This higher pressure was again the opening pressure required to identify reversal of MCA blood flow (**Fig. 1**).[8]

The requirement of a higher opening pressure (as opposed to maintenance pressure) may be related to either an increase in cerebral venous resistance as a result of the conversion from antegrade to retrograde perfusion or the need to overcome competent venous valves.[10] The concept of an opening pressure has also been described for monitoring the adequacy of antegrade selective cerebral perfusion.[11] At any rate, standard RCP flows and pressures (0.5 L/min and 25 mm Hg) may not be adequate to achieve reversed cerebral perfusion during RCP.

Many controversies still remain regarding the optimal technique for cerebral protection (RCP vs selective antegrade cerebral perfusion) and the optimal cannulation approach for the

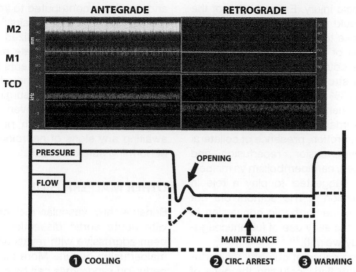

Fig. 1. Relationships of pump flow, pressure, and PMD-TCD velocity during retrograde cerebral perfusion. (1) Cooling phase: relatively constant pump flow and systemic pressure; PMD-TCD velocity may decrease. (2) Circulatory arrest phase: antegrade pump flow is discontinued; systemic pressure falls; PMD-TCD velocity disappears. RCP begins with increasing pump flow and cerebral venous pressure. Once reversed, cerebral artery flow is identified with PMD-TCD; at the corresponding opening pressure, RCP pump flow is decreased, still maintaining reversed cerebral blood flow at a maintenance pressure. (3) Warming phase: antegrade pump flow is reinitiated; systemic circulation is restarted. M1, M1 branch of the middle cerebral artery; M2, M2 branch of the middle cerebral artery.

establishment of cardiopulmonary bypass (femoral, axillary, or direct aortic) during complex aortic repairs. Regardless of the approach or technique preferred, the use of cerebral monitoring (PM-TCD, near infrared spectroscopy [NIRS], or electroencephalography [EEG]) to confirm and potentially guide cerebral perfusion during repairs of acute type A aortic dissection may improve outcomes. Therefore, cerebral monitoring equates to cerebral protection.

INDICATIONS FOR SURGICAL INTERVENTION

All patients with acute type A aortic dissection are considered for urgent surgical repair. This decision may be influenced, however, by patient-related factors and dissection-related factors. Ultimately, both factors may influence the timing of surgery.

Age

Because of poor early and late outcomes of repair for acute type A aortic dissection in octogenarians,[12] nonoperative management has been suggested for these patients. The authors have not observed worse outcomes in this patient subgroup; specifically, with the use of profound hypothermic circulatory arrest for ascending and transverse arch repair, age was not a risk factor for early mortality or stroke. Of 37 octogenarians,

13 had acute dissections. There were 2 deaths (15.5%), no acute respiratory distress syndrome, no reexploration for bleeding, no sepsis, 1 case of renal dysfunction (7.7%), and no neurologic events. The outcomes of this subgroup of octogenarians with acute type A aortic dissection did not differ significantly from those of patients younger than 80 years requiring repair.[13]

Stroke

Some have suggested that cerebral malperfusion, causing infarction or stroke, may contraindicate immediate repair.[14,15] Because surgical repair requires cardiopulmonary bypass and full anticoagulation with concurrent profound hypothermic circulatory arrest, there exists the threat of hemorrhagic conversion of the ischemic infarction as well as cerebral reperfusion leading to worsening of neurologic outcome. The urgency for repair in this setting is tempered by the concern that immediate cerebral reperfusion may worsen neurologic outcomes.

Based on earlier reports,[16] our previous management strategy for acute type A aortic dissection complicated by stroke was delayed surgical repair of the ascending aortic dissection, awaiting neurologic stabilization. The concern arose from the fear that surgical repair, which required systemic anticoagulation for cardiopulmonary bypass, would worsen the neurologic injury. Exacerbation of the neurologic injury could be caused by conversion of the ischemic stroke to a hemorrhagic stroke or by injury as a result of cerebral reperfusion. The incidence of spontaneous hemorrhagic conversion in all patients with stroke has been reported to range from 15% to 43%.[17]

The reason for hemorrhagic conversion of ischemic strokes remains multifactorial. Size of the initial cerebral infarction, presence of collateral flow, degree of hypertension, reperfusion, and cause of infarction (eg, cardioembolism vs malperfusion) have been suggested to play a role in hemorrhagic conversion.[17] The authors did not observe any case of hemorrhagic conversion in their series despite the early use of full anticoagulation (3 mg/kg body weight).[18]

The most common cause of cerebral malperfusion is the dissecting flap occluding the ostia of the great vessels. In several cases, this condition was directly visualized during operative repair. In addition, malperfusion was the probable cause of ischemia because right-hemispheric cerebrovascular events were observed in the majority of cases (81%).[18] This malperfusion was likely the result of the false lumen occluding the true lumen of the innominate artery. For this reason, prompt aortic intervention may lead to correction of cerebral malperfusion, lessening the degree of neurologic injury.[19]

Based on experience, the authors have adopted the policy of performing immediate surgical repair of acute type A aortic dissection in the setting of stroke without neurologic devastation (Glasgow Coma Scale >5). No worsening of neurologic injury from either hemorrhagic transformation or reperfusion injury was observed, and a significant improvement in neurologic outcomes was noted. Extent of recovery depended on the time to reperfusion, with patients who underwent earlier surgical repair exhibiting a higher degree of improved neurologic function. This observation was likely biased, however, because those patients who were operated on after 10 hours (4 patients transferred from outside facilities waited 3, 4, and 10 hours and 10 days for surgery) may have been beyond the window for improvement. Regardless, none of the patients' neurologic injuries was exacerbated by surgical repair with profound hypothermic circulatory arrest and full anticoagulation in this study, which may have been related to the surgical approach.[18] A multimodal approach to cerebral monitoring is used (eg, EEG, NIRS, PM-TCD), and cannulation is varied as guided by the cerebral monitoring. Pharmacologic adjuncts (aprotinin), temperature management, and pH management were all used

and may have contributed to improved neurologic recovery during these repairs.[8]

It should be emphasized that the current strategy involves immediate repair of acute type A aortic dissection in patients without neurologic devastation or coma. Although some have suggested that immediate surgical repair can be performed in patients even with coma,[20] we continue to manage such patients expectantly, awaiting any signs of neurologic recovery before performing surgical repair.

OTHER MALPERFUSION

Because any vascular malperfusion may occur with acute aortic dissection, the authors have been aggressive with revascularization when any malperfusion occurs. More than 80% of the malperfusion syndromes can be corrected with repair of the primary proximal dissection, that is, obliterate the false channel, resect the tear, and reconstruct the proximal aorta. Peripheral malperfusion occurs in 18% of the cases of acute type A aortic dissection, but after primary repair, only 4% required a subsequent peripheral revascularization (Estrera and Safi, unpublished data, 2010). Thus, the authors proceed with emergent surgery in the setting of peripheral malperfusion. Visceral and renal malperfusion will require emergent repair to prevent worsening of ischemia. After repair of the ascending aorta, the abdomen may be explored for ischemic gut if persistent uncorrectable acidosis persists. Spinal cord ischemia would also require immediate surgery, but if spontaneous recovery does not occur early during recovery then neurologic recovery is unlikely.

PREVIOUS CARDIAC SURGERY

Complicating acute type A aortic dissection is a history of PCS. Extensive adhesions, manipulating patent bypass grafts, and managing previously inserted valve prostheses are challenges encountered during these repairs and may contribute to higher mortality and morbidity.

Adhesions from PCS have been proposed to prevent rupture and tamponade, thus decreasing the mortality of acute type A aortic dissection.[21,22] Early death often occurs as a result of rupture into the pericardial space leading to tamponade. PCS and the associated adhesions may reduce the risk of tamponade and hemodynamic instability,[21] suggesting that purposeful delay should be undertaken to obtain the required coronary angiography to assess the patency of the previous grafts (in the case of prior coronary artery bypass grafting).[21] Previous aortic valve surgery may also reduce the risk of tamponade with acute type A aortic dissections.[23] The lower risks of rupture and tamponade are proposed as reasons why mortality from acute type A aortic dissection after PCS was no worse than for repair of the primary condition.[21,24]

In contrast, there was a significantly higher mortality (31% vs 16%) in patients with PCS.[25] This is corroborated in other series with mortality rates ranging from 30% to 66%.[24,26,27] Tamponade or hypotension occurred as frequently in the PCS group as the primary group. In the setting with no PCS, pericardial tamponade can develop quickly after rupture when no adhesions are present, but in the setting of extensive adhesions, the rupture may be problematic although contained by the adhesions. Mediastinal hematoma may compress mediastinal structures, most often the low-pressure, right-sided chambers of the heart. In addition, rupture directly into the pulmonary artery leading to aortopulmonary artery fistulas may also occur. This complication was associated with a mortality of 100% (2 of 2).[25]

But these events did not explain the higher mortality in patients with PCS. Differences in the cohorts (older patients, more extensive procedures, more transfusions) likely explained the higher mortality.

From the authors' perspective, mortality from acute type A aortic dissection after PCS appears to be related to expected events that occur with the dissection and is also the result of performing very complex procedures on older, more disabled patients. For this reason, urgent surgical intervention for acute type A aortic dissection after PCS is recommended, because the natural history, even in the setting of PCS, remains dismal, with an early mortality of 50% if left untreated.[24]

TYPE A INTRAMURAL HEMATOMA

Much controversy exists regarding the management of acute type A intramural hematoma (IMH). Robbins and colleagues[21] first reported an experience of 13 patients with acute aortic IMH, of which 3 patients had IMH involving the ascending and transverse arch. In this series, those with ascending IMH had an associated mortality of 66%, leading the investigators to recommend early graft replacement for these patients. Several ensuing studies of Asian cohorts with type A IMH, however, reported low early mortality with medical management alone, ranging from 0% to 8%.[15,22,28,29] Complete absorption of the IMH in as high as 67% of patients has been reported,[22] with 5-year survival as high as 80% to 85%.[15,22,28] In contrast, medical management

led to poor early outcomes, with mortalities ranging from 33% to 80%, leading to the recommendation of early surgical repair.[14,21,26,30] In an attempt to determine the optimal management for type A IMH, a meta-analysis of 12 studies involving 328 patients (9 of which were Asian cohorts) was performed.[31] This analysis ultimately reported no significant difference in early mortality between those who were medically managed (10.1% in 168 patients) and those who had surgical repair (14.4% in 160 patients), $P = .36$. In their conclusion, the investigators recommended individualization of treatment, noting that patients with progression of size, enlarged initial aortic diameter, and subadventitial wall thickness greater than 12 mm were candidates for early surgery.[31] Despite all available data regarding type A IMH, a general consensus on treatment has not been achieved.

Influenced by early studies that reported high mortality with medical management of type A IMH and acknowledged the potential for reabsorption of the hematoma in some cases, the authors adopted a strategy of initial optimal medical management with eventual or purposefully delayed surgery. Patients who underwent immediate repair were those in extremis and who clinically demonstrated progression of disease, such as conversion to typical dissection leading to malperfusion. Patients who were clinically stable, however, were admitted to the intensive care unit and initiated on anti-impulse therapy to control blood pressure and pain and were scheduled for eventual repair. In most cases, after 2 to 3 days of medical management, surgical repair was performed. In these cases, examination of the aorta revealed clot and organizing thrombus that was completely evacuated, leaving a thickened adventitial aortic wall for repair. An advantage of purposeful delay was the observation that after even a few days, the aortic wall was thicker, allowing for easier reconstruction and ultimately a more expeditious repair. Although not significant, there were no reoperations for bleeding in the type A IMH group. Another possible advantage of purposeful delay for acute type A IMH involves the avoidance of the extensive systemic inflammatory response encountered during emergent surgery. This, however, is not supported by the study and remains only hypothetical.[32]

Results of this study are comparable to the findings of other studies that compared typical type A aortic dissection with IMH. Patients with type A IMH tended to be older (63 years vs 58 years, $P = .06$) and presented with more chest pain (100% vs 88%, $P = .04$) and less frequently with hypotension (8% vs 22%, P = .07), tamponade (6% vs 16%, P = .16), and moderate or greater aortic insufficiency (11% vs 38%, P = .002). The decreased incidence of malperfusion and tamponade with IMH as compared with typical dissection is not surprising because thrombosis of the false channel should decrease the risk of these events. Conversion to typical dissection was observed in 33% (12 of 36) of cases in this study, similar to previous studies reporting conversion in up to 40% of cases. Although not demonstrated in this study, previously reported risk factors for conversion have included an initial aortic diameter greater than 5.0 cm and an adventitial thickness greater than 12 mm.[22,26,31]

Despite increasing experience with IMH, much still remains unknown. The influence of ethnicity on IMH and its management is interesting but unclear. Many studies on type A IMH have involved primarily Asian cohorts, with a majority of these series reporting good results with medical management alone. Why Asian cohorts may fare better with medical management remains unclear. It should be noted that the Asian cohort used serial scans to identify complications, which then determined the timing of operative intervention. Although the authors' cohort had a variety of ethnicities, interestingly, the single patient who was managed medically was Japanese, who refused aortic replacement and whose aorta measured 4.9 cm.

In analyzing these data before establishing a consistent strategy for the management of acute type A IMH, repair was delayed in several patients for various reasons, including poor medical status or unknown neurologic status. As such, this provided an opportunity to analyze the risk for conversion to typical aortic dissection because almost all patients eventually underwent repair and a thorough examination of the aorta could be performed. This analysis resulted in the hazard plot, which provided the instantaneous risk for conversion to typical dissection at any given time during the patient's clinical course. From this plot, it was observed that no patients converted within 3 days of symptoms when surgery was purposefully delayed, but an increasing risk of conversion up to and beyond 8 days was noted (**Fig. 2**). This strategy, however, assumed that optimal medical management was maintained. These data suggest that a significant risk of conversion to typical dissection ultimately existed in the patient population and that repair should be performed eventually. Implications of these data suggest that patients managed medically need close follow-up for at least 2 weeks and a regimen of routine long-term radiographic surveillance.

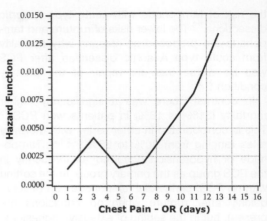

Fig. 2. Hazard plot depicting the instantaneous risk for conversion to typical dissection as a function of time (days) from the onset of symptoms.

SUMMARY

Urgent surgical intervention should be considered in all patients with acute type A aortic dissection. Immediate repair is performed for those who are hypotensive due to rupture and tamponade and who exhibit malperfusion of the coronary, cerebrovascular, visceral, or peripheral arterial systems. Selective delayed management with eventual repair may be assumed in patients with type A IMH and in those with coma (potential neurologic devastation), assuming that neurologic status improves. Urgent repair should not be precluded in patients presenting with active stroke, older age, and PCS. Ultimately, each patient should be individualized and the decision to intervene left to the surgeon.

ACKNOWLEDGMENTS

The authors acknowledge G. Ken Goodrick for editing and Chris Akers for the figures.

REFERENCES

1. Hirst AE Jr, Johns VJ Jr, Kime SW Jr. Dissecting aneurysm of the aorta: a review of 505 cases. Medicine 1958;37:217–79.
2. Crawford ES. The diagnosis and management of aortic dissection. JAMA 1990;264:2537–41.
3. Estrera AL, Huynh TT, Porat EE, et al. Is acute type A aortic dissection a true surgical emergency? Semin Vasc Surg 2002;15:75–82.
4. Elefteriades JA. What operation for acute type A dissection? J Thorac Cardiovasc Surg 2002;123: 201–3.
5. Estrera AL, Safi HJ. Repair of the transverse arch using retrograde cerebral perfusion during repair of

acute Type A aortic dissection. Operat Tech Thorac Cardiovasc Surg 2005;10:3–22.

6. Hagan PG, Nienaber CA, Isselbacher EM, et al. The International Registry of Acute Aortic Dissection (IRAD): new insights into an old disease. JAMA 2000;16(283):897–903.

7. Mehta RH, Suzuki T, Hagan PG, et al. Predicting death in patients with acute type a aortic dissection. Circulation 2002;105:200–6.

8. Estrera AL, Garami Z, Miller CC 3rd, et al. Cerebral monitoring with transcranial Doppler ultrasonography improves neurologic outcome during repairs of acute type A aortic dissection. J Thorac Cardiovasc Surg 2005;129:277–85.

9. Estrera AL, Garami Z, Miller CC 3rd, et al. Determination of cerebral blood flow dynamics during retrograde cerebral perfusion using power M-mode transcranial Doppler. Ann Thorac Surg 2003;76:704–9.

10. Okamoto H, Sato K, Matsuura A, et al. Selective jugular cannulation of safer retrograde cerebral perfusion. Ann Thorac Surg 1993;55:538–40.

11. De Vries AJ. Transcranial Doppler technique for monitoring the efficacy of selective antegrade cerebral perfusion. Anesth Analg 1999;89:1587–8.

12. Neri E, Toscano T, Massetti M, et al. Operation for acute type A aortic dissection in octogenarians: is it justified? J Thorac Cardiovasc Surg 2001;121:259–67.

13. Shah PJ, Estrera AL, Miller CC 3rd, et al. Analysis of ascending and transverse aortic arch repair in octogenarians. Ann Thorac Surg 2008;86:774–9.

14. Evangelista A, Mukherjee D, Mehta RH, et al. Acute intramural hematoma of the aorta: a mystery in evolution. Circulation 2005;111:1063–70.

15. Moizumi Y, Komatsu T, Motoyoshi N, et al. Clinical features and long-term outcome of type A and type B intramural hematoma of the aorta. J Thorac Cardiovasc Surg 2004;127:421–7.

16. Cambria RP, Brewster DC, Gertler J, et al. Vascular complications associated with spontaneous aortic dissection. J Vasc Surg 1988;7:199–209.

17. Lyden PD, Zivin JA. Hemorrhagic transformation after cerebral ischemia: mechanisms and incidence. Cerebrovasc Brain Metab Rev 1993;5:1–16.

18. Estrera AL, Garami Z, Miller CC, et al. Acute Type A aortic dissection complicated by stroke: can immediate repair be performed safely? J Thorac Cardiovasc Surg 2006;132(6):1404–8.

19. Uchino K, Estrera A, Calleja S, et al. Aortic dissection presenting as an acute ischemic stroke for thrombolysis. J Neuroimaging 2005;15:281–3.

20. Pocar M, Passolunghi D, Moneta A, et al. Coma might not preclude emergency operation in acute aortic dissection. Ann Thorac Surg 2006;81:1348–51.

21. Robbins RC, McManus RP, Mitchell RS, et al. Management of patients with intramural hematoma of the thoracic aorta. Circulation 1993;88:II1–10.

22. Song JM, Kim HS, Song JK, et al. Usefulness of the initial noninvasive imaging study to predict the adverse outcomes in the medical treatment of acute type A aortic intramural hematoma. Circulation 2003;108:II324–8.

23. Feldman M, Shah M, Elefteriades JA. Medical management of acute type A aortic dissection. Ann Thorac Cardiovasc Surg 2009;15:286–93.

24. Ehrlich MP, Ergin MA, McCullough JN, et al. Results of immediate surgical treatment of all acute type A dissections. Circulation 2000;102:III248–52.

25. Estrera A, Miller CC III, Kaneko T, et al. Outcomes of acute type A aortic dissection after previous cardiac surgery. Ann Thorac Surg, in press.

26. von Kodolitsch Y, Csosz SK, Koschyk DH, et al. Intramural hematoma of the aorta: predictors of progression to dissection and rupture. Circulation 2003;107:1158–63.

27. Kaji S, Nishigami K, Akasaka T, et al. Prediction of progression or regression of type A aortic intramural hematoma by computed tomography. Circulation 1999;100:II281–6.

28. Kaji S, Akasaka T, Horibata Y, et al. Long-term prognosis of patients with type A aortic intramural hematoma. Circulation 2002;106:I248–52.

29. Moriyama Y, Yotsumoto G, Kuriwaki K, et al. Intramural hematoma of the thoracic aorta. Eur J Cardiothorac Surg 1998;13:230–9.

30. Nienaber CA, von Kodolitsch Y, Petersen B, et al. Intramural hemorrhage of the thoracic aorta. Diagnostic and therapeutic implications. Circulation 1995;92:1465–72.

31. Kan CB, Chang RY, Chang JP. Optimal initial treatment and clinical outcome of type A aortic intramural hematoma: a clinical review. Eur J Cardiothorac Surg 2008;33:1002–6.

32. Estrera AL, Miller C 3rd, Lee TY, et al. Acute type A intramural hematoma: analysis of current management strategy. Circulation 2009;120(Suppl 11):S287–91.

Acute Type A Aortic Dissection: Surgical Intervention for All: CON

John A. Elefteriades, MD*, Marina Feldman, MD

KEYWORDS

- Type A aortic dissection • Medical management
- Surgical therapy • Dissection surgery

The time-honored dictum is that type A aortic dissection requires urgent surgery. Is medical management of aortic dissection ever more appropriate?

Certainly, medical management is part of the initial stabilization of any patient with type A dissection, during clinical and radiographic evaluation, and en route to the operating room.

There are, however, situations in which the patient's appropriate treatment continues with medical management rather than surgical therapy. This article explores those situations. Specifically considered is medical management as sole or interval therapy for the patients with the following conditions:

- completed stroke
- serious comorbid conditions (eg, cancer, advanced multiple organ dysfunction, extremely advanced age)
- prior aortic valve replacement
- presentation to the hospital beyond 48 to 72 hours of onset of aortic dissection.

STROKE IN THE SETTING OF ACUTE TYPE A AORTIC DISSECTION

Introduction of stroke into an already complicated picture of acute type A dissection results in a lower short- or long-term survival rate. Reestablishment of blood flow into the infarcted area of the brain and administration of high-dose heparin for extracorporeal circulation may induce hemorrhagic infarcts and result in intractable brain edema.[1]

Many experienced cardiac surgeons have had the misfortune of performing an impeccable aortic procedure in this setting, only to see a brain-dead patient with massive intracranial hemorrhage suffer brainstem herniation from severe mass effect upon returning to the ICU. Piccione and colleagues[2] have reported on the usefulness of intentionally delaying surgery in a patient with Marfan syndrome. Deeb and colleagues[3] reported good results with a combination of early percutaneous reperfusion and delay of surgery until reperfusion injury is resolved. Intentional delay of surgery and observation under intensive medical treatment is useful for patients who have acute type A aortic dissection with cerebral infarction (**Fig. 1**).[4]

Stroke in patients with acute type A aortic dissection should constitute only a relative contraindication to operation at most, as full neurologic recovery and acceptable outcomes are possible in some cases in which prompt surgery is performed.[5] Coma may not represent an absolute contraindication for resuscitative surgery with modern techniques in hemodynamically stable patients with acute type A aortic dissection, provided that surgery is performed expeditiously after the onset of brain malperfusion.[6] Surgical repair of acute type A aortic dissection with acceptable mortality in the setting of acute stroke was demonstrated in one recent study, without worsening of neurologic condition after surgical repair.[7]

Although additional clinical studies are needed to draw definitive conclusions, the authors believe

Section of Cardiac Surgery, Department of Surgery, Yale University School of Medicine, Yale-New Haven Hospital, PO Box 208039, New Haven, CT 06520-8039, USA
* Corresponding author.
E-mail address: john.elefteriades@yale.edu

Cardiol Clin 28 (2010) 325–331
doi:10.1016/j.ccl.2010.02.010
0733-8651/10/$ – see front matter © 2010 Elsevier Inc. All rights reserved.

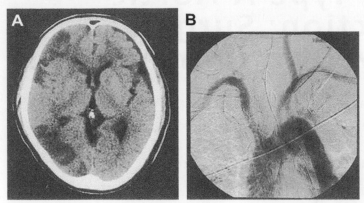

Fig. 1. (*A*) Brain CT scan demonstrating multiple low-density infarctions in the right hemisphere, with moderate cerebral edema. (*B*) Arch angiogram of the same patient, demonstrating impaired flow through the right carotid artery as a result of the dissection process. It was thought that immediate surgical intervention was not appropriate in the acute phase of the dissection. Interval medical management was undertaken, with eventual aortic replacement 3 months after initial presentation. (*From* Fukuda I, Imazuru T. Intentional delay of surgery for acute type A dissection with stroke. J Thorac Cardiovasc Surg 2003;126(1):290–1; with permission.)

that if a patient with acute type A aortic dissection presents with stroke that is in progress (the stroke is evolving), immediate surgical repair produces suitable results. On the other hand, in a completed stroke, acute type A aortic dissection is usually best managed medically, owing to the risk of devastating heparin-induced hemorrhagic infarcts occurring intraoperatively. If the infarct has been realized for 4 hours or more, or if a CT scan shows a sizable acute infarction, surgery should generally be avoided.

ADVANCED AGE AND COMORBIDITIES IN THE SETTING OF ACUTE TYPE A AORTIC DISSECTION

It is important to consider whether it is acceptable to operate for acute type A aortic dissection when the patient is at extreme advanced age. Similarly, it is important to consider whether is acceptable to operate emergently in patients with profound comorbidities, rather than taking time to provide medical treatment to relieve or optimize the comorbidities.

Mehta and colleagues[8] have shown that the risk of mortality from surgery for acute type A aortic dissection is 45% for patients 80 to 84 years of age, and 50% for those 85 or older. These formidable levels of operative risk beg the question of whether nonoperative management can produce similar results in patients with advanced age.

The authors have shown that, in those patients presenting 2 or 3 days from symptom onset, correcting comorbidities before surgery or avoiding surgery can result in acceptable outcomes. Patients presenting with acute type A aortic

dissection who were denied surgery because of their advanced age or comorbidities achieved a 30-day survival rate of 42%.[9]

DELAYED PRESENTATION OF ACUTE TYPE A AORTIC DISSECTION FOR 48 TO 72 HOURS

Immediate surgical therapy is still recommended for acceptable operative candidates with acute type A aortic dissection who seek immediate treatment.[10,11] However, patients with type A aortic dissection who are referred from outside facilities or whose conditions are diagnosed several days after presentation and have survived the initial perilous period, can safely undergo a semielective surgery.[9,11] Delayed repair after optimization of the clinical condition and detailed evaluation of concomitant diseases results in outstanding long-term results.[9] If such late-presenting patients are not considered operative candidates, they may be treated with aggressive anti-impulse therapy and accomplish suitable early and short-term outcomes with in-hospital mortality of 5.2%.[11] Specifically, if a patient has presented beyond 48 to 72 hours after onset of pain, we do not take him to the operating room in the middle of the night; rather, we operate at the next daytime slot, with our full, specialized team available. These "late presenters" have essentially "weathered the eye of the storm" without rupturing the aorta and, we find, they are unlikely to rupture during a short period until the next semielective daytime surgical slot. The authors specifically published this data to provide some legal support in the literature for surgeons who, appropriately, wait until morning to operate on a late-presenting aortic dissector.

PRIOR AORTIC VALVE REPLACEMENT

Currently, aortic resection is considered appropriate for patients undergoing aortic valve replacement for valvular disease who have coexisting moderate aortic enlargement. However, in the past, many patients underwent aortic valve replacement without concomitant resection of a moderately dilated ascending aorta. In a retrospective study, 18 out of 330 patients with previous aortic valve replacement had an ascending aorta with a diameter greater than 5 cm. Aortic dissection occurred in 4 (22%) of these 18 patients. Three of these 18 patients underwent elective replacement of the ascending aorta.[12] In another study, 8 out of 2202 patients who underwent aortic valve replacement were subsequently reoperated on because of ascending aortic dissection—5 with acute and 3 with chronic ascending aortic dissection.[13] In acknowledgment of this observed risk of late events, the authors recommend replacement of the ascending aorta during aortic valve replacement when its diameter is greater than 4.5 cm.[14]

Thus, patients present not infrequently with type A dissection, having had a prior aortic valve replacement. For such patients, we usually do not operate acutely; rather, we pursue medical therapy with the anti-impulse paradigm. We take this approach because we feel the prior aortic valve replacement provides substantial protection from the complications that make type A dissection lethal in other circumstances. Specifically, aortic insufficiency cannot occur as a consequence of type A dissection in the presence of a prosthetic aortic valve. Furthermore, dissection cannot cross a suture line, so the right coronary artery is protected by the suture line made previously for the aortic valve replacement. Finally, the periaortic adhesions from the prior operation are likely to discourage free rupture of the acute type A dissection (**Fig. 2**). This protection from dissection was confirmed in a study by Gillinov and colleagues.[15] Organ ischemia, of course, may still occur downstream and is not impacted by the prior aortic valve replacement.

Thus, in the authors view, type A aortic dissection in the setting of prior aortic valve replacement behaves more like type B dissection, and we treat it as such,[16–20] at least early on after dissection. Later, we undertake semielective or elective resection when the patient is more stable and the aorta is no longer acutely dissected. The Cleveland Clinic experience in patients with acute type A dissection in the face of prior cardiac surgery also generally supports a nonemergent approach to these patients (with angiography to identify coronary graft status), finding that rupture, tamponade, and hemodynamic instability occur infrequently.[15] Evidence from Europe also suggests that prior cardiac surgery is protective against rupture in acute type A aortic dissection, and that interval or sole medical therapy may be considered.[21]

PERMANENT NONOPERATIVE MANAGEMENT

It has always been maintained that, without surgical therapy, acute type A aortic dissection was nearly invariably lethal, with a stated mortality of 1 per hour, with an expected 90 day mortality of 70% to 90%.[20,21] With modern ICU care and anti-impulse therapy, it is becoming apparent that survival rates with sole medical management are greater than previously thought.

The authors studies found that, in patients with absolute contraindications to surgery, a better survival rate could be produced with medical management than anticipated from prior (often quite old) studies.[9] **Fig. 3** shows the flow patterns in three groups of patients from the authors' study: those treated with immediate surgery, those treated with delayed surgery, and those treated entirely nonoperatively. We were able to achieve a hospital survival rate of 88% in patients who underwent interval or permanent nonoperative management and 80% in patients who underwent entirely nonoperative management. **Fig. 4** indicates that the survival rate was essentially equivalent in the immediate surgery, delayed surgery, and exclusively medical groups. This data does not deter the authors' enthusiasm for urgent surgery as a general principle for acute aortic dissection. Rather, the authors only wish to indicate that, when necessary, interval or exclusive medical management can produce better results than previously expected.

In the authors' study of medical management, the patients were highly selected by having survived the early hours and days after acute dissection long enough to permit diagnosis and transfer from the presenting facility to our tertiary aortic center. Thus, the statistics in this study do not reflect the dismal outlook of primary presentation of acute type A aortic dissection, wherein many patients die in the field without ever reaching a hospital or succumb early after hospital arrival. These findings are focused on the survivors of the acute dissection and confirm the authors' observations from an earlier study.[11] In patients presenting later than 48 hours after the initial onset of pain, medical and surgical treatment modalities have no significant difference in the survival in a 10 year follow up study ($P = .10$)

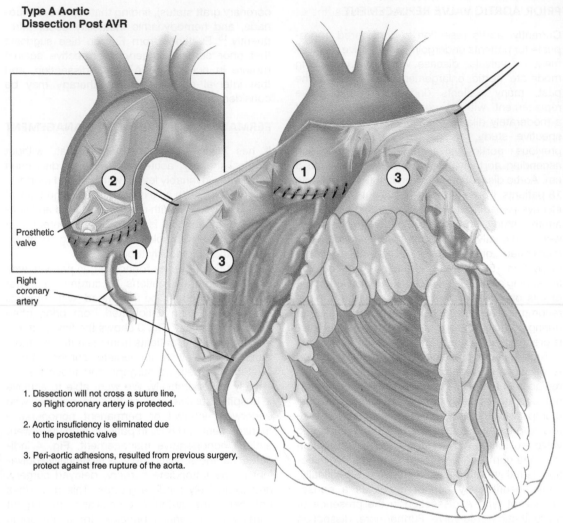

Type A Aortic
Dissection Post AVR

Prosthetic
valve

Right
coronary
artery

1. Dissection will not cross a suture line,
   so Right coronary artery is protected.

2. Aortic insuficiency is eliminated due
   to the prostethic valve

3. Peri-aortic adhesions, resulted from previous surgery,
   protect against free rupture of the aorta.

Fig. 2. Dissection cannot cross suture line, so right coronary artery protected. Aortic insufficiency is impossible with prosthetic valve; adhesions discourage free rupture into the pericardial sack. AVR, aortic valve replacement.

(see **Fig. 4**), although there is a trend toward better survival in the surgical group. These conclusions have been reached in other studies: Chan and colleagues[22] were able to achieve a survival of about 50% with medical management alone, and Masuda and colleagues[23] also reported better than expected results with medical management.

A paper from Centofanti and colleagues[24] asked an intriguing question "Is surgery always mandatory for type A aortic dissection?" The investigators found that age, coma, acute renal failure, shock, and redo operation constitute highly predictive surgical risk factors. They suggest that, when the predicted risk level exceeds 58%, surgery should be withheld, as the survival rate with medical therapy alone will be equal. They

arrive at this figure by means of the International Registry of Acute Aortic Dissection (IRAD) data, which indicate that medically treated patients can achieve a survival of 42% (ie, a mortality of 58%).[10] Thus, if predicted surgical risk exceeds this criterion, medical therapy can be considered in lieu of surgical therapy. While the Centofanti and colleagues[24] paper brings up important issues in acute type A aortic dissection, melding observations from one study to another to draw a combined statistical conclusion is fraught with difficulties. It is doubtful that the medical survivors in the IRAD study are the same patients who rate a prohibitive risk score in the Centofanti and colleagues[24] study. This recommendation remains controversial and has elicited strong contrary response.[25]

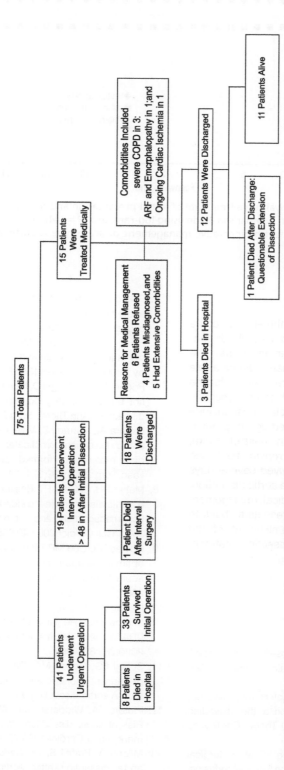

Fig. 3. Outcome of all patients treated for acute type A aortic dissection. The three main branch points represent, respectively, those patients treated with urgent surgery, patients undergoing delayed operation, and those undergoing exclusively medical management. ARF, acute renal failure; COPD, chronic obstructive pulmonary disease. (*From* Scholl FG, Coady MA, Davies R, et al. Interval or permanent nonoperative management of acute type A aortic dissection. Arch Surg 1999;134:402–6; with permission.)

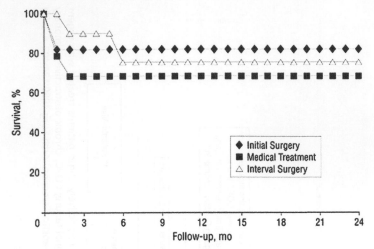

Fig. 4. Kaplan-Meier actuarial survival curve from date of initial presentation and treatment. Note that survivals over the first 2 years are equivalent. Comparison made using log-rank test ($P = .44$).[9] (*From* Scholl FG, Coady MA, Davies R, et al. Interval or permanent nonoperative management of acute type A aortic dissection. Arch Surg 1999;134:402–6; with permission.)

SUMMARY

The principles of anti-impulse therapy for acute dissection have stood the test of time. As dissection surgery has become better and better, the authors have recognized that there may be a role for interval or permanent medical therapy for the specific groups of acute type A aortic dissection patients enumerated in this article. These include patients with extremely advanced age or prohibitive comorbidities, patients with realized stroke, patients with prior aortic valve replacement, and patients who have already survived several days after onset of symptoms of acute aortic dissection. The very consideration of medical management for acute type A dissection represents a "back to the future" paradigm shift reminiscent of the earliest recommendations for dissection treatment many decades ago before surgical therapy was feasible or safe.

REFERENCES

1. Crawford ES, Svensson LG, Coselli JS, et al. Aortic dissection and dissecting aortic aneurysms. Ann Surg 1988;208:254.
2. Piccione W Jr, Hamilton IN, Najafi H. Intentional delayed repair of acute dissection of the ascending aorta complicated by stroke. J Thorac Cardiovasc Surg 1995;109:807–8.
3. Deeb GM, Williams DM, Bolling SF, et al. Surgical delay for acute type A dissection with malperfusion. Ann Thorac Surg 1997;64:1669–75.
4. Fukuda I, Imazuru T. Intentional delay of surgery for acute type A dissection with stroke. J Thorac Cardiovasc Surg 2003;126(1):290–1.
5. Fann JI, Sarris GE, Miller DC, et al. Surgical management of acute aortic dissection complicated by stroke. Circulation 1989;80(3 Suppl 1):I257–63.
6. Pocar M, Passolunghi D, Moneta A, et al. Coma might not preclude emergency operation in acute aortic dissection. Ann Thorac Surg 2006;81:1348–52.
7. Estrera AL, Garami Z, Miller CC, et al. Acute type A aortic dissection complicated by stroke: can immediate repair be performed safely? J Thorac Cardiovasc Surg 2006;132(6):1404–8.
8. Mehta RH, O'Gara PT, Bossone E, et al. Acute type A aortic dissection in the elderly: clinical characteristics, management, and outcomes in the current era. J Am Coll Cardiol 2002;40:685–92.
9. Davies RR, Coe MP, Mandapati D, et al. What is the optimal management of late-presenting survivors of acute type A aortic dissection? Ann Thorac Surg 2007;83:1593–602.
10. Hagan PG, Nienaber CA, Isselbacher EM, et al. The International Registry of Acute Aortic Dissection (IRAD): new insights into an old disease. JAMA 2000;283:897–903.
11. Scholl FG, Coady MA, Davies R, et al. Interval or permanent nonoperative management of acute type A aortic dissection. Arch Surg 1999;134:402–6.
12. Pieters FA, Widdershoven JW, Gerardy AC, et al. Risk of aortic dissection after aortic valve replacement. Am J Cardiol 1993;72:1043–7.
13. Milano A, Pratali S, De Carlo M, et al. Ascending aorta dissection after aortic valve replacement. J Heart Valve Dis 1998;70(1):75–80.

14. Friedman T, Mani A, Elefteriades J. Bicuspid aortic valve: clinical approach and scientific review of a common clinical entity. Expert Rev Cardiovasc Ther 2008;6(2):235–48.

15. Gillinov AM, Lytle BW, Kaplon RJ, et al. Dissection of the ascending aorta after previous cardiac surgery: differences in presentation and management. J Thorac Cardiovasc Surg 1999;117:252–60.

16. Estrera AL, Miller CC 3rd, Safi HJ, et al. Outcomes of medical management of acute type B aortic dissection. Circulation 2006;114(Suppl I):384–9.

17. Dalen JE, Alpert JS, Cohn LH, et al. Dissection of the thoracic aorta: medical or surgical? Am J Cardiol 1974;34:803–8.

18. Elefteriades JA, Hartleroad J, Gusbert RJ, et al. Long-term experience with descending aortic dissection: the complication-specific approach. Ann Thorac Surg 1992;53:11–20.

19. Elefteriades JA, Lovoulos C, Coady MA, et al. Management of descending aortic dissection. Ann Thorac Surg 1999;67:2002–5.

20. Green GR, Kron IL, Edmunds LH Jr. Cardiac surgery in the adult. New York: McGraw-Hill; 2003.

21. Myrmel T, Lai DTM, Miller DG. Can the principles of evidence-based medicine be applied to the treatment of aortic dissections? Eur J Cardiothorac Surg 2004;25:236–42.

22. Chan SH, Liu PY, Lin LJ, et al. Predictors of in-hospital mortality in patients with acute aortic dissection. J Cardiol 2005;105:267–73.

23. Masuda Y, Yamada Z, Morooka N, et al. Prognosis of patients with medically treated aortic dissections. Circulation 1991;84(Suppl 5): III7–III13.

24. Centofanti P, Flocco R, Ceresa F, et al. Is surgery always mandatory for type A aortic dissection. Ann Thorac Surg 2006;82:1658–64.

25. Khaladj N, Haverich A, Hagl C. Should a patient with acute aortic dissection type A go to the intensive care unit or operating room? Ann Thorac Surg 2007;84:1069.

Editorial Comment: Acute Type A Aortic Dissection: Surgical Intervention for All

John A. Elefteriades, MD

There is no clear winner here (**Fig. 1**). Both essayists leave room for exceptions in their policies (**Table 1**), and both argue for individualized decisions. Both advocate a very aggressive overall surgical approach for acute type A aortic dissection.

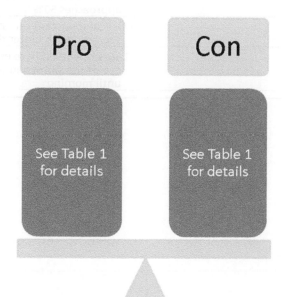

Fig. 1. There is no clear winner in this debate.

Section of Cardiac Surgery, Department of Surgery, Yale University School of Medicine, Yale-New Haven Hospital, PO Box 208039, New Haven, CT 06520-8039, USA
E-mail address: john.elefteriades@yale.edu

Cardiol Clin 28 (2010) 333–334
doi:10.1016/j.ccl.2010.02.014
0733-8651/10/$ – see front matter © 2010 Elsevier Inc. All rights reserved.

Table 1
Acute type A aortic dissection: surgical intervention for all

Pro: Surgical Intervention for All (Estrera)	Con: Consider Medical Treatment (Elefteriades)
Their policy is for routine surgical treatment for nearly all (except devastating cerebrovascular accident—Glasgow Coma Scale score >5), and they report good results even in face of • Age >80 • Stroke (no hemorrhagic conversion in their series) • Malperfusion phenomena • Prior cardiac surgery • Type A intramural hematoma	Consider medical treatment for • Completed acute stroke • Extreme age (or comorbidities) • Late presentation (>72 h) • Prior aortic valve replacement
	Stroke can undergo edema or hemorrhage after repair
	In extreme advanced age, surgical risk approaches 50%
	Medical treatment can attain 42% 30-day survival, much better than decades ago
	"Late presenters" have essentially weathered the eye of the storm and can be treated medically until morning

Extended Arch Resection in Acute Type A Aortic Dissection: PRO

Paul P. Urbanski, MD, PhD[a],*, Aristidis Lenos, MD[a],
Rainer Schmitt, MD, PhD[b], Anno Diegeler, MD, PhD[a]

KEYWORDS
- Aortic dissection • Dissection types
- Aortic arch • Aortic surgery

The number of supporters of complete arch replacement in the surgery of acute type A aortic dissection has been steadily increasing, which apparently is the result of cerebral perfusion techniques that enable the extension of safe circulatory arrest time. However, there is no agreement in the surgical community on an optimal surgical approach, especially the distal extension of aortic repair. Standardizing the surgical method or even proving the superiority of one technique over another in the therapy for acute type A aortic dissection cannot be expected for several reasons. Most importantly, patients with acute aortic dissection present different aortic and vascular pathologies, and different symptoms, from an isolated pain even to severe malperfusion. Therefore, patient randomization is not possible. Second, evidence-based analysis is also difficult because the patient population differs considerably in presented reports with respect to patient selection, surgical methods, surgical experience, and consequently surgical results. For a meta-analysis, dividing the patients into various subgroups according to the extent of dissection would be necessary. Until now, such classifications have not taken hold, although many investigators have recommended them. For these reasons, we (the authors of this article) intend to not search for evidence in the literature but report our experiences during our uniform procedures in diagnostics and surgical strategy.

DIAGNOSTICS

Surgeons' opinions on the necessity of computed tomography (CT) angiography vary extensively, and many think that emergent surgery is absolutely indicated immediately after an echocardiographic diagnosis of acute aortic dissection. In our opinion, the CT angiography is of utmost importance because it delivers crucial information about the extent of the dissection not only in the aorta but also in its branches.

The scope of the dissection can significantly influence the surgical strategy and extent of the aortic resection. The subclassification that we proposed for aortic type A dissection considers the distal extent of dissection (D: extent of dissection) and the location of the intimal tear (E: entry localization) in the 3 main segments of the aorta (a: ascending aorta, b: aortic arch, c: descending aorta).[1] Thus, there are 3 subgroups of type A dissection that are relevant from a surgical perspective. In the first group (D-a; E-a), which corresponds to the DeBakey type II classification, the dissection is limited exclusively to the ascending aorta. For the last 15 years, the prevalence of this dissection type has constantly been

[a] Department of Cardiovascular Surgery, Cardiovascular Clinic, Herz- und Gefaess-Klinik, Salzburger Leite 1, 97616 Bad Neustadt, Germany
[b] Department of Radiology, Cardiovascular Clinic, Herz- und Gefaess-Klinik, Salzburger Leite 1, 97616 Bad Neustadt, Germany
* Corresponding author.
E-mail address: p.urbanski@herzchirurgie.de

Cardiol Clin 28 (2010) 335–342
doi:10.1016/j.ccl.2010.01.007

about 25% of all acute type A dissections. In these patients, aortic arch replacement is not necessary unless there is another indication; for example, chronic aneurysm or severe atherosclerotic ulceration of the aortic arch.

A further 25% of the patients present with aortic dissection (D-ab, mostly combined with E-a) that extends from the ascending aorta through the arch, reaching approximately to the level of aortic isthmus (**Fig. 1**). In these cases, we see a clear indication for an arch replacement regardless of the entry site. In this way, a complete resection of all dissected aortic wall can be achieved (see **Fig. 1**). On the other hand, an incomplete replacement of the aortic arch is associated with leaving some parts of the dissected aortic wall, which can lead to the nolate complications (**Fig. 2**).

The information about the dissection of the arch arteries can likewise be of vital importance for selecting the operative strategy; for example, the choice of arterial cannulation and the extent of the reconstruction of the aortic arch.[2] Since 2002, if CT angiography has not already been done before admission to our clinic, we have conducted this test for every patient suspected of having an acute aortic dissection and have obtained images of the aortic arch branches, including those in the middle neck area. This examination takes only a few minutes and can be conducted on the way to the operating theater. Moreover, it provides volumetric datasets enabling 2- and 3-dimensional reconstructions of the thoracic aorta and its branches in precise, anatomic views. Of the 90 patients with acute aortic dissection who were admitted to our clinic between 2002 and 2009, 36 patients were referred without CT angiography, and we performed this examination before surgery. We even repeated the angiography on 2 additional patients because

information that was essential from a surgical standpoint was missing. None of the patients under our care died during the preoperative diagnostics. The CT angiography significantly influenced the operative strategy in many cases and contributed to the survival of all these patients, the 30-day mortality for the total population being only 4.4%. In 17 cases (20%), the CT angiography findings significantly influenced the choice of arterial cannulation site, which resulted in sufficient perfusion of all organs during the cardiopulmonary bypass in all but 1 patient. Pathologic condition in the proximal area of the arch arteries was even ascertained in 3 of the 17 patients. Had this not been considered, it could have led to a relevant impairment of the cerebral perfusion. The CT angiography enabled these pathologies to be recognized and the operative strategy to be adapted accordingly. In 1 of these 3 patients, we even had to conduct an additional magnetic resonance (MR) angiography because the CT angiography that had been done outside our facility did not include the arch arteries, and the patient showed clinical signs of cerebral malperfusion. The imaging showed a dissection of the innominate artery with severe compression of the true lumen (**Fig. 3**). To avoid insufficient cerebral perfusion through the narrowed innominate artery during cardiopulmonary bypass, we cannulated the right common carotid artery with an 8-mm Dacron side graft through a separate incision on the neck. For sufficient perfusion of the rest of the body, a second arterial line was installed in the right femoral artery and connected with a Y-shaped tube for arterial return from one pump. Because the dissection extended to the aortic isthmus (D-ab), a complete arch repair with resection of all dissected aortic walls was performed. The innominate artery showed

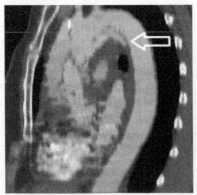 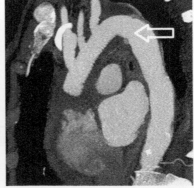

Fig. 1. Preoperative CT angiography (*left*) showing acute dissection of ascending aorta and aortic arch, and postoperative CT angiography (*right*) of the same patient after complete arch replacement. Both show the distal end of dissection and distal aortic anastomosis (*arrows*).

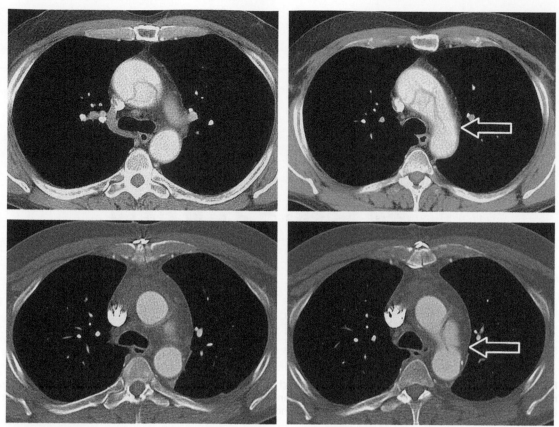

Fig. 2. Preoperative CT angiography (*upper row*) showing acute aortic dissection of ascending aorta and aortic arch (D-ab). The dissection (*arrow*) extends thorough aortic arch and ends at level of aortic isthmus. Postoperative CT (*lower row*) angiography of the same patient after incomplete arch replacement (hemiarch replacement) with remaining dissection membrane (*arrow*) in aortic arch.

multiple tears, which made anastomosis to the graft impossible. For this reason it was ligated, and the side graft that was anastomosed to the right carotid artery was used for aortocarotid bypass (see **Fig. 3**).

SURGICAL STRATEGY

The distal extent of aortic replacement and the type of proximal (aortic root) repair are not the only subjects of discussion in the surgical community. The differences of opinion concerning the surgical management of acute aortic dissection started with the choice of the optimal site for arterial cannulation. Despite a consensus that the true lumen of the arterial system should be cannulated in acute aortic dissection, the procedures to achieve this goal vary considerably, ranging from the transapical approach to the peripheral cannulation of the nondissected artery. The most tried-and-true method is cannulation of a femoral artery, which offers fast and simple establishment of cardiopulmonary bypass.[3]

In most cases, this approach enables safe and sufficient perfusion, provided the aorta is not cross-clamped before completion of distal repair and an antegrade perfusion is reestablished thereafter.[4] Because this precondition is not necessary, when an arch artery is cannulated and the aorta is still clamped during cooling, the antegrade perfusion from a cannulated arch artery is considered to improve the surgical outcome.[5] However, our reasons for changing the cannulation technique from 2002 with a cannulation of the carotid artery are more extensive and are mainly connected with the change of the cerebral protection method.[6]

Deep hypothermic circulatory arrest has been proven to be a good method of protection because it offers favorable results when its duration is limited to 30 minutes or less.[7] However, except in cases with dissection limited to the ascending aorta, distal aortic repair in acute dissection often takes more time than in elective arch surgery and frequently exceeds 30 minutes. The risk of stroke increases significantly when the duration of the

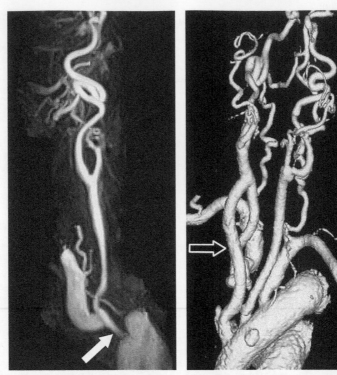

Fig. 3. Preoperative MR angiography (*left*) of aortic arch showing aortic dissection with extension into innominate artery causing severe compression of true lumen, and postoperative MR angiography (*right*) after complete arch replacement with ligation of innominate artery and right-sided aortocarotid bypass (*arrow*).

deep hypothermic circulatory arrest exceeds 40 minutes.[8] Moreover, in addition to the negative side effects of deep hypothermia on various organ systems, the duration of cardiopulmonary bypass has also been identified as an independent risk factor for an adverse outcome.[9,10] Consequently, there are 3 potential goals to improve the results in a surgery necessitating circulatory arrest—extending the safe period of cerebral protection, omitting deep hypothermia, and shortening the time of cardiopulmonary bypass. The only way to achieve all these goals is through the use of selective cerebral perfusion. Extending the safe period of circulatory arrest is especially important in surgery of acute dissection because it enables optimal repair of the aortic arch without increasing the operative risk.

Cannulation of the femoral artery in open aortic arch surgery is always associated with the necessity of circulatory arrest in deep hypothermia. Even though selective cerebral perfusion for brain protection is performed, cerebral flow must be interrupted during the placement of perfusion cannulas in the aortic arch vessels. During this manipulation, cerebrovascular injury may occur because of an air embolism or dislodgment of atherosclerotic debris.[11,12] In addition, in acute dissection of arch vessels, direct cannulation

with perfusion catheters can damage the fragile vascular wall, which can result in hemorrhagic complications or malperfusion. The damage can also be caused by a failed positioning of the perfusion catheter.[13] The risk of manipulation-related injuries can be limited by cannulating one arch artery for arterial return of cardiopulmonary bypass. In such cases, the cerebral perfusion does not have to be interrupted while placing the perfusion cannulas, and the additional manipulation on arch arteries for the completion of bilateral perfusion is consequently limited, or even completely avoided, when unilateral cerebral perfusion is used. The limitation of cerebral perfusion to one side simplifies the surgery, decreases the risk of embolism, and provides better exposure by not cluttering the surgical field with cannulas.

Although the anatomopathological conditions often limit the usefulness of the innominate artery for cannulation, numerous experiences with cannulation of the right axillary artery for arterial return have recently been reported.[14–16] The surgical approach is time consuming, especially in obese patients. Local complications with a rate of up to 14% and even dissections of the arterial system with lethal outcome have been reported.[17–19] An axillary artery of thin caliber or having a particularly fragile wall has necessitated a switch to another cannulation site in up to 11% of the cases.[19]

In contrast, the common carotid artery wall is not as delicate and not as prone to damage as the axillary artery. In a total of 90 patients with acute aortic dissection cannulated since 2002 on the carotid artery (and in our total present experience with almost 500 carotid cannulations), no local vessel alterations were observed, and a switch to another cannulation site was not necessary in any patient. Moreover, the arterial return was always sufficient. A common carotid artery in the neck can be accessed quickly and easily, even in obese patients, and is therefore suitable in an emergency.

An extension of the safe circulatory arrest time has a calming effect on the surgeon, and this facilitates an optimal repair of the arch corresponding to the anatomopathological requirement and not to surgical limitation. Possibly much, if not all, of the dissected aortic wall is resected, which is not only important for the late outcome but also for the incidence of anastomotic bleeding. This bleeding is the most feared complication during surgery and is considerably lower when nondissected vessels are anastomosed.[20] Surprisingly, even the time of circulatory arrest needed for total aortic arch replacement with anastomoses made to nondissected vessel walls is not much longer than the duration of hemiarch replacement with one complicated anastomosis to a dissected aortic wall.[1]

When performing anastomoses with nondissected arch arteries, use of a vascular prosthesis with 4 side branches, as available from various manufacturers, is recommended. The arch arteries are transected distally from their origin on the aortic arch and anastomosed end-to-end with the side branches of the arch prosthesis. When a dissection of an arch artery exists, the side branch is anastomosed to the true lumen of the dissected artery. This condition most often leads to an adaption of the dissection membrane and closure of the false lumen, because intimal tears in the distal segments of the arch arteries are rare.

Conversely, intimal tears in the distal aorta are common, and therefore the obliteration of the false lumen in the dissected descending aorta can seldom be achieved regardless of the anastomosis technique used (eg, "elephant trunk") or other adjuncts (eg, use of glue). Nevertheless, we use the elephant trunk technique for 2 reasons. This technique not only offers better hemostatic characteristics but also simplifies a second-stage surgery that could be required in the future. Use of a short elephant trunk is sufficient to fulfill the earlier mentioned purpose and facilitates the

placement of the tube, which should be similar to the inner caliber of the aorta. In cases with a difficult approach to the distal aortic arch or small diameter of the descending aorta, we do not use an invaginated tube as proposed originally by Borst and colleagues.[21] Instead, we insert a short piece (about 3–4 cm) of a straight tube into the aorta, which should adhere to the inner wall of the aorta. We then sew the descending aorta to the elephant trunk end-to-end with the aortic arch prosthesis (**Fig. 4**).

Procedures reported recently by some investigators show no relevant differences in the false-lumen obliteration rates in the thoracoabdominal aorta after use of the conventional elephant trunk and the frozen elephant trunk (stented graft). Therefore, a different influence on the long-term behavior of the false lumen in the descending aorta by using one or other techniques cannot be expected. Considering the vulnerability of a dissected aortic wall, which can even lead to the distal extension of the aortic dissection as observed after stent repair of type B aortic dissection,[22] a general recommendation for the use of the frozen elephant trunk cannot be given at this time.

Among 77 patients operated on in our facility between 1995 and 2001 with acute type A aortic dissections, there were 9 redo surgeries performed on the aorta during the follow-up period. In 4 cases it was a repair of the aortic root and in 5 cases a repair of the distal aorta, performed on average 3.5 ± 2.0 years after the primary surgery of acute dissection (**Fig. 5**). In addition, in 1 patient an early rupture of the dissected descending aorta

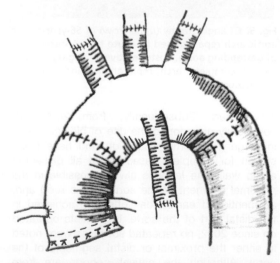

Fig. 4. Aortic arch replacement using vascular aortic arch prosthesis with 4 side branches and elephant trunk prosthesis for distal anastomosis.

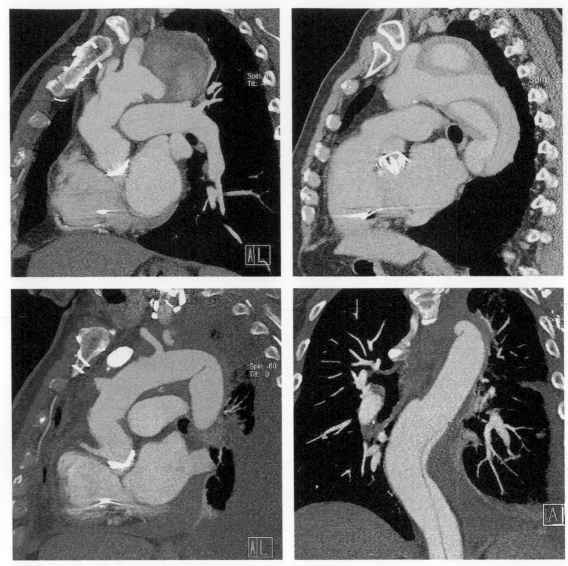

Fig. 5. CT angiography (*upper row*) of 56-year-old patient performed 6 years after ascending aorta and partial aortic arch repair caused by acute type A dissection (D-abc) showing remaining dissection with large aneurysm of descending aorta. Postoperative CT angiography (*lower row*) of the same patient after a redo surgery consisting of complete arch replacement and partial descending aorta replacement performed via clamshell thoracotomy.

was noted. Subsequently, from 2002, we completely abandoned the use of biologic glues in surgery of aortic dissection and have since striven for complete resection of all dissected aortic wall. The latter is always possible in the proximal segment of the aorta (aortic root) and, as mentioned earlier, can often be achieved in the distal part of the aorta. In patients operated on since 2002, no repeated surgeries were noted in either the proximal or distal segments of the aorta. Although the patient cohorts are from different time frames, the follow-up time of the second group of patients was almost identical

(3.5 ± 2.2 years) to the average time taken in the first group for the emergence of indications for a redo surgery on the distal aorta. In the second group, only 1 patient suffered sudden death that could have possibly been associated with the remaining dissection of the thoracoabdominal aorta. In another patient, a moderate dilatation of the dissected descending aorta (with a diameter of 5 cm) occurred within the first year after surgery and did not increase during the following 6 years.

Although reports concerning the fate of the remaining distal aortic dissection after emergent surgery due to acute type A aortic dissection

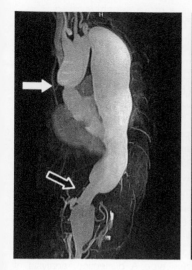 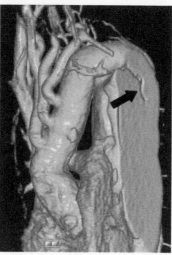

Fig. 6. MR angiography of 16-year-old patient with Marfan syndrome (*left*) performed 1 year after Bentall procedure (*upper arrow*) because of acute type A dissection, and repair of abdominal aorta (*lower arrow*) 8 weeks later caused by imminent rupture of progressive abdominal aneurysm, showing development of large aortic arch and thoracoabdominal aneurysm. MR angiography of the same patient performed after complete aortic arch replacement (*right*) with distal elephant trunk (*arrow*) using vascular aortic arch prosthesis with 4 side branches. The thoracoabdominal repair is planned.

vary considerably, there is evidence that younger patients and those having inherited aortic wall disorders are at a significantly higher risk of suffering aortic events or developing a thoracoabdominal aneurysm necessitating surgery.[23–28] To avoid the development of an aneurysm in the aortic arch and to facilitate the treatment of the consequences of dissection in the thoracoabdominal aorta, all patients with acute dissection of all 3 aortic segments (D-abc), with the exception of those at high surgical risk due to advanced age or severe comorbidities, should undergo complete aortic arch replacement. We are convinced that surgery of acute aortic dissection that is limited to only saving the patient's life is not sufficient in today's world of modern cardiac surgery. The surgery performed should also ensure the best possible life expectancy and quality of life rather than be the beginning of a painful odyssey (**Fig. 6**). In our opinion, acute type A aortic dissection frequently demands extended arch resection at the time of primary surgery, and should be performed only by experienced surgeons.

ACKNOWLEDGMENTS

The authors would like to thank Melissa Lindner and Alexandra Metz for their assistance in preparing this article.

REFERENCES

1. Urbanski PP, Siebel A, Zacher M, et al. Is extended aortic replacement in acute type A dissection justifiable? Ann Thorac Surg 2003;75:525–9.

2. Urbanski PP. Carotid artery cannulation in acute aortic dissection with malperfusion. J Thorac Cardiovasc Surg 2006;131:1398–9.

3. Fusco DS, Shaw RK, Tranquilli M, et al. Femoral cannulation is safe for type A dissection repair. Ann Thorac Surg 2004;78:1285–9.

4. Van Arsdell GS, David TE, Butany J. Autopsies in acute type A aortic dissection. Surgical implications. Circulation 1998;98:II299–304.

5. Reuthebuch O, Schurr U, Hellermann J, et al. Advantages of subclavian artery perfusion for repair of acute type A dissection. Eur J Cardiothorac Surg 2004;26:592–8.

6. Urbanski PP, Lenos A, Lindemann Y, et al. Carotid artery cannulation in aortic surgery. J Thorac Cardiovasc Surg 2006;132:1398–403.

7. Kunihara T, Grün T, Aicher D, et al. Hypothermic circulatory arrest is not a risk factor for neurologic morbidity in aortic surgery: a propensity score analysis. J Thorac Cardiovasc Surg 2005;130:712–8.

8. Gega A, Rizzo JA, Johnson MH, et al. Straight deep hypothermic arrest: experience in 394 patients supports its effectiveness as a sole means of brain preservation. Ann Thorac Surg 2007;84:759–67.

9. Kazui T, Washiyama N, Muhammad BAH, et al. Improved results of atherosclerotic arch aneurysm operations with a refined technique. J Thorac Cardiovasc Surg 2001;121:491–9.

10. Shah PJ, Estrera AL, Miller CC, et al. Analysis of ascending and transverse aortic arch repair in octogenarians. Ann Thorac Surg 2008;86:774–9.

11. Ueda T, Shimizu H, Ito T, et al. Cerebral complications associated with selective perfusion of the arch vessels. Ann Thorac Surg 2000;70:1472–7.

12. Di Eusanio M, Wesselink RMJ, Morshuis WJ, et al. Deep hypothermic circulatory arrest and antegrade

selective cerebral perfusion during ascending aorta—hemiarch replacement: a retrospective comparative study. J Thorac Cardiovasc Surg 2003;125:849–54.

13. Orihashi K, Sueda T, Okada K, et al. Malposition of selective cerebral catheter is not a rare event. Eur J Cardiothorac Surg 2005;27:644–8.

14. Strauch JT, Spielvogel D, Lauten A, et al. Axillary artery cannulation: routine use in ascending aorta and aortic arch replacement. Ann Thorac Surg 2004;78:103–8.

15. Sabik JF, Nemeh H, Lytle BW, et al. Cannulation of the axillary artery with a side graft reduces morbidity. Ann Thorac Surg 2004;77:1315–20.

16. Numata S, Ogino H, Sasaki H, et al. Total arch replacement using antegrade selective cerebral perfusion with right axillary artery perfusion. Eur J Cardiothorac Surg 2003;23:771–5.

17. Imanaka K, Kyo S, Tanabe H, et al. Fatal intraoperative dissection of the innominate artery due to perfusion through the right axillary artery. J Thorac Cardiovasc Surg 2000;120:405–6.

18. Miyatake T, Matsui Y, Suto Y, et al. A case of intraoperative aortic dissection caused by cannulation into an axillary artery. J Cardiovasc Surg (Torino) 2001;42:809–11.

19. Schachner T, Nagiller J, Zimmer A, et al. Technical problems and complications of axillary artery cannulation. Eur J Cardiothorac Surg 2005;27:634–7.

20. Massimo CG, Presenti LF, Favi PP, et al. Excision of the aortic wall in the surgical treatment of acute type A aortic dissection. Ann Thorac Surg 1990;50:274–6.

21. Borst HG, Walterbusch G, Schaps D. Extensive aortic replacement using "elephant trunk" prosthesis. Thorac Cardiovasc Surg 1983;31:37–40.

22. Urbanski PP. Retrograde extension of type B dissection after endovascular stent graft repair. Eur J Cardiothorac Surg 2002;21:767–8.

23. Ergin MA, Phillips RA, Galla JD, et al. Significance of distal false lumen after type A dissection repair. Ann Thorac Surg 1994;57:820–5.

24. Geirsson A, Bavaria JE, Swarr D, et al. Fate of the residual distal and proximal aorta after acute type A dissection repair using a contemporary surgical reconstruction algorithm. Ann Thorac Surg 2007;84:1955–64.

25. Takahara Y, Sudo Y, Mogi K, et al. Total aortic arch grafting for acute type A dissection: analysis of residual false lumen. Ann Thorac Surg 2002;73:450–4.

26. Halstead JC, Meier M, Etz C, et al. The fate of the distal aorta after repair of acute type A aortic dissection. J Thorac Cardiovasc Surg 2007;133:127–35.

27. Immer FF, Hagen U, Berdat PA, et al. Risk factors for secondary dilatation of the aorta after acute type A aortic dissection. Eur J Cardiothorac Surg 2005;27:654–7.

28. Yu HY, Chen YS, Huang SC, et al. Late outcome of patients with aortic dissection: study of a national database. Eur J Cardiothorac Surg 2004;25:683–90.

Extended Arch Resection in Acute Type A Aortic Dissection: CON

Arnar Geirsson, MD

KEYWORDS

- Acute type A aortic dissection • Aortic arch
- Aortic replacement • Ascending aorta
- Great vessels • Hypothermic circulatory arrest

Acute type A aortic dissection remains one of the most challenging diseases the cardiothoracic surgeon faces. The clinical presentation can be dramatic, and expeditious and proper clinical management is paramount to assure the best possible short- and long-term outcome for the patient. Clinical decision making has evolved significantly in the last 20 years. Improved surgical techniques and postoperative care have decreased hospital mortality, but there are still several contentious issues in managing patients with acute type A aortic dissection.

The most important fundamental issue that needs to be addressed by the surgeon in the operating room is the extent of aortic replacement. Proximal extent is defined by the need for aortic root replacement or preservation. This question is not addressed by this article, but, in general, preservation of the aortic valve by the means of commissural resuspension and local repair should be attempted and is associated with favorable outcome, unless there is preexisting aortic valve disease or coronary malperfusion.[1] The extent of distal aortic replacement is defined by how the aortic arch is addressed, and depends on where the primary aortic tear is located. It is generally believed that the primary tear (where the aortic dissection originated) needs to be resected whenever reasonably possible to depressurize the distal false lumen and decrease the risk of future development of descending aortic aneurysm in the residual dissected aorta.[2]

The distal anastomosis should be performed in an open fashion by means of hypothermic circulatory arrest. This technique allows the best visualization of the aorta and identification of the primary tear site, and also allows for optimal apposition of the dissected layers and resection of the cross-clamp site. Anything less, such as performing the distal anastomosis with an aortic cross-clamp in place, is associated with suboptimal results. In nearly all cases of acute type A aortic dissection, the goal of resecting the primary tear can be accomplished by replacing the ascending aorta and hemiarch.

Recently, some groups have advocated a more aggressive approach in which routine total arch replacement or placement of a descending aortic stent graft are promoted as the primary operative strategy.[3–5] The main argument for more aggressive distal operation is to promote occlusion of the false lumen, curtail the development of descending aortic aneurysm, decrease the risk for late distal reoperations, and thus improve long-term survival. The main counterarguments are that increased operative complexity, prolonged operative time, and increased hypothermic circulatory arrest time increases the operative risk compared with standard reconstruction at the distal ascending aorta level. There is minimal evidence in the literature to support the more aggressive approach. The information that is available supports a conservative approach, which is associated with the best outcomes.

Section of Cardiac Surgery, Yale University School of Medicine, 333 Cedar Street, Boardman 204, PO Box 208039, New Haven, CT 06520-8039, USA
E-mail address: arnar.geirsson@yale.edu

Cardiol Clin 28 (2010) 343–347
doi:10.1016/j.ccl.2010.01.008
0733-8651/10/$ – see front matter. Published by Elsevier Inc.

Aortic dissection is characterized by separation of the aortic intima and adventitia to various extents. Risk factors for aortic dissection include hypertension, thoracic aortic aneurysm, atherosclerotic disease, bicuspid aortic valve, aortic coarctation, and connective tissue disorders such as Marfan syndrome.[6] Generally, the initiating event is a hypertensive episode resulting in primary intimal tear. The inflow of blood then propagates the dissection proximally and distally, creating a false lumen that communicates with the true aortic lumen at 1 or more secondary intimal tear sites. Stanford type A dissection involves the ascending aorta and, to various extents, the descending aorta, whereas Stanford type B dissection involves only the descending aorta. In type A aortic dissection, the extent is confined to the ascending aorta (DeBakey type II) in 28% of cases, whereas 72% of cases involve the whole aorta (DeBakey type I).[1] The primary tear is located in the ascending aorta in 72% to 79% of cases, in the transverse aorta in 12% to 18%, in the descending aorta in 1% to 2%, and unknown or other in the remaining cases.[7–9]

In the early days of cardiac surgery, early mortality of type A aortic dissection without surgical treatment was considered to be 1% to 2% per hour, with less than 10% of patients surviving 3 days.[10] Current operative mortality ranges from 12.7% to 32.5%, whereas in-hospital mortality for nonoperative treatment is 58% in the International Registry of Acute Aortic Dissection (IRAD) database.[1,9,11–13] Therefore, in all patients presenting with acute type A aortic dissection, the primary intervention should be an operation unless the patient has significant comorbitities or moribund preoperative condition. Advanced age should not exclude patients from an operation.[14–17] Patients with evidence of circulatory collapse indicating rupture, pericardial tamponade, and coronary malperfusion are at high risk for mortality. Patients with evidence of malperfusion syndromes, especially cerebral malperfusion (stroke and coma) but also mesenteric, renal, and limb malperfusion, are at even higher risk, especially when combined with circulatory collapse.[14,18,19]

Contemporary surgical strategies have been developed over many years. Although interinstitutional differences exist, the general view among aortic surgeons is that acute type A aortic dissection should be considered an emergency and treated as such. If adequate expertise is not available at the initial institution, the patient should be rapidly transferred to an aortic center where the operation can be performed immediately. Cannulation strategies differ between the use of femoral artery, right axillary artery, or ascending aorta as cannulation sites. Perfusion strategies also vary between the use of hypothermic circulatory arrest, with or without adjuvant use of retrograde cerebral perfusion, or direct antegrade cerebral perfusion, under deep hypothermic circulatory arrest or with more tepid temperatures. Cannulation and perfusion strategies are contested among cardiac surgeons, and each point of view has pros and cons worthy of separate discussion.

What is generally not contested regarding distal operation in acute type A aortic dissection is that the distal anastomosis needs to be performed as open anastomosis under circulatory arrest. The dissected layers of the aorta are usually reinforced with the use of felt or biologic glue. Biologic glue, especially gelatin-resorcin-formalin–based formulations, should be used modestly because excessive application has been associated with aortic necrosis and development of pseudoaneuryms.[20] Accurate realignment of the aortic layers around the aortic arch will ensure proper cerebral perfusion and establish normal true lumen flow down the proximal descending thoracic aorta.

The separation of conservative and extensive arch resection is the level of the innominate artery. Resection of the ascending aorta and the underside of the aortic arch results in hemiarch replacement, which is defined as the conservative approach in this discussion. In more extensive operations, the aortic arch is resected and the arch vessels (innominate, left carotid, and left subclavian arteries) are anastomosed directly or as a patch to the aortic graft. In an even more aggressive approach, the residual descending aortic dissection is addressed at the time of the initial operation, by replacing the proximal descending aorta or, as has recently been described, by using an endovascular stent graft.[3,5]

Advocates for the more aggressive approach argue that more extensive arch resection improves long-term outcome without detrimental short-term outcome. The rationale proposed is that by replacing the full arch, or even placing an endovascular stent graft into the descending aorta, the residual descending aortic dissection will more likely thrombose or collapse, resulting in decreased rates of descending aortic aneurysm formation. Total arch replacement also ensures resection of primary tear, increasing the chances of false-lumen decompression. Operations for chronic descending aortic dissection-related aneurysm, it is argued, are complex and associated with high morbidity and mortality.

There are several arguments against the more aggressive approach, and these are discussed in the following sections.

NO EVIDENCE OF SURVIVAL BENEFIT

There is no evidence to support improved long-term survival with the more aggressive arch approach. There are limited data that directly compare long-term survival between patients who undergo conservative versus a more aggressive surgical approach. In a study involving few patients in which 3 different distal operations were performed (ascending aorta alone, ascending aorta and hemiarch, and total arch replacement), there was no difference in long-term survival.[21] Another report showed significantly worse 5-year survival in patients undergoing total arch replacement (44.4%) versus hemiarch replacement (91.3%).[22] Data from Stanford showed no difference in long-term survival in patients with the primary tear in the arch who underwent hemiarch or total arch replacement.[23] Late reinterventions on the distal aorta are high-risk and associated with high rates of mortality up to 31%.[1] However, the long-term survival in patients undergoing reoperations is not different from patients who do not require reoperations.[8] In addition, 2 separate reports show that long-term survival is independent of distal operative strategy.[9,24] This phenomenon may be explained by the generally low long-term survival in patients with type A aortic dissection, reported to be between 37% and 56% at 10 years. Preoperative and intraoperative predictors of decreased long-term survival include peripheral vascular disease, prior stroke, coronary artery disease, hypotension at time of presentation, preoperative cardiac arrest, cerebral malperfusion, and length of cardiopulmonary bypass.[1]

HIGHER MORTALITY WITH MORE EXTENSIVE RESECTION

Total aortic arch replacement is traditionally associated with significantly higher operative mortality. This association may have changed with improved perioperative care over the years, but older reports describe an operative mortality of 55% for patients undergoing total arch replacement versus 41% undergoing hemiarch replacement when the primary tear is located in the arch proper.[23] Various groups have shown acceptable mortality with total arch replacement, but those reports do not include comparative series of less extensive resection, making interpretation and comparison with less aggressive techniques impossible.[4,25] Operative mortality for acute type A aortic dissection is primarily dependent on hemodynamic stability, neurologic status, and presence of malperfusion syndromes.[1,18,19] Extended repair of the aortic arch, whether total arch replacement or adjuvant use of stent graft, significantly increases the length of cardiopulmonary bypass and the hypothermic circulatory arrest time.[5] Although those factors have not been clearly shown to increase the incidence of cerebral events in those particular patient groups, prolonged hypothermic circulatory arrest is undoubtedly associated with cerebral ischemia and worse neurologic outcome in elective procedures.[26,27] It is therefore paramount to minimize the extent of circulatory arrest. Additional maneuvers that do not clearly improve patient outcome but prolong circulatory arrest time should be avoided.

NO EVIDENCE OF DECREASED INCIDENCE OF LATE DISTAL ANEURYSMS

Extended arch resection probably results in increased incidence of false lumen thrombosis, but does that translate into reduced rates of descending aneurysms? Is the status of the distal false lumen the primary determinant of aneurysm formation? The Mt Sinai group calculated the growth rate of descending aortic aneurysm to be 0.8 to 1.0 mm/y. Initial size greater than 4 cm and initial diameter of less than 4 cm with a patent false lumen were the predictors of greater growth in the descending aorta.[8] Another report described more rapid and more unpredictable aortic growth of 5.3 mm/y. Patients who did not have any aneurysm enlargement were excluded.[24] The significance of a patent false lumen is not clear. The average growth rate of the proximal descending aorta seems to be greater, 1.9 mm/y in patients with patent false lumen compared with 0.7 mm/y in patients with a thrombosed false lumen. However, there was no significant difference in rates of reoperations between the 2 groups in that study.[28]

IS TEAR RESECTION REALLY NECESSARY?

Resection of the primary tear should generally be attempted. However, there are conflicting reports as to whether this produces any difference in outcome. A large series from Stanford indicated that there was no difference in survival whether primary tear was resected or not.[29] A more contemporary report showed that an unresected primary tear was associated with decreased freedom from distal reoperations.[24] The group making that observation does not advocate a more aggressive approach and prefers to leave primary tear unresected if it cannot be encompassed with hemiarch replacement. That rationale is based on increased short-term complications associated with more extensive operations.

REOPERATION RATES ARE NOT AFFECTED BY MORE EXTENSIVE RESECTION

Actuarial freedom from distal reoperations regardless of distal approach ranges from 74% to 89% at 10 years. Actual rates of reoperation at 10 years range between 3.7% and 8.9%.[1,8,9,24,28] The way the arch was approached did not affect freedom from reoperation. Also, in a series of 70 patients who underwent total arch replacement, the freedom from distal reoperation was 77% at 5 years, further supporting the belief that the distal extent of arch resection is not a significant determinant of reoperations.[4] Risk factors that have been shown to determine need for reoperation include age less than 45 years, Marfan syndrome, unresected primary tear, absence of postoperative β-blocker therapy and increased blood pressure in late follow-up.[1,24] A troublesome issue regarding rates of reoperation is that there is considerable variability between different series and institutions regarding which patients are selected for reoperation. The true freedom from reoperation is therefore unclear. Some centers are undoubtedly more aggressive than others in offering an operation for patients with descending aortic aneurysm, and size criteria for intervention can differ. Some patients are not offered operations because of comorbidities, despite meeting size criteria for operation. Those issues have not been addressed appropriately and should be kept in mind when interpreting outcome data.

ACUTE TYPE A AORTIC DISSECTION IS AN INHERENTLY LETHAL CONDITION

The first priority is to produce a live patient.[30] Survival constitutes success regardless of later onset of further aortic problems. There is no clear evidence that more aggressive aortic arch resection improves outcome or survival. It is therefore difficult to justify routine use of extended arch resection in acute type A dissection. Some aortic centers have achieved acceptable outcome with a more extended approach, but the ability to perform these complex operations may not translate into general cardiac surgery practice. DeBakey type I represent 70% of the cases. There is no evidence that patients with DeBakey type II will benefit from extensive arch resection. Furthermore, the primary tear is only located in the arch 12% to 18% of the time, and in most of those instances can be resected with aggressive hemiarch replacement. Consequently, there are few

cases that might benefit from total arch replacement. The only cases in which total arch replacement should be considered are in young patients (<45 years of age) and patients with Marfan syndrome, who are clearly at higher risk for distal reoperations even after hemiarch replacement.[1] Whether total arch replacement can prevent the need for distal reoperation in those patients has not been reported. Marfan syndrome represents only 4.5% of cases, and, in most of those, the Marfan diagnosis (Ghent criteria) is made after the acute operation. The acuity of type A dissection and the urgent need for operation do not allow for confirmatory genetic workup. It may therefore not be appropriate to perform total arch repair in patients only suspected to have Marfan disease. A commonly overlooked, but important, issue is that proper blood pressure control following the acute operation might be one of the most important factors beneficial to the patient, mitigating the requirement for distal reoperation.[24]

One of the major difficulties in determining the best surgical approaches is that the evidence in the surgical literature for any specific approach is generally weak. All experiential reviews are of necessity retrospective and nonrandomized. These are generally single-institutional case series, and comparison of outcomes between different techniques at different institutions is inherently flawed. The ideal situation would be to have randomized prospective data to support a certain argument. However, acute aortic dissection (and most surgical conditions) will never be studied in a randomized fashion. Surgical data need to be interpreted with caution; in most instances operative decision making must be based on scarce literature but also institutional tradition, anecdotal data, and prior personal experience. These issues need to be kept in mind when proposing new treatment paradigms. Cardiac surgery needs to be pushed forward to improve patient outcomes. Studies need to be done in a controlled investigational fashion so improvements in short- and long-term prognosis can be clearly shown. So far, the literature supporting extensive arch resection in acute type A aortic dissection has not been in that category.

REFERENCES

1. Geirsson A, Bavaria JE, Swarr D, et al. Fate of the residual distal and proximal aorta after acute type A dissection repair using a contemporary surgical reconstruction algorithm. Ann Thorac Surg 2007; 84:1955–64.
2. Moon MR, Sundt TM III, Pasque MK, et al. Does the extent of proximal or distal resection influence

outcome for type A dissection. Ann Thorac Surg 2001;71:1244–50.

3. Jakob H, Tsagakis K, Tossios P, et al. Combining classic surgery with descending stent grafting for acute DeBakey type I dissection. Ann Thorac Surg 2008;86:95–102.

4. Kazui T, Washiyama N, Muhammad BA, et al. Extended total arch replacement for acute type A aortic dissection: experience with seventy patients. J Thorac Cardiovasc Surg 2000;119:558–65.

5. Pochettino A, Brinkman WT, Moeller P, et al. Antegrade thoracic stent grafting during repair of acute DeBakey I dissection prevents development of thoracoabdominal aortic aneurysms. Ann Thorac Surg 2009;88:482–90.

6. Golledge J, Eagle KA. Acute aortic dissection. Lancet 2008;372:55–66.

7. David TE, Armstrong S, Ivanov J, et al. Surgery for acute type A aortic dissection. Ann Thorac Surg 1999;67:1999–2001.

8. Halstead JC, Meier M, Etz C, et al. The fate of the distal aorta after repair of acute type A aortic dissection. J Thorac Cardiovasc Surg 2007;133:127–35.

9. Kirsch M, Soustelle C, Houel R, et al. Risk factor analysis for proximal and distal reoperations after surgery for acute type A aortic dissection. J Thorac Cardiovasc Surg 2002;123:318–25.

10. Anagnostopoulos C, Prabhakar M, Kittle C. Aortic dissections and dissecting aneurysm. Am J Cardiol 1972;30:263–73.

11. Erasmi A, Stierle U, Bechtel J, et al. Up to 7 years' experience with valve-sparing aortic root remodeling/reimplantation for acute type A aortic dissection. Ann Thorac Surg 2003;76:99–104.

12. Hagan PG, Nienaber CA, Isselbacher EM, et al. The International Registry of Acute Aortic Dissection (IRAD): new insights into an old disease. JAMA 2000;283(7):897–903.

13. Sabik J, Lytle BW, Blackstone E, et al. Long-term effectiveness of operations for ascending aortic dissections. J Thorac Cardiovasc Surg 2000;119:946–62.

14. Caus T, Frapier JM, Giorgi R, et al. Clinical outcome after repair of acute type A dissection in patients over 70 years-old. Eur J Cardiothorac Surg 2002;22:211–7.

15. Chiappini B, Tan ME, Morshuis W, et al. Surgery for acute type A aortic dissection: is advanced age a contraindication? Ann Thorac Surg 2004;78:585–90.

16. Mehta RH, O'Gara PT, Bossone E, et al. Acute type A aortic dissection in the elderly: clinical characteristics, management, and outcomes in the current era. J Am Coll Cardiol 2002;40:685–92.

17. Shrestha M, Khaladj N, Haverich A, et al. Is treatment of acute type A aortic dissection in septuagenarians justifiable. Asian Cardiovasc Thorac Ann 2008;16:33–6.

18. Augoustides JG, Geirsson A, Szeto WY, et al. Observational study of mortality risk stratification by ischemic presentation in patients with acute type A aortic dissection: the Penn classification. Nat Clin Pract Cardiovasc Med 2009;6:1–7.

19. Geirsson A, Szeto WY, Pochettino A, et al. Significance of malperfusion syndromes prior to contemporary surgical repair for acute type A dissection: outcomes and need for additional revascularizations. Eur J Cardiothorac Surg 2007;32:255–62.

20. Hata H, Takano H, Matsumiya G, et al. Late complications of gelatin-resorcin-formalin glue in the repair of acute type A aortic dissection. Ann Thorac Surg 2007;83:1621–6.

21. Driever R, Botsios S, Schmitz E, et al. Long-term effectiveness of operative procedures for Stanford type A aortic dissections. Cardiovasc Surg 2003;11:265–72.

22. Ohtsubo S, Itoh T, Takarabe K, et al. Surgical results of hemiarch replacement for acute type A dissection. Ann Thorac Surg 2002;74:S1853–6.

23. Yun K, Glower D, Miller D, et al. Aortic dissection resulting from tear of transverse arch: is concomitant arch repair warranted? J Thorac Cardiovasc Surg 1991;102:355–70.

24. Zierer A, Voeller RK, Hills KE, et al. Aortic enlargement and late reoperation after repair of acute type A aortic dissection. Ann Thorac Surg 2007;84:479–87.

25. Hirotani T, Kameda T, Kumamoto T, et al. Results of a total aortic arch replacement for an acute aortic arch dissection. J Thorac Cardiovasc Surg 2000;120:686–91.

26. Fleck T, Czerny M, Hutschala D, et al. The incidence of transient neurologic dysfunction after ascending aortic replacement with circulatory arrest. Ann Thorac Surg 2003;76:1198–202.

27. Immer F, Lippeck C, Barmettler HB, et al. Improvement of quality of life after surgery on the thoracic aorta: effect of antegrade cerebral perfusion and short duration of deep hypothermic circulatory arrest. Circulation 2004;110:II250–5.

28. Kimura N, Tanaka M, Kawahito K, et al. Influence of patent false lumen on long-term outcome after surgery for acute type A aortic dissection. J Thorac Cardiovasc Surg 2008;136:1160–6.

29. Fann J, Smith J, Miller D, et al. Surgical management of aortic dissection during a 30-year period. Circulation 1995;92:II113–21.

30. Elefteriades JA. What operation for acute type A dissection? J Thorac Cardiovasc Surg 2002;123(2):201–3.

Editorial Comment: Extended Resection in Acute Type A Aortic Dissection

John A. Elefteriades, MD

In their article in this issue of *Cardiology Clinics*, Dr Paul P. Urbanski and colleagues analyze the entire spectrum of surgical options in the care of acute type A aortic dissection, from imaging to categorization, cannulation, brain protection, use of glues, aortic resection, and extent of repair. They make excellent points regarding all of these variables (**Fig. 1**). Regarding the specific topic of the debate, the authors make a reasonable case, based on their excellent recent experience, for extending resection to include the aortic arch. Their point is that extended resection permits removal of all dissected tissue and that anastomosis to nondissected branches are quite cogent.

There are, however, several weak points in their argument. First, most of their discussion refers to dissections that are confined to the ascending aorta or that extend only to the ligamentum arteriosum. Complete resection, encompassing all the dissected tissue, makes most sense for these

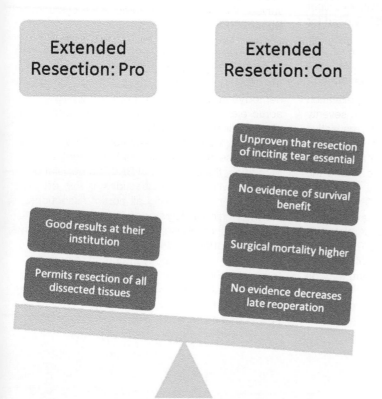

Fig. 1. Although extended resection may soon be proved superior, confirmative evidence at this point is not yet available.

Section of Cardiac Surgery, Department of Surgery, Yale University School of Medicine, Yale-New Haven Hospital, PO Box 208039, New Haven, CT 06520-8039, USA
E-mail address: john.elefteriades@yale.edu

Cardiol Clin 28 (2010) 349–350
doi:10.1016/j.ccl.2010.02.008

unusual and more limited forms of type A dissection. The authors are less sanguine, and their arguments less persuasive, regarding more common and more extensive dissections that extend all the way to the abdomen. Secondly, although their experience and results are exceptionally good, there is no control group of more limited resection, even within their single center.

The article by Dr Arnar Geirsson makes excellent points regarding the actual findings in comparative studies on extent of resection, arguing that (1) there is no evidence of survival benefit from more extensive resection, (2) surgical mortality is generally higher with more extensive resection, (3) there is no evidence that more extensive resection actually decreases the need for late reoperation, and (4) it is unproven that resection of the inciting tear is really required.

The Editor takes an intermediate approach between limited ascending resection and routine full aortic arch replacement. In a large experience at the Editor's center, traditional ascending and hemiarch replacement for acute aortic dissection has yielded excellent clinical results, with excellent early survival, good late survival, and low need for late reoperation.[1] Furthermore, reoperations that were required were well tolerated. However, the theoretical points made by Dr Urbanski are cogent, even though, as Dr Geirsson points out,

it is hard to prove benefit from the literature at this point. So, in selected cases, a tailored arch resection is performed with a specific technique: the aorta is resected to a level between the left carotid and left subclavian arteries. This resection permits a distal anastomosis that is fully and easily accessible. The distal anastomosis is done with an elephant trunk, so it is a simple circular suture line. The aorta is smaller at this site than at the hemi-arch level, so the wall tension is low. Then, the head vessels (innominate and left carotid) are re-implanted as a single patch, with the anastomosis again easily accessible. Both anastomoses are done with a single period of straight hypothermic arrest, usually of about 40 minutes. This specific technique permits the "best of both worlds," namely, a straightforward, efficient operation, with more complete resection. Furthermore, this procedure leaves an elephant trunk dangling, thus facilitating a late reoperation for the descending aorta, for the few patients in whom this becomes necessary in the very long term.

REFERENCE

1. Elefteriades JA. What operation for acute type A dissection? J Thorac Cardiovasc Surg 2002;123: 201–3.

Motor Evoked Potentials in Thoracoabdominal Aortic Surgery: PRO

T.A. Koeppel, MD[a], W.H. Mess, MD, PhD[b],
M.J. Jacobs, MD, PhD[a,c],*

KEYWORDS

- Thoracoabdominal aortic aneurysm
- Open surgical TAAA repair • Motor evoked potentials
- Spinal cord protection

The surgical management of limited as well as extensive thoracoabdominal aortic aneurysms (TAAAs), which lead to high morbidity and mortality rates, is challenging. Although minimally invasive procedures, such as hybrid or total endovascular operations, have become increasingly available in recent years, most TAAAs still require open surgical repair. Spinal cord ischemia during and after the operation, which may result in paraplegia, clearly is one of the most impairing complications of this kind of surgery. The incidence of paraplegia in patients who have undergone type II TAAA repair may be as high as 25%, especially if preventative measures are not part of the surgical protocol.[1] Therefore, prevention of paraplegia has been, and still is, a cardinal challenge in TAAA repair.

Because a variety of causes may be responsible for spinal cord lesions, several strategies for preserving spinal cord integrity have been developed. These adjunctive measures include extracorporeal circulation (ECC) for distal aortic perfusion,[2] cerebrospinal fluid (CSF) drainage,[3,4] and systemic or local hypothermia.[5] Not only do these procedures aim to maintain a sufficient blood flow to the spinal cord during the operation but they also intend to prevent irreversible ischemia-reperfusion injury. However, these neuroprotective procedures reduce the incidence of paraplegia only in a subset of patients. In a substantial remainder of the patients, an adequate blood supply to the spinal cord arteries is achieved only by active surgical intervention.[6]

SPINAL CORD BLOOD SUPPLY

In general, spinal cord ischemic injury results from temporary or permanent interruption of spinal cord blood supply. Ischemic injury caused by temporary interruption of blood flow depends on its duration, indicated by increased paraplegia rates after prolonged aortic cross-clamp times.[4,7] If a permanent interruption of blood flow occurs as a result of intercostal artery ligation during open aortic aneurysm repair, spinal cord ischemic injury is related to the variable and unpredictable anatomy of the intercostal and lumbar arteries and the extent of the aneurysm. In degenerative thoracoabdominal

Financial disclosure obligations: None.

[a] Department of Vascular Surgery, European Vascular Center Aachen-Maastricht, University Hospital of the Rheinisch-Westfälische Technische Hochschule-University Aachen, Pauwelsstrasse 30, Aachen 52074, Germany
[b] Department of Clinical Neurophysiology, European Vascular Center Aachen-Maastricht, University Hospital Maastricht, Postbus 5800, 6202 AZ-Maastricht, The Netherlands
[c] Department of Surgery, European Vascular Center Aachen-Maastricht, University Hospital Maastricht, Postbus 5800, 6202 AZ-Maastricht, The Netherlands
* Corresponding author. Department of Vascular Surgery, European Vascular Center Aachen-Maastricht, University Hospital of the RWTH-University Aachen, Pauwelsstrasse 30, Aachen 52074, Germany.
E-mail address: m.jacobs@mumc.nl

Cardiol Clin 28 (2010) 351–360
doi:10.1016/j.ccl.2010.01.013

aneurysms, most segmental arteries are occluded with mural thrombus or atherosclerotic plaques. This implies that collateral networks supply blood to the spinal cord.[8] During the operation, the surgeon has to decide whether a given artery should be reimplanted or ligated, which is a dilemma because the contribution of the patent segmental vessels to the collateral network and thus to spinal cord perfusion is unknown.

Typically, the anterior spinal artery is fed by several anterior radiculomedullary arteries, which are abundant in the cervical and upper thoracic region, where branches of the vertebral artery contribute medullary components. However, the anterior spinal artery itself becomes narrower and even discontinuous in some individuals as it courses toward the lower thoracolumbar cord. Accordingly, this region is a so-called watershed area, more prone to ischemic injury in thoracic aortic operations. The circulation to this region often depends on the largest extrinsic radiculomedullary artery, known as the Adamkiewicz artery (AKA). In turn, the AKA arises from the T8-L2 region in approximately 72% of patients[9] and originates from arborizing branches of the posterior components of (often) multiple intercostal vessels, with those on the left being more important.[10,11]

PREOPERATIVE ASSESSMENT OF SPINAL CORD CIRCULATION

Preserving spinal cord circulation during and after the repair of descending thoracic aortic aneurysms (DTAAs) and TAAAs is of utmost importance. In particular, patients with an extensive aortic aneurysm, such as type II TAAA according to the Crawford classification (**Fig. 1**), have a high risk to develop paraplegia postoperatively, because the entire thoracic aorta has to be replaced by a vascular graft.[6] Preoperative information about the location and patency of the feeding segmental artery can be important for surgical reconstruction and, in turn, may therefore strongly affect the postoperative neurologic outcome. Furthermore, the importance of lower lumbar and pelvic arteries has been well recognized. Both arteries were the major contributor to the spinal cord circulation in 16% and 8% of the cases, respectively.[12] In addition, the collateral circulation in most patients originated caudally to the distal clamp site (eg, from the pelvic arteries), which can be perfused by means of ECC during cross clamping.[8]

Computed tomography (CT) angiography and magnetic resonance angiography (MRA) have been used successfully in acquiring data about the AKA in patients with TAAAs as well as about collateral circulation in the case of segmental artery occlusion.[13,14] However, MRA is a better technique because of the higher AKA detection rate (100% in patients with TAAAs), the higher contrast-to-noise ratio, and its independence of patient obesity.[15] In most patients (68%) in whom the segmental artery supplying the AKA was cross clamped, motor evoked potentials (MEPs) were not affected, thus indicating sufficient collateral blood supply to maintain spinal cord integrity.[9] Therefore, the authors also investigated whether the preoperative and postoperative presence or absence of collateral arteries detected by

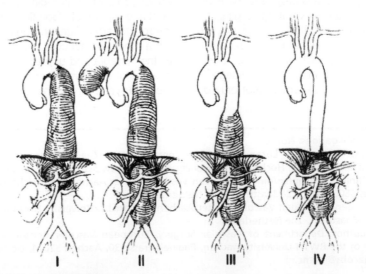

Fig. 1. Crawford classification of TAAAs.

MRA are related to spinal cord function during the intraoperative exclusion of the segmental blood supply to the AKA. This study showed that relevant collateral arteries supplying blood to the spinal cord can be visualized using MRA. Secondly, a very strong correlation could be found between the presence of collateral arteries and stable intraoperative spinal cord function, as assessed by MEPs. However, poor collateralization was associated with altered MEPs that, in turn, implied increased risk of spinal cord dysfunction.[8]

Visualizing segmental arteries by selective intercostal angiography is associated with a risk of procedure-related complications, such as spinal cord injury, renal failure, and stroke, and has a reduced sensitivity when compared with noninvasive imaging techniques.[16] Therefore, intra-arterial angiography is no longer the first choice for preoperative localization of segmental arteries in patients with TAAAs.

MONITORING OF SPINAL CORD INTEGRITY BY MEANS OF MEPS

Before the end of the last decade, it was impossible to accurately assess spinal cord function during the operation.[6] Therefore, no conclusion could be drawn whether inclusion of specific segmental arteries into the aortic reconstruction would be effective or even necessary. Whether spinal cord damage occurred during the operation could be determined only when the patient woke up from anesthesia. Consequently, the development of a reliable monitoring method was absolutely necessary to recognize threatening damage to the spinal cord early on. In this context, somatosensory evoked potentials (SSEPs), which reflect conduction in dorsal columns, have been evaluated in DTAA and TAAA surgery as a means of preventing paraplegia. However, SSEPs showed delayed ischemia detection and a high rate of false-positive results.[17] In contrast, applying MEPs that represent anterior horn motor neuron function has been proven to indicate reliably instantaneous changes of spinal cord perfusion.[18]

Basically, an electric current is applied transcranially, stimulating predominantly the motor cortex. Consequently, several action potentials travel along the pyramidal tract within the brain and the spinal cord to the alpha motor neurons in the anterior horn of the spinal cord. If an alpha motor neuron has received enough action potentials, it will fire itself and hence evokes a contraction of the muscle attached to it via the peripheral nerve (**Fig. 2**). The muscle twitch can easily be picked up by surface electrodes. The amplitude of the signal (the MEP) reflects the amount of functionally intact alpha motor neurons, which are most susceptible to ischemia. In practice, the MEPs of the tibial anterior (TA) muscle are determined. MEPs measured from the abductor pollicis brevis muscle (APB) muscle of the hand serve as reference values to rule out confounding factors not specifically related to spinal cord malfunction.

One of the confounding factors is the degree of muscle relaxation, which during the operation is maintained with vecuronium bromide. Before intubation, the amplitude of the compound muscle action potential (CMAP) of the abductor digiti V muscle on stimulation of the right ulnar nerve at the wrist is measured. During the surgical procedure, the administration of vecuronium bromide is adjusted so that a CMAP amplitude of approximately 20% as compared with the initial CMAP is achieved.

To determine a baseline level of the MEPs, measurements are first taken every 5 minutes before the aorta is cross clamped and subsequently every minute after the clamping maneuver. A reduction of the MEP amplitude of the TA muscle indicates a disturbed blood supply to the spinal cord and requires the surgeon to be attentive. If a prolonged reduction (>5 minutes) of the MEP ratio (TA/APB muscle) of more than 50% occurs, there is an impending danger of irreversible damage to the spinal cord, which makes it imperative for the surgeon to immediately initiate countermeasures to improve spinal cord perfusion.[12] In the authors' experience of more than 400 monitoring procedures, MEPs could be obtained in each patient at the start of the procedure. Furthermore, there were no false-negative or false-positive recordings, that is, the presence of TA MEPs at the end of the procedure always excluded paraplegia, whereas the absence of TA MEPs always predicted paraplegia. Taken together, assessment of MEPs during TAAA repair is a highly reliable tool in the armamentarium of the surgeon, aimed at reducing the incidence of paraplegia during open TAAA repair.

SURGICAL PROTOCOL AND ECC

The application of ECC during operations on the thoracic and thoracoabdominal aorta is fundamentally important for protecting all organ systems and tissues distal to the aortic clamp. Generally, a retrograde aortic perfusion is sufficient for repairing DTAAs. Regarding the open repair of DTAA localized directly at the origin of the left subclavian artery, and also in type I and type II TAAA, it is advantageous to perform a left heart bypass. Hereby, the left atrium or the pulmonary vein can be cannulated. In the case of TAAA,

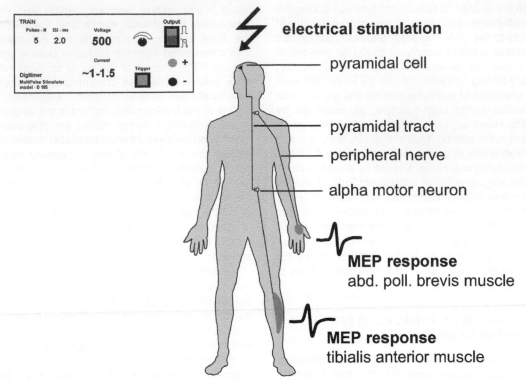

Fig. 2. For monitoring spinal cord integrity, a transcranially evoked stimulus is directed along the spinal cord pyramidal tract via the alpha motor neuron in the anterior horn of the spinal cord and the peripheral nerves. MEPs are recorded at the tibial anterior (TA) muscle as well as on both hands (abductor pollicis brevis muscle).

the retrograde aortic perfusion via the femoral artery is then combined with selective organ perfusion during reconstruction of the renal and visceral arteries. Regarding aneurysms that affect the distal or even the entire aortic arch, a total ECC with cardiac arrest and antegrade cerebral perfusion could be necessary.[19] For operations of type III and type IV TAAA, the cannulation of the femoral artery and vein has been proven favorable. In contrast to operations with total ECC, only limited amounts of heparin have to be administered to the patient for these types of repair, insofar as heparin-coated tubing systems are used that prevent coagulation.

ECC is routinely established before aortic cross clamping. In normotensive patients, the average distal aortic pressure during cross clamping is normally maintained at about 60 mm Hg. This perfusion pressure, however, may not be sufficient in particular patients having impaired collateral circulation (eg, occlusion of hypogastric arteries), especially when a relatively long segment of the lower descending aorta is cross clamped. An inadequate perfusion pressure is reflected by an amplitude decrease in the TA MEPs compared with those measured before ECC was

initiated. Thus, in these patients the pressure has to be adjusted accordingly (**Fig. 3**). Patients with hypertension and concomitant severe vascular degeneration may also need an increased perfusion pressure in the distal aorta to ensure a sufficient blood flow to the spinal cord and visceral organs.

For patients with DTAA and TAAA caused by degenerative vascular disease, most of the intercostal and lumbar arteries are already occluded by plaque or thrombi. The perfusion of the spinal cord essentially depends on sufficient collateral circulatory systems, which are fed by the remaining lumbar and hypogastric arteries (found in about 15% of the patients).[12] The presence of such collateral circulatory systems explains why most of the patients show no changes in the MEPs during the aortic cross clamping, although the blood supply to the AKA has been greatly restricted. For about one-third of the patients, however, the perfusion of the spinal cord depends on the preoperatively localized segmental artery that feeds the AKA.[18] Therefore, during the operation, it is important to localize the particular segmental artery that feeds the AKA. Inclusion of this artery during aortic reconstruction may be

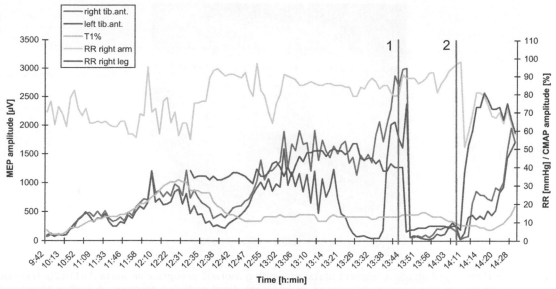

Fig. 3. Influence of distal perfusion pressure on MEP amplitude of the lower extremities. On the left Y-axis, the MEP amplitude is given in μV (red, right TA muscle; blue, left TA muscle), and on the right Y-axis the mean arterial blood pressure in the right brachial artery (*yellow*) and femoral artery (*purple*) is given in mm Hg as well as the degree of muscle relaxation (*green*). The CMAP of the right abductor digiti quinti muscle is compared with the initial situation before intubation and expressed as a percent value. At the first red vertical bar (1) the aorta is still cross clamped. The distal perfusion had to be stopped, causing a sharp decrease of blood pressure in the right femoral artery. Note that within 1 minute both MEPs of the lower extremities also showed a marked decrease, which was fully reversible after adequate perfusion was reestablished (2).

of major importance in preventing paraplegia. In practice, it has been proven effective to sequentially clamp the thoracoabdominal aorta. This technique is advantageous in localizing relevant segmental arteries by systematically excluding aortic segments and simultaneously evaluating the amplitude of the MEPs.

When the MEPs of the TA muscle consistently decrease or even disappear (despite an adequate distal perfusion pressure) after clamping an aortic segment, revascularization of intercostal or lumbar arteries is mandatory. First, the aortic segment has to be opened and relevant segmental arteries have to be identified. In the case in which no ostia of intercostal and lumbar arteries are identifiable in the opened aortic segment, a local endarterectomy is necessary, which frequently unmasks back-bleeding segmental arteries. Thereby, the target vessels can be included into the prosthesis as an onlay anastomosis, or, alternatively, they can be revascularized by using a short 8-mm bypass graft (**Fig. 4**). Depending on the progress of the work involved in aortic reconstruction, the surgeon has to decide whether selective bypass grafting or insertion of the segmental arteries by an onlay anastomosis is more practical. Once the anastomosis is completed, perfusion of the segmental

artery can be reestablished by either using a selective perfusion catheter or by antegrade or (artificial) retrograde aortic blood flow. Depending on the duration of MEP impairment, restoration of the MEP amplitude may occur immediately or after some delay. If these surgical measures are effective, a partial or even complete restoration of the MEPs ought to be noted (**Fig. 5**), reflecting an improved blood flow within the collateral vascular network.

Another situation might occur on opening of the aneurysmal sack—severe back bleeding from intercostal and lumbar arteries can frequently be observed and may be accompanied by a sudden decrease in the spinal cord perfusion pressure. As a result of the so-called steal effect, an immediate decrease or loss of MEPs can be noted, indicating critical spinal cord ischemia. In this case, it is important to control bleeding to restore the spinal cord perfusion. At this point, however, it is not clear whether revascularization of the back-bleeding arteries is necessary. Therefore, the authors prefer a temporary balloon occlusion of intercostal and/or lumbar arteries with 3F Pruitt balloon catheters. Once back bleeding is sufficiently controlled, the MEP amplitudes have to

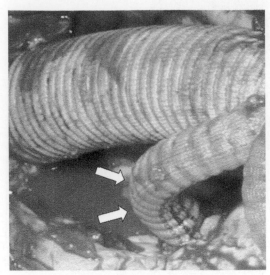

Fig. 4. After clamping of an aortic segment (distal descending thoracic to supraceliac aorta [Th11-L2]), MEPs of the TA muscle consistently disappeared (despite an adequate distal perfusion pressure). A lumbar segmental artery (level L1) was identified and revascularized by using a short 8-mm bypass graft. After revascularization, full recovery of the MEPs was noted.

be monitored carefully. In this case, it can be helpful to further increase the distal perfusion pressure. A spontaneous recovery of the MEPs indicates that a steal effect was responsible for the observed MEP alterations and a particular revascularization is not necessary (**Fig. 6**). If the MEPs show a prolonged depression and do not adequately recover, the aforementioned immediate active surgical interventions are necessary to prevent irreversible spinal cord injury. After revascularization, full or partial recovery of the MEPs should then be noted. However, in a few patients a persistent loss of the MEPs despite a technically successful revascularization was observed. This observation correlated with a postoperative paraplegia.

A somewhat different situation arises not only in patients having a chronic aortic expansion after a type B dissection (Stanford classification) but also in patients with Marfan syndrome. In both patient cohorts, most of the segmental arteries supplying the spinal cord are open. Consequently, it is recommended that segmental arteries arising between Th8 and L1 are routinely revascularized. However, one has to be very careful while suturing the anastomosis, because the aortic tissue in these patients is very vulnerable and bleeding complications may occur after revascularization. With respect to patients with Marfan syndrome, in long-term follow-up, the treating physician has to carefully examine the postoperative images

(CT, magnetic resonance imaging) to rule out aneurysm occurrence at the site of the reimplanted aortic segment (so-called island aneurysms).[20]

ADJUNCTIVE PROCEDURES TO REDUCE SPINAL CORD ISCHEMIA-REPERFUSION INJURY

With regard to the reconstruction times in complete aortic replacement, the distal aortic perfusion by means of ECC plays, as already mentioned, an essential role in the perfusion of the pelvic vasculature and/or important collateral circulatory systems for maintaining spinal cord perfusion. Moreover, ECC can be applied to induce mild hypothermia (32°–33°C), which increases the tolerance of the spinal cord against ischemia caused by a reduced metabolism. Despite these measures, spinal cord perfusion disturbances during and after repair of the aneurysm in patients with insufficient collateral circulation may still lead to spinal edema. As a result, swelling of the spinal cord may be followed by an increase in the intraspinal pressure that ultimately further impairs the spinal cord perfusion. Therefore, this complication has to be taken into account. Unstable MEPs during the operation infer a delicate balance between the spinal cord perfusion pressure and the pressure within the vertebral channel. To prevent this imbalance, the idea of draining the CSF has been introduced

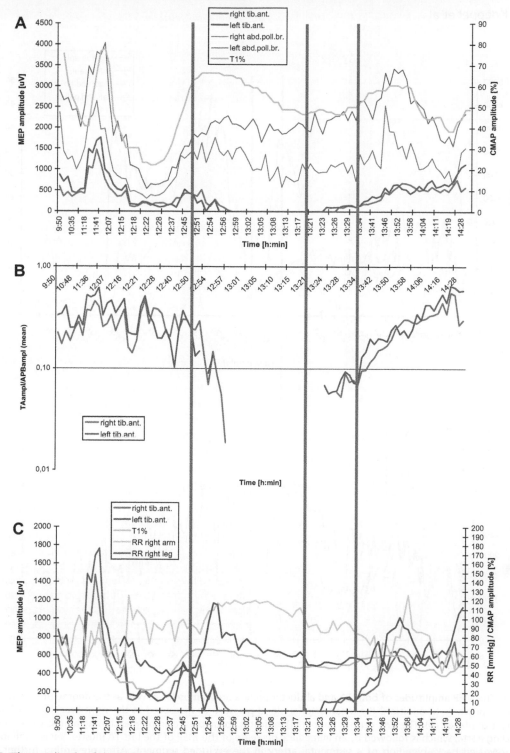

Fig. 5. The amplitude of the MEP of both TA and abductor pollicis brevis muscles as well as the degree of muscle relaxation is given in panel *A*. The ratio of the MEP of each TA muscle and the mean of both abductor pollicis brevis muscles is given in panel *B*, whereas panel *C* displays the mean arterial blood pressure as measured in the right brachial and femoral artery. The first vertical red bar indicates aortic cross clamping, which is followed by a complete loss of the MEPs of the TA muscle several minutes later. Shortly after reimplantation of 4 segmental arteries at T8/9 level (*second vertical red bar*) the MEPs of the lower extremities reappear. Possibly, reimplantation of another 2 segmental arteries (*third vertical red bar*) also contributes to a marked improvement, finally resulting in a complete normalization of the amplitude as compared with the amplitude of the abductor pollicis brevis muscle (*B*). Note the marked fluctuations of all MEP amplitudes in the beginning of the procedure, which perfectly follow the degree of muscle relaxation (*A*). Because this affects all MEPs, the ratio of leg and arm MEPs remains rather stable (*B*). Increasing the distal perfusion pressure immediately after cross clamping could not prevent the loss of the leg MEPs (*C*).

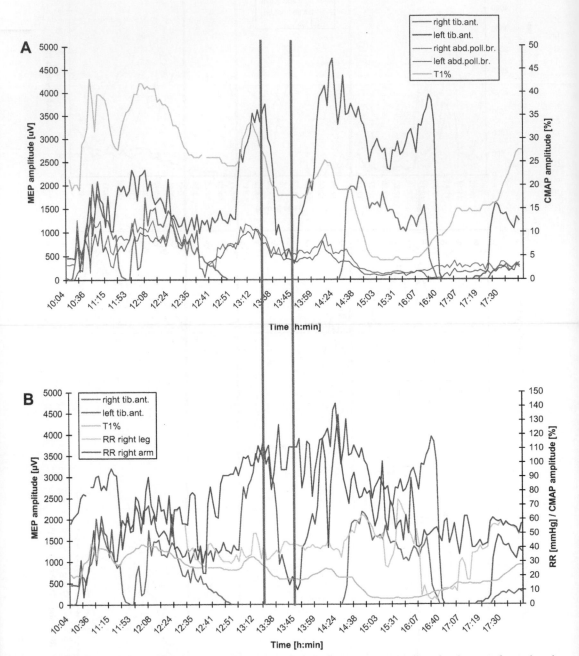

Fig. 6. The MEP amplitudes of both TA and abductor pollicis brevis muscles as well as the degree of muscle relaxation is shown *A*. In addition, the mean arterial blood pressure as measured in the right brachial and femoral artery is displayed (*B*). The first vertical red bar (1) indicates aortic cross clamping excluding almost the entire descending aorta, which is followed by an immediate decrease of the MEP of the left TA muscle. Vessel wall inspection revealed back -bleeding of a segmental artery in the excluded segment. After preventing further back -bleeding by introducing a blocking catheter (2), an immediate restoration of the MEP amplitude of the left leg can be observed. Note the relatively high distal perfusion pressure during the decline of the MEP. The MEP of the right leg had already disappeared before and recovered only later after reimplantation of several segmental arteries. Such asymmetry in spinal cord ischemia is the rare exception.

into clinical practice. Generally, CSF drainage is performed immediately before the operation, to ensure decompression during the operation. Thus, assessment of the intraspinal pressure starts intraoperatively and is continued until the third postoperative day. The drainage system is kept open so that the pressure within the vertebral channel is maintained at less than 10 mm Hg. Up to now, the effectiveness of CSF drainage for preventing neurologic complications has only been demonstrated in one prospective randomized trial.[3] Due to lack of clear data, several authors have doubted the benefit of CSF drainage as a prophylaxis against spinal cord damage in TAAA surgery.[21] Nonetheless, the authors' group and others are convinced of its effectiveness and routinely use CSF drainage in operations involving the thoracic and thoracoabdominal aorta.

DELAYED PARAPLEGIA

Preoperative risk factors for delayed paraplegia include emergency procedure, type-II–extended aortic repair, number of sacrificed segmental arteries, and renal failure. Even though the exact incidence of delayed paraplegia is unknown, centers with large experience in repairing TAAA indicate that approximately 25% of all spinal cord injuries are delayed.[22] The main postoperative risk factors include hemodynamic instability due to bleeding, atrial fibrillation, sepsis, and multiorgan failure.

Azizzadeh and colleagues[23] could not identify a single risk factor; nonetheless, the combination of lower mean arterial pressure and drain complications produced the highest odds ratio of neurologic deficit. In the authors' experience with patients developing delayed paraplegia, perioperative problems with spinal cord perfusion were already noticed by MEP recording. In some patients, complete loss of MEPs was encountered during surgery and reattachment of intercostal arteries. Yet increasing mean arterial pressure and keeping CSF pressure below 10 mm Hg restored MEP amplitudes to approximately 10% of the initial level. Prolonged hypotensive episodes during the postoperative period may cause irreversible damage to the spinal cord. This phenomenon indicates that spinal cord perfusion can be critically endangered but still sufficient to allow adequate anterior horn function, as shown by moving legs in the conscious patient. However, arterial hypotension in these circumstances can provoke definite and permanent spinal cord injury. Therefore, it is extremely important that the postoperative management includes adequate CSF drainage and optimal hemodynamic equilibrium, with elevated mean arterial pressures. However, it should be noted that CSF drainage carries significant risks itself by potentially causing intraspinal hemorrhage or subdural hematoma.[24,25]

SUMMARY

As paraplegia is clearly one of the most severe complications of open DTAA and TAAA repair, a strict protocol for neuroprotection has to be followed. This protocol includes adjunctive procedures, such as ECC for distal aortic perfusion, CSF drainage, and hypothermia, which altogether contribute to improved clinical outcome. However, spinal cord damage, which is caused by a perioperatively interrupted blood supply, is best treated with active revascularization. To guarantee a successful revascularization, it is important to first identify the segmental arteries as well as the collateral networks that contribute to spinal cord perfusion *before* the operation, so that the surgeon can incorporate this knowledge into the surgical strategy. Moreover, using MEPs to monitor spinal cord integrity provides the surgeon with an excellent tool to immediately detect impending spinal cord damage and accordingly intervene for its prevention. If revascularization is necessary, the MEPs provide real-time information about the effectiveness of the surgical intervention on the particular segmental arteries involved. The surgical strategies enumerated in this article, when applied strictly, can reduce the incidence rate of paraplegia to less than 3%.[12]

REFERENCES

1. Jacobs MJ, Mommertz G, Koeppel TA, et al. Surgical repair of thoracoabdominal aortic aneurysms. J Cardiovasc Surg (Torino) 2007;48:49–58.
2. Coselli JS, LeMaire SA. Tips for successful outcomes for descending thoracic and thoracoabdominal aortic aneurysm procedures. Semin Vasc Surg 2008;21:13–20.
3. Safi HJ, Hess KR, Randel M, et al. Cerebrospinal fluid drainage and distal aortic perfusion: reducing neurologic complications in repair of thoracoabdominal aortic aneurysm types I and II. J Vasc Surg 1996;23:223–8.
4. Coselli JS, LeMaire SA, Schmittling ZC, et al. Cerebrospinal fluid drainage in thoracoabdominal aortic surgery. Semin Vasc Surg 2000;13:308–14.
5. Cambria RP, Davison JK, Carter C, et al. Epidural cooling for spinal cord protection during thoracoabdominal aneurysm repair: a five-year experience. J Vasc Surg 2000;31:1093–102.

6. Jacobs MJ, Meylaerts SA, de HP, et al. Strategies to prevent neurologic deficit based on motor-evoked potentials in type I and II thoracoabdominal aortic aneurysm repair. J Vasc Surg 1999;29:48–57.

7. Katz NM, Blackstone EH, Kirklin JW, et al. Incremental risk factors for spinal cord injury following operation for acute traumatic aortic transection. J Thorac Cardiovasc Surg 1981;81:669–74.

8. Backes WH, Nijenhuis RJ, Mess WH, et al. Magnetic resonance angiography of collateral blood supply to spinal cord in thoracic and thoracoabdominal aortic aneurysm patients. J Vasc Surg 2008;48:261–71.

9. Nijenhuis RJ, Jacobs MJ, Schurink GW, et al. Magnetic resonance angiography and neuromonitoring to assess spinal cord blood supply in thoracic and thoracoabdominal aortic aneurysm surgery. J Vasc Surg 2007;45:71–7.

10. Thron A. Anatomy of the spinal cord blood supply. In: Thron A, editor. Vascular anatomy of the spinal cord. Heidelberg (Germany): Springer-Verlag; 1988. p. 8–12.

11. Lasjaunias P, Bernstein A. Spinal and spinal cord arteries and veins. In: Lasjaunias P, Bernstein A, editors. Surgical neuroangiography. Heidelberg (Germany): Springer-Verlag; 1990. p. 15–87.

12. Jacobs MJ, de Mol BA, Elenbaas T, et al. Spinal cord blood supply in patients with thoracoabdominal aortic aneurysms. J Vasc Surg 2002;35:30–7.

13. Yamada N, Takamiya M, Kuribayashi S, et al. MRA of the Adamkiewicz artery: a preoperative study for thoracic aortic aneurysm. J Comput Assist Tomogr 2000;24:362–8.

14. Yoshioka K, Niinuma H, Ohira A, et al. MR angiography and CT angiography of the artery of Adamkiewicz: noninvasive preoperative assessment of thoracoabdominal aortic aneurysm. Radiographics 2003;23:1215–25.

15. Nijenhuis RJ, Jacobs MJ, Jaspers K, et al. Comparison of magnetic resonance with computed tomography angiography for preoperative localization of the Adamkiewicz artery in thoracoabdominal aortic aneurysm patients. J Vasc Surg 2007;45:677–85.

16. Kieffer E, Fukui S, Chiras J, et al. Spinal cord arteriography: a safe adjunct before descending thoracic or thoracoabdominal aortic aneurysmectomy. J Vasc Surg 2002;35:262–8.

17. Meylaerts SA, Jacobs MJ, van Iterson V, et al. Comparison of transcranial motor evoked potentials and somatosensory evoked potentials during thoracoabdominal aortic aneurysm repair. Ann Surg 1999;230:742–9.

18. Jacobs MJ, Mess W, Mochtar B, et al. The value of motor evoked potentials in reducing paraplegia during thoracoabdominal aneurysm repair. J Vasc Surg 2006;43:239–46.

19. Mommertz G, Langer S, Koeppel TA, et al. Brain and spinal cord protection during simultaneous aortic arch and thoracoabdominal aneurysm repair. J Vasc Surg 2009;49:886–92.

20. Mommertz G, Sigala F, Langer S, et al. Thoracoabdominal aortic aneurysm repair in patients with Marfan syndrome. Eur J Vasc Endovasc Surg 2008;35:181–6.

21. Khan SN, Stansby G. Cerebrospinal fluid drainage for thoracic and thoracoabdominal aortic aneurysm surgery. Cochrane Database Syst Rev 2004;(1): CD003635.

22. Wong DR, Coselli JS, Amerman K, et al. Delayed spinal cord deficits after thoracoabdominal aortic aneurysm repair. Ann Thorac Surg 2007;83: 1345–55.

23. Azizzadeh A, Huynh TT, Miller CC III, et al. Postoperative risk factors for delayed neurologic deficit after thoracic and thoracoabdominal aortic aneurysm repair: a case-control study. J Vasc Surg 2003;37: 750–4.

24. Dardik A, Perler BA, Roseborough GS, et al. Subdural hematoma after thoracoabdominal aortic aneurysm repair: an underreported complication of spinal fluid drainage? J Vasc Surg 2002;36: 47–50.

25. Weaver KD, Wiseman DB, Farber M, et al. Complications of lumbar drainage after thoracoabdominal aortic aneurysm repair. J Vasc Surg 2001;34:623–7.

Motor Evoked Potentials in Thoracoabdominal Aortic Surgery: CON

Joseph S. Coselli, MD[a,b,*], Peter I. Tsai, MD[a]

KEYWORDS

- Thoracoabdominal aortic aneurysm/surgery
- Motor evoked potentials • Paraplegia
- Intraoperative monitoring

Despite improvements in the medical management of aortic aneurysms, particularly the enhanced treatment of hypertension, the natural history of thoracoabdominal aortic aneurysms (TAAAs) remains dismal.[1,2] Without operative repair, the 5-year survival rate is 54%. For aneurysms greater than 6 cm in diameter the risk of death, rupture, or dissection is 16% per year.[3] However, even with surgical repair, promoting operative survival and preventing postoperative complications such as renal failure, pulmonary insufficiency, vocal cord paralysis, visceral embolization, and poor wound healing remain challenging.[4–10] At present, operation on virtually all symptomatic aneurysms and preemptive surgery on asymptomatic aneurysms is the primary means of preventing rupture, dissection, and death.

Undoubtedly, the most devastating complication after resection and replacement of the thoracoabdominal aorta remains spinal cord ischemic injury and the development of paraplegia. Even in comparatively high-volume, highly experienced surgical centers, the risk of paraplegia ranges from 4% to 16%.[4,6–9] The mechanisms by which paraplegia and paraparesis develop are imperfectly understood; however, they are thought to be related to ischemia caused by clamping the thoracic aorta, to the loss of direct perfusion of the spinal cord through the interruption of intercostal arteries, and to reperfusion injuries. Extensive loss of intercostal arteries (as in Crawford extent II TAAA repairs) is poorly tolerated by the spinal cord and substantially increases the risk of paraplegia. Even less extensive loss may make the spinal cord ischemic and increasingly dependent on collateral circulation; in such cases, spinal cord circulation remains precarious and susceptible to malperfusion from other causes, including hypotension, cardiac dysfunction, loss of collateral circulation (such as from previous abdominal aortic aneurysm repair), thrombosis or embolism, and individual comorbidities.[11–14]

Proposed methods to reduce or eliminate the risk of spinal cord ischemia and related paraplegia are directed at either maintaining or restoring adequate spinal cord arterial perfusion. Commonly used protective adjuncts include simply maintaining adequate (ie, normal or modestly increased) proximal systemic blood pressure, distal perfusion during cross-clamping by using cardiopulmonary or left atrial-femoral bypass, reimplanting critical intercostal and lumbar arteries, and cerebrospinal fluid drainage. Additional adjuncts to protect the spinal cord from cytotoxic damage when the

[a] Division of Cardiothoracic Surgery, Michael E. DeBakey Department of Surgery, Baylor College of Medicine, One Baylor Plaza, BCM 390, Houston, TX 77030, USA
[b] The Texas Heart Institute at St Luke's Episcopal Hospital, Houston, TX 77030, USA
* Corresponding author. Division of Cardiothoracic Surgery, Michael E. DeBakey Department of Surgery, Baylor College of Medicine, One Baylor Plaza, BCM 390, Houston, TX 77030.
E-mail address: jcoselli@bcm.edu

Cardiol Clin 28 (2010) 361–368
doi:10.1016/j.ccl.2010.01.001

perfusion pressure is insufficient include local hypothermia (such as that achieved by regional lumbar epidural cooling),[15,16] systemic profound hypothermia,[17] and directed pharmacologic management with neuroprotective agents, such as free radical scavengers, barbiturates, corticosteroids, papaverine, and opioid antagonists.[18–21] As yet, no method or combination of methods has proven to be 100% effective in preventing paraplegia.

EVOKED POTENTIAL MONITORING

Traditionally, the primary limitation of paraplegia-protection strategies has been that, during surgery, spinal cord perfusion cannot be assessed rapidly and accurately enough to allow the timely modification of surgical technique to mitigate the risk that paraplegia will develop. Since the early work of Coles and colleagues[22] and Cunningham and colleagues,[23,24] which demonstrated that it was possible to detect spinal cord ischemia intraoperatively by monitoring somatosensory evoked potentials (SSEPs, generated by the stimulation of peripheral nerves), there has been great interest among cardiovascular surgeons in applying this technique to TAAA surgery. Somatosensory evoked potential monitoring might have garnered even greater interest were it not for troubling reports of the technique producing false-negative results.[25]

Since the introduction of myogenic transcranial motor evoked potential (tc-MEP) monitoring by Merton and Morton[26] in 1980, this technique has been tested as a method of guarding against the development of paraplegia. Potentially, tc-MEP monitoring can be used to assess motor tract function by recording signal amplitude and latency in the descending motor system (located in the anterior and lateral corticospinal tracts) and in the anterior horn motor neuronal system, and by measuring the function of ischemia-sensitive α motor neurons. Conceptually, tc-MEP monitoring is a highly sensitive technique for assessing spinal cord integrity in real time by promptly alerting surgeons to any critical exclusion of segmental arteries that contribute vitally to spinal cord perfusion.

ANESTHESIA DURING tc-MEP MONITORING

tc-MEP monitoring necessitates the use of specifically designed anesthetic techniques. Complete peripheral muscle relaxation and neuromuscular blockade do not allow reliable recording of MEP output signals. In addition, the use of inhalation halogenated anesthetics and nitrous oxide leads to reduced MEP signals, which limits one's ability to detect ischemic conditions. Therefore, the use of inhalation agents in patients undergoing tc-MEP monitoring is significantly curtailed. This constraint poses a significant challenge in balancing the need to provide adequate anesthesia with the need to accurately monitor the spinal cord and avoid compromising its motor signals.[26–28]

If the use of MEP monitoring is planned, administering a short-acting neuromuscular blocker is generally acceptable in the earliest stages of thoracoabdominal repair (after induction and intubation); it is done at this time to avoid any possible interference with monitoring later in the repair and in good faith that the early application will not interfere with the surgical procedure. An alternative approach is to attempt to induce incomplete muscle relaxation. This technique requires that relaxation be tightly controlled according to the continuously monitored amplitude of muscle response to peripheral nerve stimulation. Jacobs and Mess[29] have achieved graded muscle relaxation by using a closed-loop feedback system created from a Relaxograph neuromuscular transmission monitor (Datex-Ohmeda, GE Healthcare, Helsinki, Finland). This technique involves a complex set of maneuvers, including the stimulation of the ulnar nerve supramaximally at the wrist; this is done preoperatively to establish a baseline and then repeatedly after the induction of anesthesia (using an on or off application of 2 μg/kg/min vecuronium) whenever the compound muscle action potential rises to more than 20% of the maximal response. All of these tasks are well within the capabilities of a competent, experienced, and dedicated anesthesia team.

Pelosi and colleagues[30] compared the effects of mixed intravenous-inhalation anesthesia (with isoflurane and nitrous oxide) and purely intravenous anesthesia (with propofol and opioids) on MEP results and found that the use of isoflurane/nitrous oxide was associated with less consistent, smaller, and more variable MEP signals. In contrast, opioids have minimal impact on MEP recording.[28] Quinones-Hinojosa and colleagues[31] confirmed that the combination of 0.5 minimum alveolar concentration desflurane and propofol/opioid infusion allowed satisfactory measurement of tc-MEP. Clearly, because the signal amplitudes of MEP recordings can be small, the effect of inhalation agents can limit the ability of anesthesiologists and neurologists to detect significant changes in real time. Kakimoto and colleagues,[32] in an attempt to mitigate the possibility of weak signals, found that applying 2 to 5 seconds of tetanic stimulation to the peripheral muscles 1 to 5 seconds before sending the tc-MEP signal effectively augments MEP monitoring by increasing the signal.

However, restricting inhalation agents to 0.5 of the minimum alveolar concentration could conceivably increase the incidence of intraoperative recall, although this possibility is primarily theoretical. In addition, one must consider that if only intravenous anesthesia is used (because of the depressive effects of inhalation agents on the strength of MEP signals), continuous infusion pumps are generally required, because any sudden change in dosage can cause MEP signal changes and confound interpretation; however, the use of continuous infusion pumps increases the complexity of anesthetic management.

Anesthesiologists must also be concerned with the possibility of blockade potentiation, which can occur with the administration of commonly used intravenous pharmacologic agents that can depress MEP amplitudes. These agents include magnesium and antihypertensive drugs, such as α_2 receptor antagonists.[33]

RISKS ASSOCIATED WITH TC-MEP MONITORING
Thermal Injury

Safety standards for monitoring equipment have been set by the International Electrotechnical Commission (IEC). For one, the electrical stimulator output should not exceed 50 mJ through 1000-Ω load resistance.[34] The primary concern about excess electrical stimulation is that it may cause thermal injury to either the scalp or the brain. Although virtually all clinical applications do not involve exceeding these limits, for unclear reasons, intraoperative skin burns at monitoring electrode sites can still occur. In addition, it is possible that an equipment malfunction could cause a brief, high-intensity electrosurgical radiofrequency current or a sustained, low-intensity direct current to be delivered to the patient.[35,36] Short-pulse stimulators also pose a risk of exceeding the IEC limit and causing scalp burns unless low scalp electrode impedance is assured to avoid needlessly high current.[37]

Electrochemical Injury

At the electrode-tissue interface, direct cortical monophasic pulse trains can begin to transfer charge through faradic current involving electrochemical reactions, resulting in a local accumulation of a variety of toxic products.[38] To obviate this problem, biphasic pulse trains were introduced in the 1950s. These consist of 2 phases of opposite polarity that drive electrochemical reactions in opposite directions and consequently minimize the accumulation of potentially toxic by-products.[39] However, biphasic stimulation is generally less effective for inducing neuronal activation. Thus, in the clinical setting, MEP monitoring usually involves monophasic direct cortical trains. Generally, because the pulses are extremely brief (<1 second), the faradic current is limited. Fortunately, MEP monitoring in aortic surgery does not involve direct cortical stimulation; rather, stimulation is applied transcranially. Although there is a paucity of clinical evidence of either the safety or the toxicity of current approaches, they appear to be reasonably safe. Further investigation would prove valuable in confirming this apparent safety.

Excitotoxic Injury to the Brain

The development of cerebral excitotoxicity during clinical MEP monitoring seems to be highly unlikely. To date there are no reports of any signs or symptoms of such an injury, although histologic data that could confirm the absence of injury are lacking. Animal experiments have tested the safety of repeated direct cortical stimulation with continuous 50-Hz biphasic pulse trains for several hours at a time. Under these extreme conditions, excitotoxic neuronal damage has been confirmed histologically.[40] However, in a human study, Gordon and colleagues[41] found no evidence of tissue damage after 50-Hz intermittent biphasic pulse trains lasting up to 5 seconds. To date, no experiments have evaluated the safety of brief, intermittent pulse trains analogous to those used intraoperatively. Nonetheless, provided that the charge and charged density values are kept below experimental injury thresholds, the risk of excitotoxic injury should remain minimal. However, most clinicians favor larger electrodes, which produce lower charged density and consequently avoid the risk of a needlessly high charge.

Seizure Activity

Clinical use and experience in orthopedic and aortic surgery have indicated that seizures related to MEP monitoring are exceedingly rare. It is well known that direct cortical stimulation with 50- to 60-Hz pulse trains lasting 1 to 5 seconds induces clinical seizure in 5% to 20% of patients.[42] Again, in aortic surgery, MEPs performed in a transcranial fashion substantially reduce any potential risk. It remains possible that pulse-train brain stimulation could provoke a clinical seizure; however, no intraoperative seizures have yet been reported during single-pulse transcranial stimulation. Regardless, it may be difficult to separate the influence of cerebral stimulation from that of anesthesia should seizure activity develop.

Cardiovascular Issues

The development of cardiac arrhythmia and hypertension remains a theoretical possibility during any operation in which MEP monitoring and pulse-train stimulation are used. Although hard evidence is lacking, it has been hypothesized that deep current penetration to the hypothalamus or brain stem could cause these complications. To reduce this potential risk, the use of high-intensity signals or widely spaced electrodes is largely avoided. Certainly, one needs to differentiate any electrocardiographic artifacts stemming from transcranial electrical stimulation from actual cardiac arrhythmias, and such confounds may further complicate the anesthesiologist's job.[35,37,43,44]

Movement-Induced Injuries

In the absence of neuromuscular blockade, patient movement presents a clinical nuisance, but it also may pose at least a theoretical danger to the patient intraoperatively. Partial neuromuscular blockade may dampen, but not necessarily eliminate, movement. Movement-induced injuries include any bite injury arising from a contraction of the jaw muscle during electrical stimulation. This risk is low (the estimated incidence of bite injuries is approximately 0.2% with transcranial sublingual stimulation), but such injuries can be severe, and they have included significant tongue and lip lacerations and at least one mandibular fracture.[44,45] Using a soft bite block or packing gauze between the molars may reduce the risk of these complications and of endotracheal tube damage, the occurrence of which necessitates emergency reintubation under extremely difficult circumstances; repositioning a double-lumen endotracheal tube in the lateral position is a challenging task that may distract the surgeon from the job at hand and, ultimately, affect the success of the procedure.

Hypothermia

Hypothermia has long been understood to provide protection to the spinal cord.[46] Hypothermic conditions in standard TAAA repair are generally mild and passive, because core body temperature is permitted to drift downward during the course of repair. However, profound total hypothermia (such as that used by Kouchoukos and colleagues[17]) or moderate hypothermia related to regional epidural lumbar cooling[15,16] may be used in TAAA repair. There is scarce literature regarding the impact of hypothermia on MEP monitoring. However,

hypothermia is generally thought to adversely affect MEP monitoring because decreasing temperature slows the rate of electrical conduction and diminishes signal amplitude, thereby altering the stimulation threshold such that MEP monitoring becomes unreliable. Additional confounders include neurophysiologic changes that affect resting potential, duration of action potential, and depression of synaptic transmission.[28,47,48]

In animal models, it appears that moderate hypothermia (approaching 28°C) may diminish MEPs in certain settings. In rabbits that were surface-cooled to esophageal temperatures of 28°C to 35°C, Sakamoto and colleagues[49] explored the effect of decreasing temperature on single-pulse, 3-pulse, and 5-pulse trains. Compared with rabbits at normothermic temperatures of 38°C, rabbits cooled to 28°C had significantly reduced MEP amplitudes after single-pulse stimulation. However, when 3- and 5-pulse trains were used, MEP amplitude was not affected by decreasing temperature. In addition, decreasing temperatures were shown to linearly increase MEP latency in this model, with the lowest temperature (28°C) almost doubling the latency. In a porcine 5-pulse train model, Meylaerts and colleagues[47] examined the influence of moderate hypothermia (28°C) achieved by regional spinal cord cooling on MEPs after the clamping of previously identified key intercostal arteries. No significant difference was found between MEP amplitudes recorded under moderately hypothermic (28°C) and normothermic conditions. Although the investigators determined that MEP latencies increased linearly with decreasing temperature, at 28°C this change was small.

Meylaerts and colleagues[47] also examined the impact of profound cooling (to temperatures as low as 4°C) on signal amplitude by assessing the amplitude every minute during cooling. It was hoped to find a temperature threshold associated with a 25% loss in MEP amplitude, which was considered to indicate ischemic spinal cord dysfunction. With extensive cooling (to temperatures as low as 10°C), MEP amplitudes decreased and reached the 25% threshold at an average temperature of 14°C. This relationship was not linear; rather, it followed a quadratic regression curve. The investigators concluded that at cerebrospinal fluid temperatures below 25°C, MEP monitoring may become unreliable because of significant decreases in the MEP response (false-positives) that may be difficult to distinguish from actual spinal cord ischemia.

In an attempt to examine the specificity and sensitivity of monitoring, Shine and colleagues[16] analyzed retrospective data from a series of 58 consecutive TAAA repairs performed at the Mayo clinic in which MEP and SSEP monitoring were used. Regional lumbar epidural cooling was used to cool the patients to between 26°C and 28°C. Paraplegia developed in 10 of the patients. When these patients' monitoring data were compared with data recorded from the 48 patients without paraplegia, the investigators found that the negative predictive value of monitoring was high (84%–100%), but the positive predictive value was low (22%–35%). Thus, although the likelihood of developing paraplegia when the MEP signal is present is very low, the overall specificity is also low, so that patients may be subjected to needlessly prolonged repairs. In addition, these investigators observed that paraplegia was more likely to develop when the MEP signal was lost quickly; they noted that the median time to signal loss was 10 minutes for patients with paraplegia and 31 minutes for patients without paraplegia. In a case report of a TAAA repair performed after regional epidural lumbar cooling, Denda and colleagues[50] noted persistent loss of MEPs during the repair but no subsequent paraplegia. These investigators suggest that this false positive may have been related to narrowed subarachnoid space during cooling, or by the particular anesthetic agents used.

Peripheral Ischemia

Thoracoabdominal aortic repair frequently involves cannulating the femoral artery to provide a site for circulation return. Such cannulation generally creates a usually well-tolerated ischemia of the involved leg. However, it is not completely clear how this ischemia may affect motor function and MEP monitoring. Jacobs and colleagues[51] mention that lower-limb ischemia could affect MEP readings by altering the responsiveness of the muscle tissue in that area, and at times these investigators have inserted a second, antegrade femoral artery cannula.

POSTOPERATIVE MONITORING

Delayed paraplegia can develop after the patient initially awakens with intact neuromuscular function. The mechanism of delayed paraplegia is not clearly understood, but postoperative hypotension probably plays a role in its development. Kieffer and colleagues'[52] report on their experience with thoracoabdominal aortic repair stated that 3 of 8 (38%) cases of paraplegia had a delayed onset. Likewise, in a previously reported review of 2368 TAAA repairs at the authors' own site,[53] 37% (34/93) of all cases of paraplegia were delayed; paraplegia manifested between 13 hours and 91

days after the operation. Because only 26% of patients with delayed paraplegia had episodes of hypotension, other, as yet unidentified factors must also play a role in the development of postoperative spinal cord ischemia. However, in published outcomes of TAAA repair, it is not often clear what proportion of the reported cases of paraplegia had a delayed onset. Nonetheless, there is anecdotal evidence that delayed paraplegia is a not an insignificant or uncommon event after open, endovascular, and hybrid repairs.[54–57]

This late complication is devastating and frustrating. However, preventing it by the use of MEP monitoring in the postoperative period is simply not practical, because the electrical stimulation is too painful to use on conscious patients.[58] Furthermore, MEPs are generally considered unreliable in sedated patients. Postoperative SSEP monitoring is similarly unreliable, because even if sedation is sufficient, movement may occur that affects monitoring.

CONTRAINDICATIONS TO MEP MONITORING

Relative contraindications include existing patient comorbidities such as epilepsy, cortical lesions, convexity skull defects, raised intracranial pressure, proconvulsant medications or anesthetics, intracranial electrodes, vascular clips or shunts, and cardiac pacemakers or other implanted biomedical devices. Admittedly, this may be an incomplete listing of contraindications, because there is a lack of published outcomes of MEP use. In addition, some of the listed contraindications are theoretical and may be inferred from direct cortical stimulation experience. Moreover, one should be mindful that the use of multiple signals, as in pulse trains, greatly increases the possibility of confounded results, particularly as pertains to nonsynaptic and synaptic corticomotor neuron excitation, synaptic transfer, spontaneous variability, peripheral and spinal cord tract conduction, and neuromuscular transmission.[37]

SUMMARY

Paraplegia remains the nemesis of both surgeon and patient. Such a devastating complication necessitates the continued development of mitigating strategies and the refinement of existing ones. Here, the authors have played the role of "devil's advocate" in exploring the practical and theoretical limitations of MEP monitoring as used to prevent the development of spinal cord ischemia and its related complications, paraplegia and paraparesis. Although the proper application of MEPs in the intraoperative monitoring of spinal cord function remains a considerable challenge, there are highly experienced institutions that have developed expertise in this application and that can use it effectively to prevent paraplegia after aortic repair.[29,59,60] However, in less experienced centers, surgeons may rely too much on MEP monitoring to guide intercostal artery reattachment or ligation strategy during highly complex anatomic and surgical repairs. Such overreliance on this difficult-to-implement technique could cause harm if surgical missteps are taken on the basis of monitoring information (or misinformation). These missteps include not restoring crucial intercostal arteries or needlessly extending the duration of operative repair.

Reflective of the difficulties generally encountered in the routine use of MEP monitoring in aortic surgery, Jacobs and colleagues[60] found that MEP fluctuations of up to 50% commonly occur during TAAA procedures, and that most of these fluctuations are not related to any intervention. It is fortunate that the authors now have several tools in their armamentarium to monitor for and attempt to lower the risk of paraplegia in those patients who undergo thoracoabdominal aortic resection. The use of preoperative magnetic resonance angiography mapping to identify vital feeding arteries or any possible collateral circulation of the spinal cord can be a crucial step in planning the repair. Intraoperative blood pressure manipulation and cerebrospinal fluid drainage to optimize spinal cord perfusion, and the use of MEPs to guide the aggressiveness with which surgeons reattach intercostal/lumbar segmental vessels (including debridement and endarterectomy), have definitely protected some patients from paraplegia.

Again, this article only serves to bring to attention the intraoperative limitations of using MEP monitoring during complex aortic repair, which are the confounding effects of anesthesia, the need for short-acting neuromuscular blockade, the potential for thermal or electrochemical injury to the skin, the possibility of excitotoxic injury to the brain or the development of seizures, the confounding effects of hypothermia, and potential cardiovascular arrhythmic or neuromuscular complications, as well as the need to be aware of the complexities of signal delivery and how single-pulse delivery can differ from pulse-train delivery. In addition to these limitations, surgeons must be familiar with the various contraindications to the use of MEP monitoring. Further research is warranted to improve the clinical use of MEP monitoring, particularly by developing methods to eliminate false-negative signals associated with subsequent delayed paraplegia. Possible mitigating strategies include the use of cold blood

aortic infusion as an adjunct to MEP monitoring, which has been shown to accelerate MEP changes and facilitate the identification of critical intercostal arteries.[61]

Centers of excellence with vast experience in thoracoabdominal aortic repair will continue to drive the incidence of associated paraplegia downward. The proportion of paraplegia cases that are delayed-onset, rather than immediate-onset, demands further study, particularly regarding the influence of postoperative episodic hypotension on the development of delayed-onset paraplegia. Understanding the limitations of MEP monitoring will no doubt improve its clinical application and assist in further reducing paraplegia rates.

ACKNOWLEDGMENTS

The authors express gratitude to Stephen N. Palmer, PhD, ELS, of the Texas Heart Institute, as well as Susan Y. Green, MPH, for editorial assistance.

REFERENCES

1. Elefteriades JA. Natural history of thoracic aortic aneurysms: indications for surgery, and surgical versus nonsurgical risks. Ann Thorac Surg 2002; 74(5):S1877–80 [discussion: S1892–8].
2. Griepp RB, Ergin MA, Galla JD, et al. Natural history of descending thoracic and thoracoabdominal aneurysms. Ann Thorac Surg 1999;67(6):1927–30 [discussion: 1953–8].
3. Davies RR, Goldstein LJ, Coady MA, et al. Yearly rupture or dissection rates for thoracic aortic aneurysms: simple prediction based on size. Ann Thorac Surg 2002;73(1):17–27 [discussion: 27–8].
4. Coselli JS, Bozinovski J, LeMaire SA. Open surgical repair of 2286 thoracoabdominal aortic aneurysms. Ann Thorac Surg 2007;83(2):S862–4.
5. LeMaire SA, Carter SA, Volguina IV, et al. Spectrum of aortic operations in 300 patients with confirmed or suspected Marfan syndrome. Ann Thorac Surg 2006;81(6):2063–78.
6. Chiesa R, Melissano G, Civilini E, et al. Ten years experience of thoracic and thoracoabdominal aortic aneurysm surgical repair: lessons learned. Ann Vasc Surg 2004;18(5):514–20.
7. Conrad MF, Crawford RS, Davison JK, et al. Thoracoabdominal aneurysm repair: a 20-year perspective. Ann Thorac Surg 2007;83(2):S856–61.
8. Svensson LG, Crawford ES, Hess KR, et al. Experience with 1509 patients undergoing thoracoabdominal aortic operations. J Vasc Surg 1993; 17(2):357–68.

9. Schepens MA, Heijmen RH, Ranschaert W, et al. Thoracoabdominal aortic aneurysm repair: results of conventional open surgery. Eur J Vasc Endovasc Surg 2009;37(6):640–5.

10. Misfeld M, Sievers HH, Hadlak M, et al. Rate of paraplegia and mortality in elective descending and thoracoabdominal aortic repair in the modern surgical era. Thorac Cardiovasc Surg 2008;56(6):342–7.

11. Acher CW, Wynn MM, Hoch JR, et al. Cardiac function is a risk factor for paralysis in thoracoabdominal aortic replacement. J Vasc Surg 1998; 27(5):821–8.

12. Coselli JS, LeMaire SA, Miller CC III, et al. Mortality and paraplegia after thoracoabdominal aortic aneurysm repair: a risk factor analysis. Ann Thorac Surg 2000;69(2):409–14.

13. Kawanishi Y, Munakata H, Matsumori M, et al. Usefulness of transcranial motor evoked potentials during thoracoabdominal aortic surgery. Ann Thorac Surg 2007;83(2):456–61.

14. Schlosser FJ, Mojibian H, Verhagen HJ, et al. Open thoracic or thoracoabdominal aortic aneurysm repair after previous abdominal aortic aneurysm surgery. J Vasc Surg 2008;48(3):761–8.

15. Cambria RP, Davison JK, Carter C, et al. Epidural cooling for spinal cord protection during thoracoabdominal aneurysm repair: a five-year experience. J Vasc Surg 2000;31(6):1093.

16. Shine TS, Harrison BA, De Ruyter ML, et al. Motor and somatosensory evoked potentials: their role in predicting spinal cord ischemia in patients undergoing thoracoabdominal aortic aneurysm repair with regional lumbar epidural cooling. Anesthesiology 2008;108(4):580–7.

17. Kouchoukos NT, Masetti P, Rokkas CK, et al. Safety and efficacy of hypothermic cardiopulmonary bypass and circulatory arrest for operations on the descending thoracic and thoracoabdominal aorta. Ann Thorac Surg 2001;72(3):699–707.

18. Acher CW, Wynn M. A modern theory of paraplegia in the treatment of aneurysms of the thoracoabdominal aorta: an analysis of technique specific observed/expected ratios for paralysis. J Vasc Surg 2009;49(5):1117–24 [discussion: 1124].

19. Coles JC, Ahmed SN, Mehta HU, et al. Role of free radical scavenger in protection of spinal cord during ischemia. Ann Thorac Surg 1986;41(5):551–6.

20. Kunihara T, Matsuzaki K, Shiiya N, et al. Naloxone lowers cerebrospinal fluid levels of excitatory amino acids after thoracoabdominal aortic surgery. J Vasc Surg 2004;40(4):681–90.

21. Lim KH, Connolly M, Rose D, et al. Prevention of reperfusion injury of the ischemic spinal cord: use of recombinant superoxide dismutase. Ann Thorac Surg 1986;42(3):282–6.

22. Coles JG, Wilson GJ, Sima AF, et al. Intraoperative detection of spinal cord ischemia using somatosensory cortical evoked potentials during thoracic aortic occlusion. Ann Thorac Surg 1982; 34(3):299–306.

23. Cunningham JN Jr, Laschinger JC, Spencer FC. Monitoring of somatosensory evoked potentials during surgical procedures on the thoracoabdominal aorta. IV. Clinical observations and results. J Thorac Cardiovasc Surg 1987;94(2):275–85.

24. Laschinger JC, Cunningham JN Jr, Cooper MM, et al. Monitoring of somatosensory evoked potentials during surgical procedures on the thoracoabdominal aorta. I. Relationship of aortic cross-clamp duration, changes in somatosensory evoked potentials, and incidence of neurologic dysfunction. J Thorac Cardiovasc Surg 1987;94(2):260–5.

25. Crawford ES, Mizrahi EM, Hess KR, et al. The impact of distal aortic perfusion and somatosensory evoked potential monitoring on prevention of paraplegia after aortic aneurysm operation. J Thorac Cardiovasc Surg 1988;95(3):357–67.

26. Merton PA, Morton HB. Stimulation of the cerebral cortex in the intact human subject. Nature 1980; 285(5762):227.

27. Jellinek D, Platt M, Jewkes D, et al. Effects of nitrous oxide on motor evoked potentials recorded from skeletal muscle in patients under total anesthesia with intravenously administered propofol. Neurosurgery 1991;29(4):558–62.

28. Wang AC, Than KD, Etame AB, et al. Impact of anesthesia on transcranial electric motor evoked potential monitoring during spine surgery: a review of the literature. Neurosurg Focus 2009;27(4):E7.

29. Jacobs MJ, Mess WH. The role of evoked potential monitoring in operative management of type I and type II thoracoabdominal aortic aneurysms. Semin Thorac Cardiovasc Surg 2003;15(4):353–64.

30. Pelosi L, Lamb J, Grevitt M, et al. Combined monitoring of motor and somatosensory evoked potentials in orthopaedic spinal surgery. Clin Neurophysiol 2002;113(7):1082–91.

31. Quinones-Hinojosa A, Lyon R, Zada G, et al. Changes in transcranial motor evoked potentials during intramedullary spinal cord tumor resection correlate with postoperative motor function. Neurosurgery 2005;56(5):982–93 [discussion: 982–93].

32. Kakimoto M, Kawaguchi M, Yamamoto Y, et al. Tetanic stimulation of the peripheral nerve before transcranial electrical stimulation can enlarge amplitudes of myogenic motor evoked potentials during general anesthesia with neuromuscular blockade. Anesthesiology 2005;102(4):733–8.

33. de Haan P, Kalkman CJ. Spinal cord monitoring: somatosensory- and motor-evoked potentials. Anesthesiol Clin North America 2001;19(4):923–45.

34. International Electrotechnical Commission. Medical electrical equipment—Part 2-40: particular requirements for the safety of electromyographs and evoked

response equipment. IEC 60601-2-40 ed1.0, Available at: http://webstore.iec.ch/webstore/webstore.nsf/artnum/022837. Accessed December 10, 2009.

35. MacDonald DB, Deletis V. Safety issues during surgical monitoring. In: Nuwer MR, editor. Intraoperative monitoring of neural function: handbook of clinical neurophysiology. Boston: Elsevier; 2008. p. 882–98.

36. Russell MJ, Gaetz M. Intraoperative electrode burns. J Clin Monit Comput 2004;18(1):25–32.

37. MacDonald DB. Intraoperative motor evoked potential monitoring: overview and update. J Clin Monit Comput 2006;20(5):347–77.

38. Merrill DR, Bikson M, Jefferys JG. Electrical stimulation of excitable tissue: design of efficacious and safe protocols. J Neurosci Methods 2005;141(2):171–98.

39. Girvin JP. A review of basic aspects concerning cerebral stimulation. In: Cooper IS, editor. Cerebellar stimulation in man. New York: Raven Press; 1978. p. 1–12.

40. McCreery DB, Agnew WF, Yuen TG, et al. Charge density and charge per phase as cofactors in neural injury induced by electrical stimulation. IEEE Trans Biomed Eng 1990;37(10):996–1001.

41. Gordon B, Lesser RP, Rance NE, et al. Parameters for direct cortical electrical stimulation in the human: histopathologic confirmation. Electroencephalogr Clin Neurophysiol 1990;75(5):371–7.

42. Sartorius CJ, Wright G. Intraoperative brain mapping in a community setting—technical considerations. Surg Neurol 1997;47(4):380–8.

43. Journee HL. Electrical safety in intraoperative monitoring. In: Proceedings of the Symposium on Intraoperative Neurophysiology. Ljubljana, Slovenia, October 17–18, 2003. p. 65–8.

44. MacDonald DB. Safety of intraoperative transcranial electrical stimulation motor evoked potential monitoring. J Clin Neurophysiol 2002;19(5):416–29.

45. Calancie B, Harris W, Broton JG, et al. "Threshold-level" multipulse transcranial electrical stimulation of motor cortex for intraoperative monitoring of spinal motor tracts: description of method and comparison to somatosensory evoked potential monitoring. J Neurosurg 1998;88(3):457–70.

46. Pontius RG, Brockman HL, Hardy EG, et al. The use of hypothermia in the prevention of paraplegia following temporary aortic occlusion: experimental observations. Surgery 1954;36(1):33–8.

47. Meylaerts SA, De Haan P, Kalkman CJ, et al. The influence of regional spinal cord hypothermia on transcranial myogenic motor-evoked potential monitoring and the efficacy of spinal cord ischemia detection. J Thorac Cardiovasc Surg 1999;118(6):1038–45.

48. Seyal M, Mull B. Mechanisms of signal change during intraoperative somatosensory evoked potential monitoring of the spinal cord. J Clin Neurophysiol 2002;19(5):409–15.

49. Sakamoto T, Kawaguchi M, Kakimoto M, et al. The effect of hypothermia on myogenic motor-evoked potentials to electrical stimulation with a single pulse and a train of pulses under propofol/ketamine/fentanyl anesthesia in rabbits. Anesth Analg 2003;96(6):1692–7.

50. Denda S, Taneoka M, Honda H, et al. Prolonged loss of leg myogenic motor evoked potentials during thoracoabdominal aortic aneurysm repair, without postoperative paraplegia. J Anesth 2006;20(4):314–8.

51. Jacobs MJ, Meylaerts SA, de Haan P, et al. Strategies to prevent neurologic deficit based on motor-evoked potentials in type I and II thoracoabdominal aortic aneurysm repair. J Vasc Surg 1999;29(1):48–57 [discussion: 57–9].

52. Kieffer E, Chiche L, Godet G, et al. Type IV thoracoabdominal aneurysm repair: predictors of postoperative mortality, spinal cord injury, and acute intestinal ischemia. Ann Vasc Surg 2008;22(6):822–8.

53. Wong DR, Coselli JS, Amerman K, et al. Delayed spinal cord deficits after thoracoabdominal aortic aneurysm repair. Ann Thorac Surg 2007;83(4):1345–55 [discussion: 1355].

54. Backes WH, Nijenhuis RJ, Mess WH, et al. Magnetic resonance angiography of collateral blood supply to spinal cord in thoracic and thoracoabdominal aortic aneurysm patients. J Vasc Surg 2008;48(2):261–71.

55. Chiesa R, Melissano G, Marrocco-Trischitta MM, et al. Spinal cord ischemia after elective stent-graft repair of the thoracic aorta. J Vasc Surg 2005;42(1):11–7.

56. Lawlor DK, Faizer R, Forbes TL. The hybrid aneurysm repair: extending the landing zone in the thoracoabdominal aorta. Ann Vasc Surg 2007;21(2):211–5.

57. Tshomba Y, Bertoglio L, Marone EM, et al. Visceral aortic patch aneurysm after thoracoabdominal aortic repair: conventional vs hybrid treatment. J Vasc Surg 2008;48(5):1083–91.

58. Guerit JM, Dion RA. State-of-the-art of neuromonitoring for prevention of immediate and delayed paraplegia in thoracic and thoracoabdominal aorta surgery. Ann Thorac Surg 2002;74(5):S1867–9 [discussion: S1892–8].

59. Jacobs MJ, de Mol BA, Elenbaas T, et al. Spinal cord blood supply in patients with thoracoabdominal aortic aneurysms. J Vasc Surg 2002;35(1):30–7.

60. Jacobs MJ, Mess W, Mochtar B, et al. The value of motor evoked potentials in reducing paraplegia during thoracoabdominal aneurysm repair. J Vasc Surg 2006;43(2):239–46.

61. Hamaishi M, Orihashi K, Takahashi S, et al. Transcranial motor-evoked potentials following intra-aortic cold blood infusion facilitates detection of critical supplying artery of spinal cord. Eur J Cardiothorac Surg 2008;33(4):695–9.

Editorial Comment: Motor Evoked Potentials in Thoracoabdominal Aortic Surgery

John A. Elefteriades, MD

Dr Jacobs beautifully describes his surgical techniques and the conduct of motor evoked potential (MEP) monitoring. The results are excellent in his hands, and potentially paralysis-preventing modifications can be made in cases of diminution in MEPs.

Dr Coselli emphasizes the complexity and dangers of MEP monitoring as well as pointing out that in his hands and the experience of others, false-positive and false-negative results do occur.

Our Yale team formerly did not use MEPs. We have started using them in the past 2 years. We find them generally unobtrusive and helpful, but we have seen false-positive results (**Fig. 1**).

See **Table 1** for details about the arguments for and against MEPs.

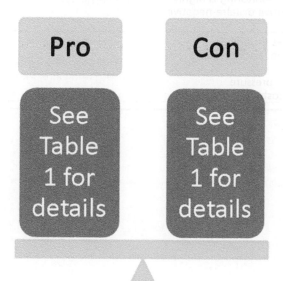

Fig. 1. Final impression: this one is a toss-up, with perhaps the world's 2 most experienced surgeons taking opposing stances, each supporting his point of view with cogent arguments.

Section of Cardiac Surgery, Department of Surgery, Yale University School of Medicine, Yale-New Haven Hospital, PO Box 208039, New Haven, CT 06520-8039, USA
E-mail address: john.elefteriades@yale.edu

Cardiol Clin 28 (2010) 369–370
doi:10.1016/j.ccl.2010.02.019

Table 1
Arguments for and against monitoring MEPs during thoracoabdominal aortic surgery

Pro: MEPs Should Be Monitored (Jacobs)	Con: MEPs Should Not Be Monitored (Coselli)
Paraplegia may still occur in up to 25% of cases in the highest risk groups	Anesthesia is complicated by MEP monitoring • No muscle relaxants • No inhalation agents
It is useful to identify the artery of Adamkiewicz by preoperative CT or MRI	Direct dangers • Burns at scalp electrodes • Neuronal injury due to continued stimulation • Possibility of seizures • Possibility of movement injury (extremities, face/jaw, endotracheal tube)
Discussion presumes all other techniques to prevent paraplegia are applied as well: left atrial–femoral artery bypass, spinal fluid drainage, relatively high blood pressure	Inaccuracy • High sensitivity (no false negative) • Low specificity (high false positive) • Perfused leg commonly loses signals • Hypothermia leads to decreased signals • Late paraplegia is not detected
Reduction of MEP amplitude indicates disturbed spinal cord blood supply and requires corrective measures	
In their experience, MEP monitoring is highly accurate—no false-positive or false-negative results	
Responses to restore MEPs include • Controlling steal from back-bleeding intercostals • Increasing perfusion pressure • Reimplanting intercostals	

What is the Best Method for Brain Protection in Surgery of the Aortic Arch? Retrograde Cerebral Perfusion

Yuichi Ueda, MD

KEYWORDS

- Aortic arch surgery • Brain protection
- Retrograde cerebral perfusion
- Hypothermic circulatory arrest
- Aortic arch replacement

Significant advances in aortic arch surgery have been made over the past several decades; however, aortic arch surgery is still challenging for surgeons. Surgery on the aortic arch requires systemic organ protection. Brain protection is the most critical because the brain is the most vulnerable organ during the interval in which normal circulation is interrupted. In addition to preventing ischemic injury, the prevention of stroke due to embolization of thrombus or atheromatous debris, which can escape into the cerebral circulation during the cooling phase of cardiopulmonary bypass and immediately after a graft replacement, is of overriding importance.

Antegrade cerebral perfusion and hypothermic circulatory arrest (HCA) are the 2 bypass techniques that were used for organ protection during aortic arch surgery in the past. HCA has been widely used, with acceptable surgical results since the 1970s.[1–9] HCA can be used by itself in most operations in which the duration of arrest is not expected to exceed 30 to 45 minutes.[1–4] The clinical application of continuous retrograde cerebral perfusion (RCP) combined with HCA for aortic arch surgery was first shown in a substantial series of reports starting in 1988.[10] Before 1990, RCP had been used for the aortic arch surgery mainly in Japan. Thereafter, many clinical articles demonstrated the efficacy of RCP and identified a reduction in early mortality and morbidity.[11–23] HCA with RCP was then routinely used as an adjunct for prolonged HCA in the 1990s.

In 1980, Mills and Ochsner[24] originally used RCP to treat accidental air embolisms during cardiopulmonary bypass. In 1982, Lemole and colleagues[25] reported the use of intermittent RCP for the treatment of an acute type A dissection using an intraluminal sutureless graft. They described the RCP method only briefly in a part of the discussion section, with a schema of the perfusion circuit. RCP into the superior vena cava (SVC) was used every 20 minutes during HCA. RCP was introduced independently in the author's department without notice of Lemole's article. This procedure was later extended from an intermittent administration to continuous administration.[10–12] RCP flow was always regulated to maintain a pressure of less than 20 mm Hg in the internal jugular vein, which was found to provide satisfactory RCP flow in experimental animal models.[26] Flow-regulated RCP is not recommended, but pressure-regulated RCP is favored to reduce the risk of

Division of Cardiac Surgery, Department of Surgery, Nagoya University Graduate School of Medicine, 65 Tsurumai-cho, Showa-ku, Nagoya 466-8550, Japan
E-mail address: yueda@med.nagoya-u.ac.jp

Cardiol Clin 28 (2010) 371–379
doi:10.1016/j.ccl.2010.01.006

brain edema with sustained high jugular vein pressure of more than 20 mm Hg.

However, there are several drawbacks in RCP with HCA, such as the requirement of an extended duration of cardiopulmonary bypass for cooling and rewarming, hemorrhagic tendencies, and a high incidence of postoperative delirium. There has been a question of whether efficient cerebral blood flow is provided by RCP.

This article discusses the clinical results and published data of aortic arch surgery using RCP and HCA. Experimental studies of RCP are also reviewed.

CLINICAL EXPERIENCE

The surgical techniques and results of aortic arch surgery in the author's department were published several times in the early 1990s.[10–12] In addition, a retrospective analysis of 249 patients who underwent aortic arch surgery at 3 Japanese cardiovascular centers where HCA with RCP was a routine adjunct was reported in 1999.[23] The subjects came from 3 Japanese hospitals, Tenri Hospital, National Cardiovascular Center, and Tokyo Women's Medical College, between January 1994 and December 1996. The pathology of the aortic arch was atherosclerotic aneurysm in 133 patients and dissection in 116. Seventy patients had surgery on an emergency basis. The hospital mortality was 25 of 249 (10%). Stroke developed in 11 patients (4%). The median duration of RCP was 46 minutes (range, 5–95 minutes). A multivariate logistic analysis revealed that pump time ($P = $ .0001), age ($P = $ .0001), and RCP time ($P = $ .052) are the most significant risk factors. The risk factors for mortality and neurologic morbidity are pump time ($P = $ .0001), age ($P = $ .0002), urgency of surgery ($P = $ .07), and RCP time ($P = $ .15). The relationship between mortality and the duration of RCP time is shown in **Fig. 1**.

A total of 207 patients who underwent aortic arch surgery using RCP and HCA at Tenri Hospital (138 patients) from 1988 to 1999 and at Nagoya University Hospital (69 patients) from 1990 to 2000 were retrospectively analyzed.[27] The pathology of the aorta included aortic dissection in 103 patients (50%) and atherosclerotic aneurysm in 104 patients (50%) (**Table 1**). The HCA times were 44 ± 20 minutes (**Table 2**). Hospital mortality was 12% (25 patients) overall (**Table 3**). A cardiopulmonary bypass time of longer than 6 hours, low cardiac output syndrome, respiratory failure, and central nervous system (CNS) dysfunction contributed to the hospital deaths (**Table 4**). Late mortality was 16% (34 patients). The predictors of late death were age (>70 years), total arch

replacement, HCA time longer than 60 minutes, nondissecting aneurysm, and postoperative CNS injury.

The results of aortic arch surgery using RCP and HCA were generally satisfactory in patients who underwent elective surgery. However, the long-term results of total arch replacement for patients older than 70 years, in particular for emergent aortic arch surgery, and patients suffering from postoperative CNS injury were poor (**Fig. 2**). Although the prolonged duration of HCA may contribute to these poor results, other factors such as emergency surgery, late death due to aging, and systemic atherosclerosis with severe aortic atheroma are considered to be major risk factors.

ARCH-FIRST TECHNIQUE

The arch-first technique (reconstruction of arch vessels first and distal anastomosis second) was adopted in 1999 instead of the distal anastomosis first technique, for total arch replacement in Nagoya University Hospital. The aim is to reduce the period of HCA and RCP time. Rokkas and Kouchoukos[28] originally advocated the arch-first technique. Details of the surgical technique using RCP were published in 2005 and 2007 (**Fig. 3**).[29,30] Total arch replacement using this procedure was performed in 91 cases (61 men and 30 women), with an average age of patients being 67 years. There were 66 cases of atherosclerotic arch aneurysms and 25 cases of aortic dissections. Mean HCA time was 31 ± 9 minutes, including RCP time of 14.5 ± 9 minutes. The cardiopulmonary bypass time was 225 ± 69 minutes. Surgical mortality occurred in 4 patients (4.4 %), and late death in 2 (2.2 %). Stroke was a complication in 7 cases (7.7%). The 5-year survival rate was 89.1%. The arch-first technique is superior to the conventional distal first technique for several reasons, such as less surgical mortality and morbidity, better neurologic outcomes, a higher survival rate, and a better quality of life. The arch-first technique is an excellent method for total arch replacement using RCP and HCA.

PUBLISHED CLINICAL STUDIES

In 1997, Safi and colleagues[19] demonstrated that the overall 30-day mortality rate was 6% and the incidence of stroke was 4% in 161 patients who underwent surgery for aneurysms of the ascending aorta and transverse arch using HCA and RCP. The use of RCP had a protective effect against stroke (3 of 120 patients or 3%) in comparison to the absence of RCP (4 of 41 patients or 9%;

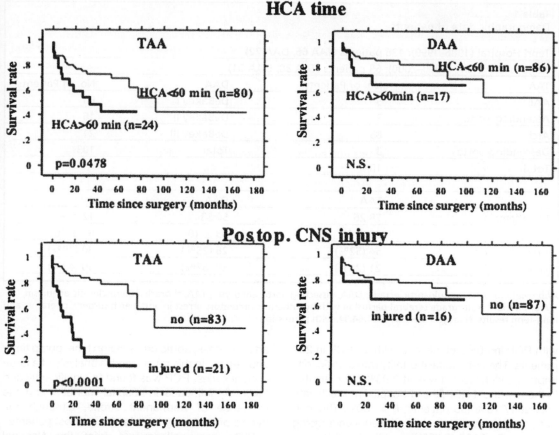

Fig. 1. Survival rates in patients with TAA and DAA: HCA time of more than 60 minutes and less than 60 minutes, and with or without postoperative CNS injury. DAA, dissecting aortic aneurysm; TAA, thoracic atherosclerotic aneurysm. (*From* Ueda Y. Retrograde cerebral perfusion with hypothermic circulatory arrest in aortic arch surgery: operative and long-term results. Nagoya J Med Sci 2001;64:98; with permission.)

$P<.049$), and this phenomenon was most significant in patients older than 70 years. The cardiopulmonary bypass time was the sole factor found to be associated with an increased risk of stroke and mortality.

These investigators revised their surgical results in 2008.[31] They performed 1107 repairs of the ascending and transverse aortic arch between August 1991 and June 2007. RCP was used in 82% of the cases (907 of 1107). Thirty-day mortality was 10.4% (115 of 1107). Stroke occurred in 2.8% (31 of 1107) of patients. The risk factors for stroke were an emergency status ($P<.009$) and hypertension ($P<.05$). RCP showed a protective effect against mortality and stroke. They concluded that the use of RCP with profound HCA was associated with a reduction in mortality and stroke. The use of RCP thus remains warranted during repairs of the ascending and transverse aortic arch. The use of RCP was also identified to be an independent factor that protected against early mortality, stroke, major

morbidity, and late death, although these results were not noted in previous animal experimental studies.

Safi's group also described the detection of RCP flow in the middle cerebral arteries during surgery.[31] The RCP flow rate will vary depending on the information obtained from bilateral power mode transcranial Doppler ultrasound and bilateral near-infrared spectroscopy (cerebral oximetry). The adequacy of RCP flow was determined by the presence of reversed blood flow in the middle cerebral arteries when power mode transcranial Doppler ultrasound was used. Although a higher "opening" pressure is required, the maintenance flow rate is often less than 500 mL/min, maintaining the SVC line pressure at less than 25 mm Hg. The information obtained from power mode transcranial Doppler ultrasound was correlated with information obtained from near-infrared spectroscopy (cerebral oximetry).

Coselli[20] also published results of aortic arch surgery from July 1987 to March 1997 using HCA

Table 1
Demographic data of patients

Tenri Hospital (1986–1999): 138 patients (TAA 66, DAA 72)

Nagoya University (1990–2000): 69 patients (TAA 38, DAA 31)

TAA	No. of Patients	DAA	No. of Patients
AAE	5	DeBakey I	66
Ascending aorta	3	DeBakey II	16
Arch	88	DeBakey III	21
Descending aorta	3	Total	103
Total	104		

	TAA	DAA	All
Male/female	78:26	50:53	128:79
Age (y)	69 ± 9	63 ± 10	66 ± 10
Age>70 y	54 (52%)	26 (25%)	80 (39%)
Emergency	21 (20%)	69 (67%)	90 (43%)

Abbreviations: AAE, annuloaortic ectasia; DAA, dissecting aortic aneurysm; TAA, thoracic atherosclerotic aneurysm.
From Ueda Y. Retrograde cerebral perfusion with hypothermic circulatory arrest in aortic arch surgery: operative and long-term results. Nagoya J Med Sci 2001;64:94; with permission.

with RCP in 305 patients and without RCP in 204 patients. The in-hospital mortality rate significantly improved with RCP; it was at 3.93% (12 patients). In those without RCP, the in-hospital mortality rate was at 17.16% (35 patients; P = .001). The incidence of permanent stroke in patients undergoing RCP was 8 of 305 (2.62%), and the incidence for those without RCP was 13 of 204 (6.37%, P = .037). The variables that were associated with early mortality in the patients with RCP were atherosclerotic heart disease, concurrent coronary artery bypass, aortic cross clamp time, pump time, and sepsis. In this retrospective analysis of a large clinical series, RCP was found to significantly and favorably influence in-hospital mortality and the incidence of permanent stroke, although the period of HCA may be tolerable in most patients.

Okita and colleagues[22] from the National Cardiovascular Center of Japan reported similar results and concluded that prolonged HCA and RCP for longer than 60 minutes was not a risk factor for mortality or stroke in patients who

Table 2
Operative data

	TAA	DAA	All
CPB time (min)	218 ± 106	209 ± 102	213 ± 104
CPB >6 h	6 (6%)	7 (7%)	13 (6%)
Operation (min)	457 ± 154	455 ± 244	456 ± 199
Operation >12 h	6 (6%)	8 (8%)	14 (7%)
HCA (min)	45 ± 19	43 ± 22	44 ± 20
HCA >60 min	24 (24%)	17 (17%)	41 (20%)
Aorta replaced			
Ascending aorta	4	23	27
Hemiarch	13	38	51
Aortic arch	30	25	55
Distal arch	49	9	58
Descending aorta	13	8	21

Abbreviations: CPB, cardiopulmonary bypass; DAA, dissecting aortic aneurysm; TAA, thoracic atherosclerotic aneurysm.
From Ueda Y. Retrograde cerebral perfusion with hypothermic circulatory arrest in aortic arch surgery: operative and long-term results. Nagoya J Med Sci 2001;64:95; with permission.

Table 3
Hospital and late death

	TAA	DAA	All
No. of patients	104	103	207
Hospital death	12 (11%)	13 (12%)	25 (12%)
Operative death	9 (9%)	6 (6%)	15 (7%)
Late death	22 (21%)	12 (12%)	34 (16%)
Lost follow-up	1 (1%)	4 (4%)	5 (2%)

Abbreviations: DAA, dissecting aortic aneurysm; TAA, thoracic atherosclerotic aneurysm.

underwent aortic arch surgery. However, the prevalence of transient delirium necessitates further investigation. Their logistic regression analysis showed that the risk factors for mortality were ruptured aneurysm, chronic obstructive pulmonary disease, arterial cannulation in the ascending aorta, and stroke.

In 2001, Reich and colleagues[32] published a review concerning RCP during thoracic aortic surgery. They summarized a large number of studies that demonstrated a spectrum of beneficial, neutral, and detrimental effects of RCP in humans and experimental animal models. They concluded that it remains unclear whether RCP provides effective cerebral perfusion, metabolic support, the washout of embolic material, and improved neurologic and neuropsychological outcomes.

ANIMAL EXPERIMENTAL STUDIES

Various experimental studies on animals have been performed to evaluate the efficacy or the

limitations of RCP.[32–39] The venous return route from the brain in animals, such as the dog or pig, differs much from that in humans. In humans, internal jugular veins, which have jugular bulbs with a remnant of venous valve, are the main venous drainage route from the brain. On the other hand, the external jugular veins, which have many venous valves, are the main venous route from the head in animals. Therefore, those animals can eat and drink while lowering their heads without difficulty, because the venous regurgitation to the head is regulated by the venous valves in the external jugular veins. Therefore, maintaining RCP flow is difficult in experimental animal models, and the pressure of RCP can become considerably high because of the competent venous valves in the animals.[37] RCP blood flow goes into rich collateral circulation to whole body. Furthermore, there were several controversial factors in the experimental protocols, such as an extended HCA with RCP time up to 90 to 120 minutes and body temperature of 20°C

Table 4
Predictors of hospital deaths

TAA	Univariate		Multivariate	
	Odds	P value	Odds	P value
Emergency surgery	5.534	0.0089		NS
CPB >6 h	21.74	0.0011		NS
Operation >12 h	1124	0.0075		NS
Bleeding	5.050	0.0235		NS
LOS	9.523	0.0111		NS
CNS injury	4.926	0.0131		NS
DAA				
CPB >6 h	6.060	0.0330		NS
Respiratory	3.817	0.0029		NS

Abbreviations: CPB, cardiopulmonary bypass; DAA, dissecting aortic aneurysm; LOS, low cardiac output syndrome; NS, not significant; TAA, thoracic atherosclerotic aneurysm.

From Ueda Y. Retrograde cerebral perfusion with hypothermic circulatory arrest in aortic arch surgery: operative and long-term results. Nagoya J Med Sci 2001;64:96; with permission.

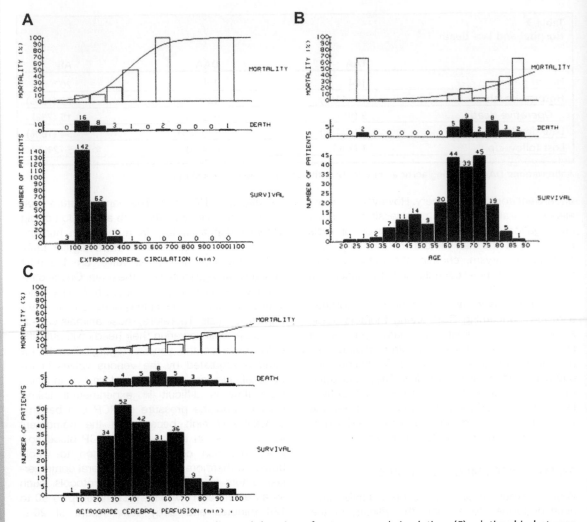

Fig. 2. (*A*) Relationship between mortality and duration of extracorporeal circulation, (*B*) relationship between mortality and the age of the patient, and (*C*) RCP times. (*From* Ueda Y, Okita Y, Aomi S, et al. Retrograde cerebral perfusion for aortic arch surgery: analysis of risk factors. Ann Thorac Surg 1999;67:1880; with permission.)

instead of 18°C. Those experiment protocols seemed to be designed to lead the conclusion of the inferiority of RCP for brain protection in comparison to antegrade cerebral perfusion. However, it should be appreciated that RCP combined with HCA, even in those abnormal protocols, revealed a better neuroprotective effect than HCA alone.[33–36]

Safi and colleagues[33] used a pig model of RCP. They established 3 groups of 5 pigs each; group A (control) underwent cardiopulmonary bypass and normothermic circulatory arrest for 1 hour, group B underwent cardiopulmonary bypass and profound HCA (15°C nasopharyngeal) for 1 hour, and group C underwent the same procedure as group B along with RCP. None of the animals awoke in group A (normothermia). In group B (HCA only), 2 of 5 did not awake, whereas 3 of 5

awoke but were unable to stand; 2 showed perceptive hind limb movement, and 1 was able to move all extremities. All of the group C (HCA with RCP) animals awoke, 4 of 5 were able to stand, and 1 of 5 was unable to stand, but could move all limbs. The neurologic evaluation of group B showed significantly lower Tarlov scores than group C ($P = .009$). Group B had a mean wake-up time of 124.6 ± 4.6 minutes versus 29.2 ± 5.1 in group C ($P = .009$). The late phase circulatory arrest brain oxygenation decreased $46.0\% \pm 13.9\%$ in group B, but it increased $26.1\% \pm 5.4\%$ in group C ($P = .0013$). This difference was reduced somewhat during rewarming (B, $-21.2\% \pm 14.9\%$; C, $16.4\% \pm 4.7\%$; $P = .043$). The group B rewarming jugular venous oxygen saturation was $30.8\% \pm 2.5\%$ versus $56.0\% \pm 4.4\%$ in group C ($P = .0011$). They concluded

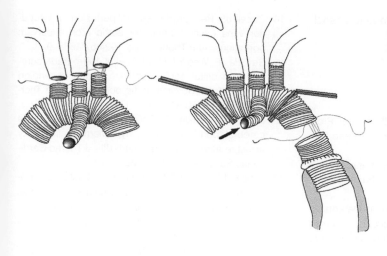

Fig. 3. Surgical procedure of the arch-first technique. The arch vessels were transected at their orifice, and each vessel was reconstructed with a 4-branched arch graft under RCP in the following sequence: left subclavian artery, left carotid artery, brachiocephalic artery. The antegrade cerebral perfusion was resumed through the 4-branched arch graft, with clamping at both ends. Distal anastomosis was performed with another graft, using the elephant trunk technique. (*From* Sasaki M, Usui A, Yoshikawa M, et al. Arch-first technique performed under hypothermic circulatory arrest with retrograde cerebral perfusion improves neurological outcomes for total arch replacement. Eur J Cardiothorac Surg 2005;27:822; with permission.)

that RCP combined with profound HCA significantly reduces neurologic dysfunction, providing superior brain protection in pigs.

Juvonen and colleagues[35] developed a chronic porcine model to evaluate RCP. They demonstrated that RCP resulted in a small amount of nutritive flow and provided cerebral protection that seemed to be superior to simple prolonged HCA. Yerlioglu and colleagues[34] also designed a study to evaluate the efficacy of RCP in mitigating the effects of particulate cerebral embolism occurring during cardiac surgery. They speculated that RCP, in addition to its usefulness as an adjunct to HCA, is attractive as a potential means of preventing air and particulate emboli, which are the major causes of permanent neurologic injury after cardiac and aortic surgeries in adults. They concluded that some animals recover after embolization and RCP with either minimal or no cerebral injury. The complete recovery of these animals, without any histopathologic evidence of cerebral injury, in contrast to the almost invariable neurologic impairment and histopathologic abnormalities in the antegrade embolism group, suggests that RCP provides some degree of cerebral protection after embolization in the ascending aorta. As a result, gradually instituting RCP and maintaining the SVC pressures at a level less than 40 mm Hg seem to improve the results.

Recently, Kawata and colleagues[38,39] introduced a novel RCP method with intermittent pressure augmentation for cerebral protection during aortic surgery. In an animal study, the effect of such brain protection was reinforced by raising the RCP pressure intermittently (every 30 seconds) to 45 mm Hg from 15 mm Hg in less than 120 minutes HCA at 18°C. Intermittent augmented

pressure effectively dilates the cerebral vessels, thereby enabling an adequate blood supply to reach the brain, while also minimizing brain damage from edema. The authors extended this RCP with intermittent pressure augmentation to clinical use with favorable results.

SUMMARY

The current results of aortic arch surgery using RCP and HCA are generally satisfactory in patients who undergo elective surgery. However, the long-term results of total arch replacement for elderly patients tend to be poor, particularly for patients undergoing emergency surgery for either an atherosclerotic aneurysm or acute dissection, and for patients suffering from postoperative CNS injury. Although a prolonged duration of HCA may contribute to these poor results, other factors such as emergency surgery, late death due to aging, and progressive systemic atherosclerosis with severe aortic atheroma are considered to be major risk factors.

RCP potentially reduces the risk of stroke related to embolic materials. After a period of HCA, although short, RCP eliminates the air or atheromatous debris, and thereafter the cardiopulmonary bypass should be resumed.

The technical simplicity of RCP together with a highly favorable effect on both the stroke rates and survival after aortic arch surgery justifies the continued clinical use of RCP in patients requiring HCA, especially in patients with either dissecting or atheromatous arch branches. RCP is therefore considered to provide effective brain protection during HCA lasting about 40 to 60 minutes, although there are some time limitations associated with its effectiveness.

REFERENCES

1. Griepp RB, Stinson EB, Hollingsworth JF, et al. Prosthetic replacement of the aortic arch. J Thorac Cardiovasc Surg 1975;70:1051–63.
2. Crawford ES, Snyder DM. Treatment of aneurysm of the aortic arch. A progress report. J Thorac Cardiovasc Surg 1983;85:237–46.
3. Coselli JS, Crawford ES, Beall AC, et al. Determination of brain temperature for safe circulatory arrest during cardiovascular operation. Ann Thorac Surg 1988;45:638–42.
4. Crawford ES, Svensson LG, Coselli JS, et al. Surgical treatment of aneurysm and/or dissection of the ascending aorta, transverse aortic arch, and ascending aorta and transverse aortic arch. Factors influencing survival in 717 patients. J Thorac Cardiovasc Surg 1989;98:659–74.
5. Svensson L, Crawford ES, Hess KR, et al. Deep hypothermia with circulatory arrest. Determinants of stroke and early mortality in 656 patients. J Thorac Cardiovasc Surg 1993;106:19–31.
6. Kouchoukos NT, Abbound N, Klausing WR. Perfusion for thoracic aortic surgery. In: Gravlee GP, Davis RE, Utley JR, editors. Cardiopulmonary bypass. Principles and practice. Baltimore (MD): Williams & Wilkins; 1993. p. 636–54.
7. Borst HG, Laas J. Surgical treatment of thoracic aortic aneurysms. Adv Card Surg 1993;4:47–87.
8. Ergin MA, Griepp EB, Lansman SL, et al. Hypothermic circulatory arrest and other methods of cerebral protection during operations on the thoracic aorta. J Card Surg 1994;9:525–37.
9. Kouchoukos NT, Dougenis D. Surgery of the thoracic aorta. N Engl J Med 1997;336:1876–88.
10. Ueda Y, Miki S, Kusuhara K, et al. Surgical treatment of aneurysm or dissection involving the ascending aorta and aortic arch, utilizing circulatory arrest and retrograde cerebral perfusion. J Cardiovasc Surg 1990;31:553–8.
11. Ueda Y, Miki S, Kusuhara K, et al. Deep hypothermic systemic circulatory arrest and continuous retrograde cerebral perfusion for surgery of aortic arch aneurysm. Eur J Cardiothorac Surg 1992;6:36–41.
12. Ueda Y, Miki S, Kusuhara K, et al. Protective effect of continuous retrograde cerebral perfusion on the brain during deep hypothermic systemic circulatory arrest. J Card Surg 1994;9:584–95.
13. Takakamoto S, Matsuda T, Harada M, et al. Simple hypothermic retrograde cerebral perfusion during aortic arch replacement. J Thorac Cardiovasc Surg 1992;104:1106–9.
14. Coselli JS. Retrograde cerebral perfusion via a superior vena caval cannula for aortic arch aneurysm operations. Ann Thorac Surg 1994;57:1668–9.
15. Bavaria JE, Woo YJ, Hall RA, et al. Retrograde cerebral and distal aortic perfusion during ascending and thoracoabdominal aortic operations. Ann Thorac Surg 1995;60:345–53.
16. Deeb GM, Jenkins E, Bolling SF, et al. Retrograde cerebral perfusion during hypothermic circulatory arrest reduces neurologic morbidity. J Thorac Cardiovasc Surg 1995;109:259–68.
17. Lytle B, McCarthy P, Meanly K, et al. Systemic hypothermia and circulatory arrest combined with arterial perfusion of the superior vena cava: effective intraoperative cerebral protection. J Thorac Cardiovasc Surg 1995;109:738–43.
18. Usui A, Abe T, Murase M. Early clinical results of retrograde cerebral perfusion for aortic arch operations in Japan. Ann Thorac Surg 1996;62:94–103.
19. Safi H, Letsou G, Iliopoulos D, et al. Impact of retrograde cerebral perfusion on ascending aortic and arch aneurysm repair. Ann Thorac Surg 1997;63:1601–7.
20. Coselli JS. Retrograde cerebral perfusion in surgery for aortic arch aneurysms. In: Ennker J, Coselli JS, Hetzer R, editors. Cerebral protection in cerebraovascular and aortic surgery. Darmstadt: Steinkopf Verlag; 1997. p. 239–49.
21. Bavaria JE, Pochettino A. Retrograde cerebral perfusion (RCP) in aortic arch surgery: Efficacy and possible mechanisms of the brain protection. Semin Thorac Cardiovasc Surg 1997;9:222–32.
22. Okita Y, Takamoto S, Ando M, et al. Mortality and cerebral outcome in patients who underwent aortic arch operations using deep hypothermic circulatory arrest with retrograde cerebral perfusion: no relation of early death, stroke, and delirium to the duration of circulatory arrest. J Thorac Cardiovasc Surg 1998;115:129–38.
23. Ueda Y, Okita Y, Aomi S, et al. Retrograde cerebral perfusion for aortic arch surgery: analysis of risk factors. Ann Thorac Surg 1999;67:1879–82.
24. Mills NL, Ochsner JL. Massive air embolism during cardio-pulmonary bypass. Causes, prevention, and management. J Thorac Cardiovasc Surg 1980;80:708–17.
25. Lemole GM, Strong MD, Spagna PM, et al. Improved results for dissecting aneurysms. Intraluminal sutureless prosthesis. J Thorac Cardiovasc Surg 1982;83:249–55.
26. Usui A, Oohara K, Liu T, et al. Determination of optimum retrograde cerebral perfusion conditions. J Thorac Cardiovasc Surg 1994;107:300–8.
27. Ueda Y. Retrograde cerebral perfusion with hypothermic circulatory arrest in aortic arch surgery: operative and long-term results. Nagoya J Med Sci 2001;64:93–102.

28. Rokkas CK, Kouchoukos NT. Single-stage extensive replacement of the thoracic aorta: the arch-first technique. J Thorac Cardiovasc Surg 1999; 117:99–105.

29. Sasaki M, Usui A, Yoshikawa M, et al. Arch-first technique performed under hypothermic circulatory arrest with retrograde cerebral perfusion improves neurological outcomes for total arch replacement. Eur J Cardiothorac Surg 2005;27:821–5.

30. Usui A, Ueda Y. Arch first technique under deep hypothermic circulatory arrest with retrograde cerebral perfusion. MMCTS, January 2, 2007. DOI:10.1510/mmcts.2006.001974.

31. Estrera AL, Miller CM, Madisetty J, et al. Ascending and transverse aortic arch repair. The impact of retrograde cerebral perfusion. Circulation 2008; 118:S160–6.

32. Reich DL, Uysal S, Ergin MA, et al. Retrograde cerebral perfusion as a method of neuroprotection during thoracic aortic surgery. Ann Thorac Surg 2001;72:1774–82.

33. Safi HJ, Iliopoulos DC, Gopinath SP, et al. Retrograde cerebral perfusion during profound hypothermia and circulatory arrest in pigs. Ann Thorac Surg 1995;59:1107–12.

34. Yerlioglu ME, Wolfe D, Mezrow CK, et al. The effect of retrograde cerebral perfusion after particulate embolization to the brain. J Thorac Cardiovasc Surg 1995;110:1470–85.

35. Juvonen T, Zhang N, Wolfe D, et al. Retrograde cerebral perfusion enhances cerebral protection during prolonged hypothermic circulatory arrest: a study in a chronic porcine model. Ann Thorac Surg 1998;66:38–50.

36. Anttila V, Kiviluoma K, Pokela M, et al. Cold retrograde cerebral perfusion improves cerebral protection during moderate hypothermic circulatory arrest: a long-term study in a porcine model. J Thorac Cardiovasc Surg 1999;118:938–45.

37. Ehrlich MP, Hagl C, McCullough JN, et al. Retrograde cerebral perfusion provides negligible flow through brain capillaries in the pig. J Thorac Cardiovasc Surg 2001;122:331–8.

38. Kawata M, Takamoto S, Kitahori K, et al. Intermittent pressure augmentation during retrograde cerebral perfusion under moderate hypothermia provides adequate neuroprotection: an experimental study. J Thorac Cardiovasc Surg 2006;132:80–8.

39. Kawata M, Sekino M, Takamoto S, et al. Retrograde cerebral perfusion with intermittent pressure augmentation provides adequate neuroprotection: diffusion- and perfusion-weighted magnetic resonance imaging study in an experimental canine model. J Thorac Cardiovasc Surg 2006;132:933–40.

What is the Best Method for Brain Protection in Surgery of the Aortic Arch? Straight DHCA

John A. Elefteriades, MD

KEYWORDS
- Aortic arch • Brain perfusion • Deep hypothermic arrest
- Hypoperfusion

There are 3 techniques available for brain preservation during deep hypothermic arrest in aortic arch replacement: (1) retrograde cerebral perfusion, (2) antegrade cerebral perfusion, and (3) straight deep hypothermic circulatory arrest (DHCA). A decade or two ago, straight deep hypothermic arrest was the most popular technique. More recently, surgeons have been more inclined to use some brain perfusion adjunct, either antegrade or retrograde perfusion, and fewer centers apply straight DHCA.

At our center, we practice nearly entirely straight DHCA. We prefer this technique for various reasons. Straight DHCA is simple; no extra cannulas or tubings are required and there is no diversion of the surgeon's attention for perfusion matters. Straight DHCA provides an entirely uncluttered field, totally dry and without any mechanical encumbrances in the way of exposure or suturing. Basically, the aortic replacement remains the operation; the perfusion system does not become primary, relegating the surgical replacement of the aorta to an ancillary importance (this sentence is taken somewhat in jest). Straight DHCA is also quick and simple, an advantage in the case of aortic dissections being operated in the middle of the night.

With straight DHCA, one avoids certain dangers inherent in the perfusion techniques. First and foremost, one does not know how fast to flow, either for antegrade or for retrograde perfusion. Flowing too slow risks hypoperfusion and flowing too fast risks cerebral edema or other problems. Further, there is serious concern about whether retrograde perfusion really reaches the brain. Also, with antegrade perfusion, cannulas must be placed in the vessels, risking intimal injury or embolization. As well, with antegrade perfusion, there is the question of the subclavian artery. Ideally, proponents say, the subclavian artery should be clamped to prevent steal of perfusion into the open aortic arch, but it appears this step is often omitted in clinical practice. Also, there is the question of how many branches need to be perfused with the antegrade technique; does the innominate and left carotid suffice? Perfusion of less than all 3 head vessels anticipates a complete circle of Willis, which may not always obtain. All of these issues are obviated by straight DHCA.

This does not imply that we do not think that blood flow is good; rather, the opposite. Our team intrinsically favors provision of blood flow, especially to the brain.

However, it happens that historically ours has been a straight DHCA institution and we have never changed; this provides a large clinical experience for analysis. We have looked at outcomes carefully (including specialized neurologic analyses), and they are good. For this reason, we have continued to practice straight DHCA, as have multiple institutions specializing in aortic surgery. In fact, as mentioned later, the general

Section of Cardiac Surgery, Department of Surgery, Yale University School of Medicine, Yale-New Haven Hospital, PO Box 208039, New Haven, CT 06520-8039, USA
E-mail address: john.elefteriades@yale.edu

Cardiol Clin 28 (2010) 381–387
doi:10.1016/j.ccl.2010.02.004
0733-8651/10/$ – see front matter © 2010 Published by Elsevier Inc.

and neurologic results achieved by straight DHCA are unsurpassed by any other techniques recorded in the literature.

First, it is worth reviewing the details of our straight DHCA routine.

> *Cannulation.* We use femoral cannulation if the preoperative studies and the intraoperative transesophageal echo show a clean descending aorta appropriate for perfusion from below. Most patients with ascending aortic pathology have clean arteries; in fact, in a recent article, we were able to show evidence of a genetic protection from arteriosclerosis in patients with annuloaortic ectasia or ascending aortic dissection.[1]
>
> *Temperature.* We use a temperature of 19°C for hemiarch and 18°C for full arch replacements. We monitor mainly the bladder temperature as our index of core temperature. We do not use electroencephalography for confirmation of electrical silence; this can fairly be expected at these temperatures.
>
> *Cooling/warming.* It takes us about 35 minutes to cool (during which time we work on the aortic root) and about 60 minutes to rewarm.
>
> *pH management.* We use alpha-stat management.
>
> *Topical cooling.* We apply ice to the head, to augment local cooling.
>
> *Medications.* We give steroids routinely, but no barbiturates or other agents aimed at decreasing cerebral metabolic rate. So, in essence, this is a simple system.

Coagulation. Many of these cases were done during the era when aprotinin was available, and it was used liberally. In addition, most patients preemptively received 2 units of fresh frozen plasma and a 4-pack of platelets.

Our results were recently reported regarding nearly 400 patients operated on at our institution with straight DHCA over a 10-year period. Mean duration of circulatory arrest was 31 minutes (range 10–66 minutes) (**Fig. 1**). Ninety percent of the cases were ascending, 22% were urgent, and 23% involved aortic dissection. For ascending and arch cases, total mortality was 2.2% (including elective and urgent cases). Reexploration for bleeding was required in only 4.5% of the cases. During this time interval, we did in a small handful of cases apply antegrade cerebral perfusion for exceptionally complex arch cases requiring difficult resection or complex, multiple vascular anastomoses; our preference for these cases is antegrade perfusion via the axillary, with or without left carotid perfusion.

In terms of brain results, among the ascending and arch cases, the stroke rate was 2.3%. There was a trend toward increased stroke rate at DHCA times exceeding 40 minutes. Sixty-two percent of strokes were judged to be embolic based on brain distribution on computed tomography scan and thus not caused by generalized hypoperfusion.

Now, how do these data compare with those that are published on antegrade or retrograde perfusion? We reviewed 20 excellent case series performed with a variety of techniques (**Table 1**). Although it is difficult to compare series directly

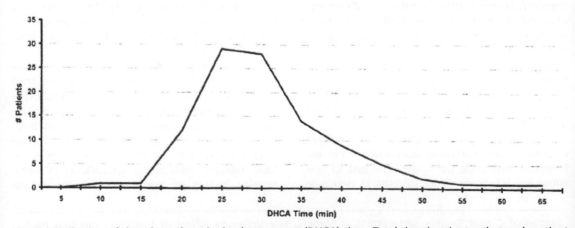

Fig. 1. Distribution of deep hypothermic circulatory arrest (DHCA) time. Total time in minutes that each patient was exposed to straight DHCA at our institution (mean, 31 minutes; range, 10–61 minutes). (*From* Gega A, Rizzo JA, Johnson MH, et al. Straight deep hypothermic arrest: experience in 394 patients supports its effectiveness as a sole means of brain preservation. Ann Thorac Surg 2007;84(3):759–66; with permission.)

Table 1
Review of pertinent literature

First Author	Year	Patients (n)	Mortality (%)	Stroke (%)	Comments
RCP					
Safi[2]	1993	11	0	9.1	
Ueda[3]	1994	33	12.1	6.1	
Deeb[4]	1995	35	8.6	2.9	
Lytle[5]	1995	43	9.3	9.3	
Bavaria[6]	2002	163	9.8	5.0	
Appoo[7]	2003	79	7.6	3.8	Confined to elective cases unlike most other reports
ACP					
Matsuda[8]	1989	34	9.0	2.9	
Bachet[9]	1991	54	13.0	1.8	
Kazui[10]	1992	8	0	0	Type A dissections
Ando[11]	1994	42	7.1	7.0	Type A dissections (acute and chronic)
Kazui[12]	1994	80	16.3	1.3	
Tabayashi[13]	1994	77	1.0	5.0	
Kazui[14]	2000	220	12.7	3.3	
DiEusanio[15]	2002	403	9.4	3.7	
DHCA (straight)					
Svensson[16]	1993	656	12.0	7	DHCA >45 min correlated with stroke DHCA >65 min correlated with death

(continued on next page)

Table 1
(continued)

First Author	Year	Patients (n)	Mortality (%)	Stroke (%)	Comments
Geja [this study]	2007	394	6.3 2.2 for asc/arch	4.8 3.1 for asc/arch	Includes ruptured/extensive descending and thoracoabdominal aneurysms; other series confined to ascending pathologies
Comparison studies					
Alamani[17]	1995	DHCA = 19 ACT = 16	DHCA = 26.3 ACP = 18.7	DHCA = 15.7 ACP = 12.5	Compared straight DHCA to ACP
Okita[18]	2001	RCP = 30 ACP = 30	RCP = 6.6 ACP = 6.6	RCP = 3.3 ACP = 6.6	No straight DHCA patients
Dong[19]	2002	DHCA = 15 RCP = 50	DHCA = 20 RCP = 2.0	DHCA = 25 RCP = 2.0	
Moon[20]	2002	DHCA = 36 RCP = 36	DHCA = 8.0 RCP = 11.0	DHCA = 11 RCA = 6.0	
Matalanis[21]	2003	DHCA = 14 RCP = 23 ACP = 25	DHCA = 7.1 RCP = 0 ACP = 16.0	DHCA = 0 RCP = 4.3 ACP = 12.0	
Immer[22]	2004	DHCA = 322 ACP = 41	Overall mortality = 9.6	DHCA = 6.5 ACP = 1.0	No comparisons of DHCA vs ACP were significant

Abbreviations: ACP, antegrade cerebral perfusion; RCP, retrograde cerebral perfusion.
From Gega A, Rizzo JA, Johnson MH, et al. Straight deep hypothermic arrest: experience in 394 patients supports its effectiveness as a sole means of brain preservation. Ann Thorac Surg 2007;84(3):759–66; with permission.

because of different patient profiles, aneurysm extent, acuities, and complexities. Mortality and stroke rates in other series are not generally superior to those realized in our series of patients operated with straight DHCA.

We believe this comparison with other published data further demonstrates that adjunctive perfusion techniques are largely unnecessary.

We now describe a follow-up study that we performed.[23] Our DHCA patients seemed to function well in their home and work environments. However, our team wished to look at the functional issue in more detail. We reasoned that individuals with high cognitive demands for their work—doctors, nurses, lawyers, surgeons, administrators, college deans, artists, musicians, and the like—would be more likely to manifest any subtle postoperative defects. We applied standard metrics, tailored specifically to detect postoperative changes, to a subgroup of 45 such patients. The metric (Jorm's Short Form IQCODE) uses information from patients and their family observers, conferring a better reflection of patients' functional status. In this metric, a score of 3 represents no change in level of function from preoperative status. A score of 1 indicates much worse and 5 indicates much improved. As can be seen in **Fig. 2**, our high-cognitive patients functioned at exactly the same level, using this

specific neurologic metric, as they did before surgery with DHCA. In fact, they functioned just as well as a control group undergoing simpler aortic surgery without DHCA.

One technical point important in this analysis has to do with our technique for arch replacement (**Fig. 3**). Acute dissection cases, with a single distal arch anastomosis, and hemiarch cases are easily accommodated within the safe period of DHCA. Even in more complicated cases, our particular arch surgical technique permits comfortable performance of formal arch replacement within the 40- to 45-minute period of high safety with DHCA. For formal arch replacement, we prefer anastomosis of the head vessels as a pedicle to the main aortic graft. We often chose to anastomose only the innominate and left carotid arteries during DHCA, leaving the anastomosis of the left subclavian artery to be performed with a separate sidearm graft after resuming circulation (during rewarming) or even after terminating cardiopulmonary bypass. With this technique, the distal (descending aortic) anastomosis can be performed in about 20 minutes and the arch anastomosis in about 20 minutes, leading to a total DHCA time of approximately 40 minutes. We believe that use of this technique goes hand-in-hand with the application of straight deep hypothermic arrest.

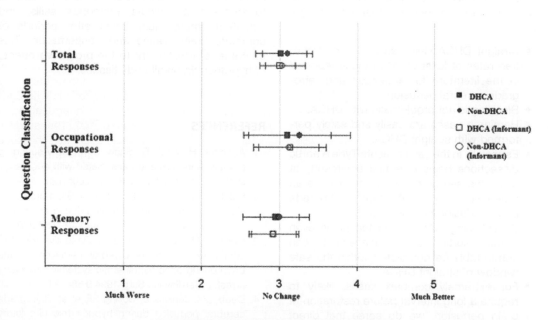

Fig. 2. Depiction of questionnaire results (see text). Note near identity of response grades for DHCA and non-DHCA groups, according to both patient and informant. (*From* Percy A, Widman S, Rizzo JA, et al. Deep hypothermic circulatory arrest in patients with high cognitive needs: full preservation of cognitive abilities. Ann Thorac Surg 2009;87:117–23; with permission.)

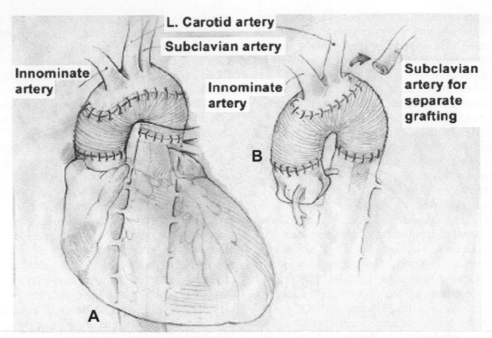

Fig. 3. Alternate technique (shown on *right, B*) that facilitates aortic arch replacement by limiting the arch anastomosis to a single, small pedicle. The left subclavian artery is connected with a separate small caliber graft during rewarming or after bypass (*arrow*). We find this alternative technique more expedient than the traditional method shown on the left (*A*). (*From* Gega A, Rizzo JA, Johnson MH, et al. Straight deep hypothermic arrest: experience in 394 patients supports its effectiveness as a sole means of brain preservation. Ann Thorac Surg 2007;84(3):759–66; with permission.)

Based on our extensive clinical experience, we make the following points regarding straight DHCA:

- Straight DHCA yields survival and stroke-free rates at least equal to those reported in the literature for antegrade and retrograde cerebral perfusion.
- Bleeding is not problematic with DHCA.
- Hemiarch cases are easily and safely performed with straight DHCA.
- Especially in the case of acute Type A aortic dissections being operated emergently at night, we see no reason to complicate an urgent situation by antegrade or retrograde brain perfusion techniques.
- With the single Carrel patch technique, even formal aortic arch replacement can comfortably be completed within the safe window of straight DHCA.
- For extremely complex cases, likely to require a long interval before restoration of brain perfusion, we do agree that direct cerebral perfusion via the right axillary artery is indicated.

The technique of straight DHCA, popularized by Griepp and colleagues,[24] is an extraordinary method in the medical sciences. It never ceases to amaze that instincts, memories, skills, and cognition emerge fully intact after periods of complete brain silence and nonperfusion. This outcome is a testament to the protective effects of hypothermia on all body tissues.

REFERENCES

1. Achneck H, Modi B, Shaw C, et al. Ascending thoracic aneurysms are associated with decreased systemic atherosclerosis. Chest 2005;128:1580–6.
2. Safi HJ, Brien HW, Winter JN, et al. Brain protection via cerebral retrograde perfusion during aortic arch aneurysm repair. Ann Thorac Surg 1993;56:270–6.
3. Ueda Y, Miki S, Okita Y, et al. Protective effect of continuous retrograde cerebral perfusion on the brain during deep hypothermic systemic circulatory arrest. J Cardiovasc Surg 1994;9:584–94.
4. Deeb GM, Jenkins E, Bolling SF, et al. Retrograde cerebral perfusion during hypothermic circulatory arrest reduces neurologic morbidity. J Thorac Cardiovasc Surg 1995;109:259–68.
5. Lytle BW, McCarthy PM, Meaney KM, et al. Systemic hypothermia and circulatory arrest combined with arterial perfusion of the superior vena cava. Effective

intraoperative cerebral protection. J Thorac Cardiovasc Surg 1995;109:738–43.

6. Bavaria JE, Brinster DR, Gorman RC, et al. Advances in the treatment of acute type A dissection: an integrated approach. Ann Thorac Surg 2002;74:S1848–52 [discussion: S1857–63].

7. Appoo JJ, Augoustides JG, Pochettino A, et al. Perioperative outcome in adults undergoing elective deep hypothermic circulatory arrest with retrograde cerebral perfusion in proximal aortic arch repair: evaluation of protocol-based care. J Cardiothorac Vasc Anesth 2006;20:3–7.

8. Matsuda H, Nakano S, Shirakura R, et al. Surgery for aortic arch aneurysm with selective cerebral perfusion and hypothermic cardiopulmonary bypass. Circulation 1989;80:1243–8.

9. Bachet J, Guilmet D, Goudot B, et al. Cold cerebroplegia. A new technique of cerebral protection during operations on the transverse aortic arch. J Thorac Cardiovasc Surg 1991;102:85–93.

10. Kazui T, Yamada O, Komatsu S. Emergency graft replacement of the aortic arch for acute type A aortic dissection. J Cardiovasc Surg (Torino) 1992;33:211–5.

11. Ando M, Nakajima N, Adachi S, et al. Simultaneous graft replacement of the ascending aorta and total aortic arch for type A aortic dissection. Ann Thorac Surg 1994;57:669–76.

12. Kazui T, Kimura N, Yamada O, et al. Surgical outcome of aortic arch aneurysms using selective cerebral perfusion. Ann Thorac Surg 1994;57:904–11.

13. Tabayashhi K, Ohmi M, Togo T, et al. Aortic arch aneurysm repair using selective cerebral perfusion. Ann Thorac Surg 1994;57:1305–10.

14. Kazui T, Washiyama N, Muhammad BA, et al. Total arch replacement using aortic arch branched grafts with the aid of antegrade selective cerebral perfusion. Ann Thorac Surg 2000;70:3–8 discussion 8–9.

15. DiEusanio M, Schepens MAAM, Morshuis WJ, et al. Antegrade selective cerebral perfusion during operations on the thoracic aorta: factors influencing survival and neurologic outcome in 413 patients. J Thorac Cardiovasc Surg 2002;124:1080–6.

16. Svensson LG, Crawford ES, IHess KR, et al. Deep hypothermia with circulatory arrest. Determinants of stroke and early mortality in 656 patients. J Thorac Cardiovasc Surg 1993;106:19–28.

17. Alamanni F, Agrifoglio M, Pompilio G, et al. Aortic arch surgery: pros and cons of selective cerebral perfusion. A multivariable analysis for cerebral injury during hypothermic circulatory arrest. J Cardiovasc Surg (Torino) 1995;36:31–7.

18. Okita Y, Minatoya K, Tagusari O, et al. Prospective comparative study of brain protection in total aortic arch replacement: deep hypothermic circulatory arrest with retrograde cerebral perfusion or selective antegrade cerebral perfusion. Ann Thorac Surg 2001;72:72–9.

19. Dong P, Guan Y, He M, et al. [Clinical application of retrograde cerebral perfusion for brain protection during surgery of ascending aortic aneurysm—a report of 50 cases]. Zhonghua Wai Ke Zhi 2003; 41:109–11 [in Chinese].

20. Moon MR, Sundt TM 3rd. Influence of retrograde cerebral perfusion during aortic arch procedures. Ann Thorac Surg 2002;74:426–31; discussion 431.

21. Matalanis G, Hata M, Buxton BF. A retrospective comparative study of deep hypothermic circulatory arrest, retrograde, and antegrade cerebral perfusion in aortic arch surgery. Ann Thorac Cardiovasc Surg 2003;9:174–9.

22. Immer FF, Lippeck C, Marmettler H, et al. Improvement of quality of life after surgery on the thoracic aorta: effect of antegrade cerebral perfusion and short duration of deep hypothermic circulatory arrest. Circulation 2004;110(11 Suppl 1):II250–5.

23. Percy A, Widman S, Rizzo JA, et al. Deep hypothermic circulatory arrest in patients with high cognitive needs: full preservation of cognitive abilities. Ann Thorac Surg 2009;87:117–23.

24. Griepp RB, Stinson EB, Hollingsworth JF, et al. Prosthetic replacement of the aortic arch. J Thorac Cardiovasc Surg 1975;70:1051–63.

What is the Best Method for Brain Protection in Surgery of the Aortic Arch? Selective Antegrade Cerebral Perfusion

Jean Bachet, MD, FEBTCS

KEYWORDS

- Aortic arch surgery • Cerebral protection
- Antegrade selective perfusion • Hypothermia
- Circulatory arrest

Despite the considerable progress made in recent decades in the operative management of lesions involving the transverse aortic arch, replacement of this portion of the vessel remains a surgical challenge and is still associated with a certain rate of mortality and morbidity. This situation is due not only to the technical difficulties of the procedure but, often, to the unsatisfactory preservation of the integrity of the central nervous system during the period of arch exclusion.

Indeed, the surgical treatment of aortic arch lesions is characterized by 2 specific peculiarities:

- The presence on this aortic segment of the origin of the vessels irrigating the superior limbs and, more importantly, the whole cerebrum, which strictly requires that a method of brain protection be implemented to obviate the ischemic consequences of exclusion of those vessels during the time of aortic repair.
- The difficulty or even the danger of cross-clamping the aorta (in particular the distal aorta) in many situations, which makes the use of circulatory arrest mandatory during the performance of the distal anastomoses.

Ischemic lesions of the central nervous system are induced rapidly. As soon as they are triggered, several types of metabolic alterations participate in their worsening, because lesions of excitotoxicity and apoptosis are soon added to the lesions induced by the interruption of the necessary supply of metabolites. Even when the cerebral blood flow (CBF) is reestablished and the metabolic supply restored, the neuronal structures can be jeopardized by definitive alterations linked to the reperfusion and consequent liberation of deleterious radicals.

The techniques of cerebral protection during surgery of the aortic arch can be divided into those aimed at suppressing the metabolic demand of the central nervous system and those aimed at maintaining the metabolic supply during the time of exclusion of the cerebral vessels.

The first group is mostly represented by the techniques based on profound hypothermia, whereas the second group is represented by the various modes of selective antegrade cerebral perfusion (SACP).

Whichever technique is used, it must maintain the normal metabolism of the central nervous system or, at least, allow restoration of the physiological conditions of its function.

METABOLIC REQUIREMENTS OF THE BRAIN

In a normal human adult, the brain weighs about 1400 g, representing 4% to 5% of the body weight. By contrast, the mean CBF is about 750 mL/min at

Department of Cardiovascular Surgery, Zayed Military Hospital, Abu Dhabi, UAE
E-mail address: jean.bachet@dms.mil.ae

Cardiol Clin 28 (2010) 389–401
doi:10.1016/j.ccl.2010.01.014
0733-8651/10/$ – see front matter © 2010 Elsevier Inc. All rights reserved.

37°C, representing about 16% of the total cardiac output and resulting in a perfusion of 55 mL/min/100 g of brain tissue. These figures emphasize the enormous metabolic demand of the brain and the absolute necessity to preserve this metabolic activity to avoid any irreversible ischemic injury.

The pressure in the intracranial carotid arteries is normally 60 to 70 mm Hg, whereas it decreases to 15 mm Hg in the cortical veins and to 0 or less in the jugular veins.

Autoregulation of the CBF is important in maintaining a stable environment in the brain. Under physiological conditions, the autoregulation of the cerebral flow is maintained for a wide spectrum of mean arterial pressures (50 to 150 mm Hg), and there is no relationship between the CBF and the level of the mean arterial pressure. Several reports[1-3] have suggested that in deep hypothermic situations (20°C), autoregulation of the CBF is maintained and prevents cerebral ischemia or hypoperfusion for perfusion pressures ranging from 30 to 100 mm Hg. If the perfusion flow rate is reduced, the total brain flow decreases, but even at lowest perfusion flow rates, all areas of the brain seem to remain perfused. This autoregulation disappears at very low temperatures (6–12°C), at which there is a direct relation between flow and perfusion pressure.

Normally, individual cerebral structures are perfused in proportion to their metabolic demands. At 37°C, oxygen consumption of the brain is 2.90 mL/gm/min. At 25°C, oxygen consumption is reduced to 0.90 mL/g/min, and, at 20°C, to one-fifth of that at normothermia. Even at very low temperatures, the cerebral oxygen consumption rate is never reduced to nil.

Those data are modified by general anesthesia or by the use of drugs such as pentobarbital that are intended to reduce metabolic demand and increase tolerance to hypoxemia.

In the cerebral tissues, ischemic phenomena are observed at 37°C, when the CBF decreases to less than 18 mL/min/100 g. A sudden interruption or dramatic reduction of the CBF leads to rapid interruption of the oxygen and glucose supply. This event stops active phosphorylation in the brain cell and exhausts the adenosine triphosphate reserves indispensable for its normal function and, in particular, for maintaining membrane integrity, ionic transfer, lipogenesis, and the reactions of deacylation-reacylation necessary for the renewal of the phospholipids. The pH decreases dramatically and membrane exchanges are discontinued. The normal electric polarity is reduced, and K^+ ions are expelled from the cell, whereas Na^+ and Ca^+ channels open widely, allowing massive influx of those ions into the intracellular space. The cell swells. Several enzymatic systems are activated, leading to the degradation of proteins and cell membranes, permitting production of peroxinitrite radicals and endonucleases, which degrade DNA. This cascade rapidly leads to cell death.

Three associated processes worsen those direct phenomena of cell necrosis: excitotoxicity, apoptosis, and eventually reperfusion injuries, if the CBF is restored.

CURRENT TECHNIQUES OF CEREBRAL PROTECTION

Since the first replacement of the aortic arch by De Bakey and Cooley in 1955,[4] various techniques of brain protection have been described and used during the time of arch exclusion.[5-8] According to the results obtained and the evolution of the medical and surgical environment, some of those techniques have disappeared, whereas others have achieved wide acceptance and are still in use.

Those latter techniques can be classified into 2 main groups:

1. Methods aimed at dramatically reducing or suppressing the metabolic demands of the cerebral tissue. These methods are mainly based on the use of deep or profound core hypothermia.
2. Techniques aimed at providing the cerebrum with its metabolic requirements despite vascular exclusion. This category groups together all the techniques of selective antegrade perfusion of the brain through the arterial network.

Deep Hypothermia Associated With Circulatory Arrest

Deep hypothermia associated with circulatory arrest (DHCA) was first used at the beginning of cardiac surgery to treat congenital defects before the routine availability of cardiopulmonary bypass (CPB).[9,10] This technique had been abandoned because of the occurrence of postoperative neurological disorders and in particular lesions of the central gray nuclei in about 5% of patients.

However, a major breakthrough occurred in 1975, when Griepp and colleagues[11] proposed using a similar technique during the replacement of the aortic arch. Many improvements have been made to the original technique. DHCA continues to be 1 of the most frequently used methods of cerebral protection. Currently, for Griepp and coworkers, DHCA is achieved through

CPB, the temperature is lowered to less than 15°C, the head of the patient is packed in ice, and the circulatory arrest is initiated when the jugular vein oxygen saturation is more than 95%. Many upholders of the method, however, do not lower the temperature to less than 18°C or even 20°C.

This technique has obvious advantages. It necessitates no brachiocephalic cannulation, and it can be used in almost any circumstances with a regular CPB circuit. The main advantage, however, is to allow a total circulatory arrest and, thus, the possibility of performing an open blood-less replacement of the aortic arch without cross-clamping the vessel.

Conversely this method has some drawbacks. Mostly efficient when temperature gradients between organs are absent or reduced, DHCA requires a long time to decrease the patient's temperature to an appropriate level and a longer time to increase it back to its physiological value. Besides, the time required on CPB to avoid excessive thermal gradients during rewarming of the patient (about 5 minutes per degree centigrade) has been held responsible for generating important coagulation and inflammatory disorders and, consequently, for high morbidity and mortality.

It has been proposed that total circulatory arrest be performed at moderate hypothermia to reduce the rate of those complications.[12] The time allowed then to perform the distal aortic repair is severely limited and calls the surgeon's skill into play.

In 2002, Ehrlich and colleagues[13] showed experimentally on pigs that, even at very low temperatures, the cerebral metabolism is never completely interrupted and that at 8°C (a temperature that is never reached in clinical practice) the cerebral oxygen consumption (CMR_{O_2}) is still 11% of the baseline. These investigators concluded that "The presence of significant residual metabolic activity at 18°C suggests that this degree of hypothermia may provide incomplete cerebral protection during prolonged interruption of CBF."

Therefore, the most important unresolved question is the limit of time allowed for circulatory arrest. This limit of time has not been clearly defined. Several experimental studies have been undertaken to estimate the maximum duration of circulatory arrest that could safely be applied to animals. Despite the various methods and techniques of analysis used, these studies generally agree that the limit is about 60 minutes when temperature is less than 18°C.[14] It seems that in man the safe limit of time is shorter and that the risk of neurological disturbance becomes serious if the period of circulatory arrest exceeds 45 minutes. Although most distal aortic repairs can be performed within this time, it can never be assured that a longer time would not be required, either in extended and complex anatomic lesions or if there are unforeseen difficulties.

For all these reasons the results associated with circulatory arrest at profound hypothermia vary widely in the literature.[15-17] Gega and colleagues[18] have recently published a report on 394 patients operated on in a 10-year period in whom only DHCA was used. The overall hospital mortality was 6.3% and the rate of neurologic disorders was 8%. The investigators concluded: "Straight DHCA without adjunctive perfusion suffices as a sole means of cerebral protection. Stroke and seizure rates are low. Cognitive function, by clinical assessment, is excellent. Especially for straightforward ascending/arch reconstructions, there is little need for the added complexity of brain perfusion strategies."

However, in this experience the mean duration of the circulatory arrest was short (31 minutes) and remained within the proven safety limits of the method. In the 61 patients in whom the circulatory arrest time exceeded 40 minutes the stroke rate was 13%, which can hardly be considered as a low rate.

The authors used DHCA between 1977 and 1986 in 34 patients (including 10 acute type A dissections) with a hospital mortality of 44% (15 patients).

In addition to this high mortality, this experience has been disappointing.[19] Many surviving patients, especially elderly individuals, had postoperative awakening times exceeding the usual few hours. Transient or permanent neurological complications were not rare and were responsible for death in several instances. Our experience is in accordance with some reports in the literature but it contrasts sharply with the results obtained by other groups. This disparity might be explained because in most patients the temperature was not lower than 20°C, the patient's head was not packed in ice, and, despite the permanent monitoring of esophageal and rectal temperatures, temperature gradients between organs might have been generated by rapid cooling and the brain might not have been as cold and protected as we wanted it to be.

Retrograde Cerebral Perfusion Through the Superior Vena Cava at Deep Hypothermia

To improve the protective efficacy of deep hypothermia, in 1992 Ueda and colleagues[20] proposed the use of retrograde perfusion of oxygenated blood through the superior vena cava associated with deep hypothermia. The idea was to perfuse the brain retrogradely through the venous and capillary systems on the analogy of retrograde cardioplegia. The perfused flow was adjusted to maintain a pressure of about 20 to 25 mm Hg into the superior vena cava.

This technique rapidly gained wide acceptance and has been used routinely in many centers. However, the efficiency of retrograde cerebral perfusion (RCP) remains controversial on experimental and clinical grounds:

- One of the main criticisms is linked to the association of the method with deep hypothermia. It has been shown that deep hypothermia alone, provided it is performed properly, is efficient in protecting the central nervous system when circulatory arrest lasts less than 30 to 40 minutes. Because in most reported experiences the mean duration of circulatory arrest is within this limit of time, it is not clear whether the brain is protected by profound hypothermia or retrograde perfusion or by their combination.
- Anatomically, the presence of valves in the human jugular system has been proved, and this is a major impediment to proper distribution of the perfusate to the brain.[21,22]
- DeBrux and coworkers[23] have shown on cadavers that most of the liquid retrogradely perfused into the superior vena cava irrigates the perivertebral venous system through the azygos vein.
- Ehrlich and colleagues[24] have shown in pigs that only 3% to 5% of the oxygenated perfusate flowing through the superior vena cava reappears as a backflow through the carotid and subclavian arteries, and that, thus, the perfusion of the brain is extremely poor.
- Midulla and coworkers[25] have shown in pigs that the aortic backflow was less than 5% of the total retrograde inflow.
- Katz and colleagues[26] have also shown by using technetium[99]-labeled albumin that little of the injected retrograde flow passes through the brain.
- Boeckxstaens and Flameng[27] showed that retrograde perfusion does not protect the brain in baboons.
- Bonser and colleagues[28] showed more recently that RCP is unable to attenuate the metabolic changes induced in the brain by deep hypothermia.

Clinical studies are more difficult to interpret, and some articles have reported good outcomes with the technique.[29–31] On the other hand, studies by groups advocating the method have reported rates of postoperative neurological injury (strokes and neurocognitive disorders) as high as 24%.[32,33]

In the author's opinion, it is impossible to conclude in favor of this method. It is likely that RCP, by ensuring a better distribution of cold to the brain, enhances the protective effect of profound hypothermia, therefore allowing longer times of circulatory arrest.

ANTEGRADE SELECTIVE PERFUSION

Because of adverse experiences, the surgical community was looking for a technique that had the advantages of deep hypothermia and antegrade perfusion but avoided their drawbacks.

In particular it seemed worthwhile:

- to eliminate the unnecessary general deep hypothermia
- to keep the advantage of the distal open anastomosis
- to obtain a safe cerebral protection without limit of time.

For those reasons, the technique of SACP was developed. In principle this consists of perfusing the brain through the brachiocephalic arteries with oxygenated blood at physiological flow and pressure, independently of the rest of the body, while the core temperature of the patient is lowered to a level of moderate hypothermia. CPB is discontinued and the cerebral perfusion is maintained during the open distal aortic repair.

In most patients, as soon as the distal anastomosis and the arch vessel reimplantation are completed, the aortic arch is carefully de-aired, the aortic prosthesis is cross-clamped, the selective perfusion is discontinued, and CBP is resumed at full flow while rewarming of the patient is started. The proximal anastomosis or the necessary proximal procedures are then performed during the rewarming time. This system has the advantage of synchronizing the time necessary for those procedures with the duration of the CPB and not needlessly prolonging the duration of hypothermia.

During the last 2 decades several modes of selective antegrade perfusion have been described. They are all based on the same principles but differ mainly on 3 features:

- the level of the patient's core temperature
- the temperature of the brain perfusate
- the mode of cannulation of the cerebral vessels.

The Core Temperature

Although they have adopted the technique of SACP, many groups, nevertheless, continue to associate it with deep core hypothermia. They consider that this association provides a better protection to the spinal cord and the viscera during the time of distal circulatory arrest and allows, if the need arises, discontinuation of the cerebral perfusion for a given time. We consider that this is inappropriate and useless for several reasons:

1. It associates the major drawbacks of deep hypothermia with the potential drawbacks of SACP.
2. A distal circulatory arrest of up to 60 minutes at moderate temperature (23–25°C rectal) can be performed without ischemic complications for the viscera and the spinal cord.[34,35]
3. Most distal anastomoses and supra-aortic vessel reimplantations can be performed within 30 to 45 minutes, with CPB being resumed as soon as their completion is achieved. This situation is particularly true if a femoral artery has been cannulated or if CPB is resumed through a lateral branch of the aortic prosthesis. The prosthesis can indeed be cross-clamped upstream after the completion of the distal anastomosis and the cerebral vessels reimplanted during CPB.

The Perfusate Temperature

As early as 1986, Guilmet and our group proposed the technique of SACP with cold blood (cold blood cerebroplegia) while maintaining the patient's core temperature at moderate hypothermia.[36,37] A few years later Kazui and coworkers[38] proposed a similar technique, in which, however, brain perfusion and CPB were performed at the same level of moderate hypothermia. Since then, both techniques have gained wide acceptance and have had excellent results in hospital mortality and neurological outcome. We have personally successfully used the technique of cold blood cerebroplegia for more than 15 years. In recent years we have used the Kazui technique.

Antegrade Selective Perfusion With Cold Blood: Cold Blood Cerebroplegia

This technique was aimed at cooling the brain through a selective perfusion of the brachiocephalic arteries with cold blood (10–12°C) using the analogy of cold blood cardioplegia, maintaining the patient at moderate core hypothermia (25–28°C).

We considered that only antegrade selective cerebral perfusion could permit an even distribution of the cold perfusate to the brain despite the nonpreservation of the CBF regulation. In addition, we believed that the necessity of reducing the metabolic demands of the brain through selective cooling was of some importance.

A regular CPB circuit is modified by addition, beyond the oxygenator, of a heat exchanger usually dedicated to cold blood cardioplegia and a roller pump. By means of the heat exchanger, blood derived from the oxygenator can be cooled down to 10 to 12°C. A perfusion line distributes cold blood to the brachiocephalic arteries and the coronary arteries through a quadrifurcated connector. Specially designed cannulas are available in several diameters to perfuse the carotid arteries. The cannulas are bent at a right angle to allow their proper placement and position during operation.

Arterial pressure is measured in the right radial artery to allow monitoring pressure in the right carotid artery during perfusion. The rectal and esophageal temperatures are recorded permanently throughout the procedure, as well as the electroencephalogram, if possible.

CPB is established between the right atrium (2-stage single cannula) and 1 femoral artery. Cooling of the patient is initiated. During cooling, the brachiocephalic arteries are dissected free and encircled with snares.

When the rectal temperature reaches 28°C (which corresponds in many patients to a nasopharyngeal temperature of 24–25°C), cannulas are inserted in the innominate and left carotid arteries, and held by means of adventitial 5-0 polypropylene purse-string sutures. The brachiocephalic arteries are then cross-clamped, and selective cold perfusion is initiated. The main CPB is discontinued and the aortic arch opened. Myocardial protection is achieved by perfusing cold blood through selective cannulation of the coronary ostia or the ascending aorta, if this segment is not replaced.

During circulatory arrest selective perfusion of the cerebral and coronary arteries is maintained at a flow rate of about 7 mL/kg/min. The pressure in the carotid arteries is kept between 60 and 70 mm Hg because, at this level of temperature, there is a direct pressure-flow relation. During cerebral perfusion and circulatory arrest, no adjuncts, such as barbiturates or steroids, are used to enhance cerebral protection.

Withdrawal of the cannulas is easy, hemostasis being achieved by tightening the adventitial purse-string sutures.

We have used this method successfully in more than 200 patients.[39] However, it has some drawbacks:

- It requires a sophisticated perfusion circuit.
- Lateral cannulation of the brachiocephalic vessels may be uneasy or even dangerous in

case of deeply atheromatous lesions or in some cases of aortic dissection.

- The technique was described to be used with femoral artery cannulation. The almost systematic cannulation of the right axillary or innominate artery makes its use less easy.

SACP in Moderate Hypothermia: Kazui Technique

This method differs from the technique described by Guilmet in the temperature of the cerebral perfusate and the mode of cannulation of the epiaortic vessels.

The usual CPB circuit is slightly modified. An extra-arterial line is derived from the main arterial line. On this line a specific pump is dedicated to brain perfusion. The same heat exchanger is used for the whole circuit because CPB and cerebral perfusion are performed at the same temperature.

After cannulation and heparinization, the core temperature (nasopharyngeal) of the patient is lowered to 25°C, which generally corresponds to a rectal temperature of 28°C. When this temperature is reached, CPB is discontinued.

When reimplantation of the epiaortic vessels is performed en bloc, the aortic arch is opened; cannulas are inserted into the ostia of the innominate and left common carotid arteries; SACP is established.

When reimplantation of the cerebral vessels is performed separately, the vessels are cross-clamped near their origin, divided, and selectively cannulated.

Autoinflatable balloon cannulas such as the ones used for retrograde cardioplegia or specially designed cannulas may be used. In any case it may be useful to maintain the cannulas in proper position by snares put around the vessels and tied with a tourniquet.

A total flow of 10 mL/kg is perfused through both cannulas. Such a flow is sufficient to adequately satisfy the metabolic demand of the cerebrum at this level of hypothermia. Assessment of the perfusion flow has been proposed by measuring the pressure in the carotid arteries.[40] This does not seem useful as those elements are closely linked and, because of the cerebral flow autoregulation, the pressure in the carotid arteries sets generally between 50 and 70 mm Hg at a flow of 10 mL/kg/min.

When the distal anastomosis on the aorta is completed, the prosthesis is cross-clamped proximally and CPB may be resumed through a lateral branch of the aortic prosthesis. By doing so, the duration of circulatory arrest in the lower part of the body is reduced to the time of the distal anastomosis. Reimplantation of the cerebral vessels is then performed.

If the right axillary or the innominate artery is cannulated, CBP is resumed only after reimplantation of the epiaortic vessels. However, the duration of distal circulatory arrest seldom exceeds 40 minutes.

Cannulas of the cerebral vessels are withdrawn in succession at the end of the reimplantation anastomosis (or anastomoses) after reducing but without discontinuing the perfusion flow to avoid any air embolism during withdrawal.

Because of its simplicity and the easy mode of cannulation of the cerebral vessels, this technique of SACP has gained large acceptance in the last few years.

THE ISSUES
Is the Use of SACP Easy?

Selective perfusion of the brachiocephalic arteries might seem a complicated technique: it requires that the cephalic arteries be dissected free and cannulated; it necessitates specific equipment and the presence of several perfusion lines in an already encumbered surgical field. Any obstruction (kinking, malposition) of the supplying line or cannula may result in cerebral ischemia.

With properly chosen and placed cannulas, this difficulty can be easily managed. Specially designed cannulas are available in several diameters to perfuse the carotid arteries. The blunt tip of the cannulas avoids traumatization of the cannulated vessel. The cannulas can be bent at a right angle and, in general, their proper placement and positioning during operation are not a concern.

Some investigators have suggested that the carotid cannulation may be the cause of atheromatous or gas emboli.[41,42] We have observed such a complication in 3 of 249 patients (1.2%) and we believe that it can be easily avoided by taking care in de-airing and not interrupting completely the flow during removal of the cannulas.

In addition, in the last decade the techniques of cannulation of the right axillary artery or the innominate artery have gained acceptance and have become a standard mode of arterial return during CPB. By definition, they allow full antegrade arterial inflow during the whole duration of CPB. They make useless any kind of cannula switch after completion of the aortic repair. They allow antegrade perfusion of the brain through the right carotid artery during the time of arch repair and distal circulatory arrest. In this case, only 1 additional cannula needs to be inserted into the left common carotid to achieve full flow bilateral cerebral perfusion.

Is the Use of SACP Safe?

During the last 2 decades, SACP has had some important experimental support:

- In an article published in 1991 by Swain and colleagues[43] there is a striking difference in favor of selective antegrade deep hypothermic perfusion at moderate flow, which shows no alteration of any of the energetic components of the cerebral tissues.
- Ye and colleagues[44] performed a comparative experimental study of neuronal damage after hypothermic circulatory arrest (HCA), RCP, and SACP. They concluded that retrograde perfusion provided some brain protection but was unable to prevent moderately severe neuronal alteration and that only SACP safely prevents ischemic damage to the brain.
- Similarly, Sakurada and coworkers[45] performed a comparative study of the 3 techniques. They, too, concluded that retrograde perfusion had some advantage for cerebral protection compared with DHCA but could not supply sufficient blood flow to maintain brain function and that SACP was the safest method of brain protection during arch exclusion.
- In 1995, Filgueras and colleagues,[46] comparing the 3 methods of brain protection, showed by means of P magnetic resonance that only SACP was able to preserve the integrity of the cerebral metabolism.
- More recently, Hagl and coworkers[47] have compared in pigs the neurological and metabolic evolution after cold SACP and deep HCA. They concluded "Cold SACP is associated with better neurophysiological recovery and less cerebral edema, indicated by lower intracranial pressure (ICP) during perfusion. Neuropsychological recovery correlated well with the rise in ICP. HCA alone causes prolonged acidosis in the brain tissue during reperfusion."

Clinically, there are no randomized controlled studies comparing DHCA associated or not with RCP or SACP. Such a randomized study would be difficult to carry out and would be questionable from an ethical standpoint. However, during the last decade, numerous observational retrospective studies have reported favorable results and outstanding improvements in the outcome of the patients with the use of SACP.[39,48–54] It seems that those clinical reports tend more and more to confirm the hierarchy established experimentally between DHCA alone, DHCA associated with RCP, and SACP (under its various modes).[55] So, SACP has become the preferred method of cerebral protection in most groups dealing with aortic arch surgery.

Between April 1986 and November 2009 we used SACP associated with moderate core hypothermia (25°C) in 249 patients, including 71 patients (27%) operated on in emergency, mainly for acute type A dissection. Sixty-six patients had already undergone 1 or several procedures on the thoracic aorta. In 217 patients the brain was perfused with cold blood (Guilmet technique) and in the remaining 32 patients the brain was perfused at the core temperature (Kazui technique). Mean duration of CPB, cerebral perfusion, and distal circulatory arrest were 121 minutes (65–248 minutes), 53 minutes (15–90 minutes), and 34 minutes (10–57 minutes), respectively. The overall hospital mortality was 16% (40 patients) (10% in elective surgery and 22% in emergency surgery). Fatal new neurologic injuries were observed in 12 patients (5%) but only in 3% patients after elective surgery. Nonlethal new neurological disorders have been observed in 12 patients (7% of survivors) and, again, in only 3% of patients operated on electively. In the 32 patients operated on according to the Kazui technique there were 2 deaths (6%) and 2 transient new neurologic disorders (6%). Emergency, age greater than 65 years, and extension of the aortic repair to the descending aorta were the risk factors for mortality and neurologic disorders on multivariate analysis. No correlation could be established between the duration of CPB, distal circulatory arrest, and cerebral perfusion and the rate of mortality or neurological complications.

What is the Best Perfusate Temperature?

The choice of a very low temperature (10–12°C) of the blood perfusate irrigating the brain has been questioned. We were convinced at the beginning of our experience that, at this level of temperature, the metabolic demands of the brain were suppressed, whereas the integrity of the energetic components and the pH of the cell were maintained through the use of oxygenated blood.

At this level of hypothermia, the dissociation curve of hemoglobin is displaced toward the left. The oxygen delivered to the tissues is, therefore, mainly transported in the dissolved form. The main advantage of using oxygenated blood consists, thus, in the buffer capacity of the imidazole nucleus of the hemoglobin molecule. Those factors constituted the basic reasons for the beneficial effect of permanently perfusing the brain at a very low temperature.

The well-founded rationale of this technique was confirmed by several experimental studies.

Strauch and colleagues[56] compared in pigs the CBF, the cerebral vascular resistance, the ICP, and the CMR_{O_2} at 2 levels of perfusate temperature (10–15°C and 20–25°C) as well as the neurological behavior of the animals in the aftermath of the experiment. They concluded that "The study suggests that SCP [selective cerebral perfusion] at 10°C to 15°C results in profound metabolic suppression lasting several hours after SCP, thus permitting faster neurological recovery at lower CBF than SCP at higher temperatures. In addition to providing better cerebral protection, SCP at lower temperature, by reducing CBF, also minimizes the risk of cerebral injury from embolization during arch surgery."

Clinically, in addition to our experience, several articles have confirmed the safety and usefulness of perfusing the brain with cold blood.[57,58]

As our clinical results were rewarding compared with the other methods, we did not change our protocol, but we acknowledged that the perfusate temperature could be higher, as reported in many experimental and clinical experiences.

Khaladj and colleagues,[59] in a study comparing several levels of temperature of perfusate in pigs, concluded that "Regarding the optimal temperature for SACP, it seems that 20°C provides adequate brain protection in comparison to the potential detrimental effects of moderate (30°C) or profound (10°C) temperatures."

After the initial report by Kazui and colleagues[38] in 1992, the Kazui technique of perfusing the cerebrum at the same level of moderate hypothermia (23–25°C) as the CPB was adopted by many groups. Although there are no clinical randomized controlled studies comparing several levels of perfusate temperature, studies and reports abound proving that this technique is safe and that the results are similar to those obtained when perfusing the brain at low temperatures.[48–54]

Both methods are equally safe and efficient and their results are comparable. However, as already stated, the Kazui technique seems to be simpler and more surgeon-friendly. For those reasons, we decided a few years ago to start using the Kazui technique of SACP associated with the cannulation of the right axillary or innominate artery. It is now our technique of choice for any kind of procedure involving the aortic arch (**Fig. 1**).

However, there is a present trend to increase the temperature of the perfusate during SACP. Recently, Touati and colleagues[60] have proposed carrying out SACP in normothermia. As this technique precludes any possibility of distal circulatory arrest, these investigators perfused the lower part of the body during the time of the arch repair by means of a balloon cannula placed into the descending aorta through the arch opening. Although the results reported were satisfactory we believe that such a technique has important drawbacks and is questionable, from a physiological and a purely surgical standpoint:

1. It eliminates the protection of the brain, viscera, and spinal cord provided by hypothermia. The preservation of organ homeostasis relies entirely and solely on CPB and the cerebral perfusion system. Any technical defect or unexpected malfunction in those features results immediately in deleterious ischemic disorders.
2. The proper flow necessary to maintain the cerebral homeostasis is not well defined. There is, hence, a risk of hypo- or hyperperfusion, as observed in the early experience of DeBakey and colleagues.[42]
3. The presence of an extra cannula in the descending aorta may be cumbersome and can unduly complicate the completion of the distal anastomosis.
4. In chronic dissection, when there is a discrepancy between the diameters of the false and true lumens of the descending aorta, how and where is the balloon cannula placed?

Is Unilateral Antegrade Cerebral Perfusion Equivalent to Bilateral Cerebral Perfusion?

To simplify the technique of SACP, it has been proposed to perfuse the brain unilaterally only, on the assumption that the vascular connections between both cerebral hemispheres are numerous and functional.

For many years we have considered that this method was unsafe. At least 10% to 15% of human beings have anatomic abnormalities of the circle of Willis and therefore incomplete connections between the cerebral hemispheres or between the anterior and posterior structures of the brain. We believed that unilateral perfusion could then result in prolonged ischemia of some parts of the brain and in severe postoperative neurological disorders. In our opinion, this method could be used only for short times of brain perfusion or when the assessment of the vascularization of the brain had been performed preoperatively and had shown a perfectly functional circle of Willis.

However, in the last decade, many articles have reported satisfactory clinical results with unilateral perfusion, even in emergency situations or in aged patients.[51,61–66]

CANNULATION OF THE RIGHT AXILLARY and MEDIAN STERNOTOMY

or

MEDIAN STERNOTOMY and CANNULATION OF THE INNOMINATE ARTERY

Cannulation of the Right atrium

Rectal Temperature: 25-28°C.

Naso-pharyngeal Temperature: 23-25°C

Dissection of the arch and supra aortic vessels

DISTAL CIRCULATORY ARREST

Cross clamping of the origin of the innominate artery

Right Axillary or Innominate Artery perfusion: 10ml/kg/min

Opening of the aortic arch.

CANNULATION OF THE LEFT COMMON CAROTID ARTERY

Cross clamping or occlusion of the left sub clavian artery

Cannulation of the left common carotid artery (balloon catheter)

BILATERAL PERFUSION : 10ML/KG/MIN; (50-70 mm Hg)

Resection of the aortic arch.

Division of the supra aortic vessels (en bloc or separately)

DISTAL ANASTOMOSIS (regular or "Elephant trunk")

Reimplantation of the supra aortic vessels (en bloc or separately)

De-airing

RESUMPTION OF FULL FLOW CPB AND RE-WARMING

Rewarming

PROXIMAL ANASTOMOSIS OR REPAIR

Fig. 1. Our current technique for transverse aortic arch replacement.

In general, unilateral perfusion of the brain is performed through the right axillary or the innominate arteries. Urbanski and colleagues[67] proposed using of 1 common carotid artery as the only site of arterial return and cerebral perfusion during surgery of the aortic arch. After a small cervicotomy is performed, the artery is perfused through a side graft sewn in an end-to-side fashion on the artery. These investigators have mainly used the right common carotid artery, but also the left carotid artery in some instances. They have reported outstanding results with low mortality and neurological complications. In a recent report they preoperatively studied the quality of the circle of Willis in patients operated on electively and found that 40% had an abnormal circle of Willis. Unilateral cerebral perfusion was used in all patients. Only 1 death (1%) and 1 stroke (1%) occurred. They concluded that "The anatomic status of the circle of Willis assessed with cranial CT [computed tomography] angiography does not correlate with functional and intraoperative tests examining the cerebral cross-perfusion. [We] do not recommend cranial CT angiography as a preoperative standard examination before open arch surgery in which unilateral cerebral perfusion is scheduled."[68]

However, in this study the average times of cerebral perfusion and circulatory arrest were short (18 minutes), which is less than generally reported and could explain the innocuity of the technique. It is not known whether such a technique would be safe in longer times of perfusion.

In addition, our experience has shown that, when using perfusion at moderate hypothermia through the right side and after starting the perfusion unilaterally, it takes a short time (a few seconds) to place a balloon cannula into the left common carotid artery through the opened arch and to achieve bilateral perfusion. We therefore consider that there are few reasons for not doing so and for putting the patient at undue risk.

Should the Left Subclavian Artery be Perfused?

In most reported experiences of SACP, only the right axillary or the innominate arteries and the left common carotid artery are cannulated and perfused. Apparently, not perfusing the left subclavian artery has no harmful clinical consequences.

It seems that this is true under several conditions:

1. If the left subclavian artery is not selectively perfused, it is important that it be cross-clamped or occluded by a small Foley catheter to avoid any possible steal syndrome and consequent ischemia of the posterior cerebrum.
2. If the preoperative investigations have shown that the left vertebral artery is largely dominant or single, left subclavian artery perfusion may prove indispensable.
3. As has been shown, in particular by Griepp and Biglioli,[69–71] the left subclavian artery participates in the anterior spinal arterial network. Its suppression or the absence of proper perfusion may result in spinal cord injury when this network is already jeopardized (eg, chronic dissection, occlusion of the intercostal arteries, previous replacement of the abdominal aorta).

In our experience we have observed 5 cases (2%) of oculomotor nerve palsy. All patients had undergone a difficult redo procedure in which the left subclavian artery could not be occluded or perfused because of anatomic abnormalities or technical difficulties and 2 cases of paraplegia in patients with chronic dissection in whom the left subclavian artery had been ligated.

It seems therefore that in selected cases (eg, expected difficult redo procedures, previous surgery on the distal aorta, particularly dominant left vertebral artery), perfusion of the left subclavian artery, when possible, represents an important element in the safety of SACP.

SUMMARY

Surgery of the aortic arch has benefited from various improvements during the last 3 decades, especially in brain protection and neurological outcome. Several techniques are available that allow the surgeon to perform the aortic repair with a fair certainty of success. The analysis of the literature shows that, when all sensory-motor alterations are reported, the rate of postoperative neurological injury may reach 25% with DHCA with or without RCP, although this latter technique seems to increase the tolerated time of ischemia.

Conversely, whatever the modifications described since the initial reports proposing SACP, its basic principles and rationale have not changed. The technique provides the cerebrum with its basic oxygen and metabolic demands and preserves the energetic components of the neurons. Clinically, perfusing the brain either with cold blood (10–12°C) or at moderate hypothermia (23–25°C) has proved to be equally efficacious.

The safety provided by SACP during a nonlimited time of arch exclusion makes it the gold standard in brain protection during arch surgery. This opinion has been strengthened by the publication of numerous clinical studies reporting excellent results with SACP associated with core moderate hypothermia (23–25°C). In addition to our own experience, all those publications have reinforced our conviction that perfusing the cerebrum antegradely represents the best and safest way of preserving the complete integrity of the neurologic functions in terms of sensory-motor and cognitive faculties, as acknowledged recently by Griepp.[72] This is particularly true in frail and aged patients or in patients requiring a long and difficult surgical procedure.

REFERENCES

1. Fox LS, Blackstone EH, Kirklin JW, et al. Relationship of brain blood flow and oxygen consumption to perfusion flow rates during profoundly hypothermic cardiopulmonary bypass. J Thorac Cardiovasc Surg 1984;87:658–64.
2. Neri E, Sassi C, Barabesi L, et al. Cerebral autoregulation after hypothermic circulatory arrest in operations on the aortic arch. Ann Thorac Surg 2004;77: 72–9.
3. Tanaka J, Shiki J, Asai T, et al. Cerebral autoregulation during deep hypothermic non pulsatile cardiopulmonary bypass with selective cerebral perfusion in dogs. J Thorac Cardiovasc Surg 1988; 95:124–32.
4. Cooley DA, Mahaffey DE, De Bakey ME. Total excision of the aortic arch for aneurysm. Surg Gynecol Obstet 1955;10:667–72.
5. De Bakey ME, Crawford ES, Cooley DA, et al. Successful resection of fusiform aneurysm of aortic arch with replacement by homograft. Surg Gynecol Obstet 1957;105:657–64.
6. Hou YL, Shang TY, Wu YK. Surgical treatment of aneurysm of the thoracic aorta. Chin Med J 1964; 83:740–9.
7. Guilmet D, Scetbon V, Ricordeau G, et al. Memoires de l'Académie de chirurgie. Mem Acad Chir (Paris) 1966;92:479–87 [in French].

8. Fontan F, Beaudet E, Mounicot FB, et al. Résection-greffe d'un anévrysme de la crosse de l'aorte (segment 1) à cœur battant et sous shunt pulsé partiel. Ann Chir Thorac Cardiovasc 1971;10:59–63 [in French].

9. Bigelow WG, Lindsay WK, Greenwood WF. Hypothermia; its possible role in cardiac surgery: an investigation of factors governing survival in dogs at low body temperatures. Ann Surg 1950;132:849–66.

10. Borst HG, Shaudig A, Rudolph W. Arteriovenous fistula of the aortic arch: repair during deep hypothermia and circulatory arrest. J Thorac Cardiovasc Surg 1964;48:443–7.

11. Griepp RB, Stinson EB, Hollingsworth JF, et al. Prosthetic replacement of the aortic arch. J Thorac Cardiovasc Surg 1975;70:1051–63.

12. Cooley DA, Ott DA, Frazier OH, et al. Surgical treatment of aneurysms of the transverse aortic arch: experience with 25 patients using hypothermic techniques. Ann Thorac Surg 1981;32:260–72.

13. Ehrlich MP, McCullough JN, Zhang N. Effect of hypothermia on cerebral blood flow and metabolism in the pig. Ann Thorac Surg 2002;73:191–7.

14. O'Connor JV, Wilding T, Farmer P, et al. The protective effect of profound hypothermia on the canine central nervous system in surgery of the ascending aorta and the aortic arch. Ann Thorac Surg 1986;41:255–9.

15. Crawford ES, Saleh EB. Transverse aortic arch aneurysm: improved results of treatment employing new modifications of aorta reconstitution and hypothermic cerebral circulatory arrest. Ann Surg 1981;194:180–8.

16. Ergin AM, O'Connor J, Guinto R, et al. Experience with profound hypothermia and circulatory arrest in the treatment of aneurysm of the aortic arch. J Thorac Cardiovasc Surg 1982;84:649–55.

17. Livesay JJ, Cooley DA, Reul GJ, et al. Resection of aortic arch aneurysms: a comparison of hypothermic techniques in 60 patients. Ann Thorac Surg 1983;36:19–28.

18. Gega A, Rizzo JH, Johnson MH, et al. Straight deep hypothermic arrest: experience in 394 patients supports its effectiveness as a sole means of brain preservation. Ann Thorac Surg 2007;84:759–67.

19. Guilmet D, Diaz F, Roux PM, et al. Anévrysmes de la crosse aortique: traitement chirurgical: 60 observations. Nouv Presse Med 1986;15:2191–5 [in French].

20. Ueda Y, Miki S, Kusuhara OY, et al. Deep hypothermic systemic circulatory arrest and continuous retrograde cerebral perfusion for surgery of aortic arch aneurysm. Eur J Cardiothorac Surg 1992;6:36–42.

21. Dresser LP, Mc Kinney WM. Anatomic and pathophysiologic studies of the human internal jugular valves. Am J Surg 1987;154:220–4.

22. Künzli A, Zingg PO, Zünd G, et al. Does retrograde cerebral perfusion via superior vena cava cannulation protect the brain? Eur J Cardiothorac Surg 2006;30:906–9.

23. De Brux JL, Subayi JB, Pegis JD, et al. Retrograde cerebral perfusion: anatomic study of the distribution of blood to the brain. Ann Thorac Surg 1995;60:1294–8.

24. Ehrlich MP, Hagl C, McCullough JN, et al. Retrograde cerebral perfusion provides negligible flow through brain capillaries in the pig. J Thorac Cardiovasc Surg 2001;122:331–8.

25. Midulla PS, Gandsas A, Sadeghi AM, et al. Comparison of retrograde cerebral perfusion to antegrade cerebral perfusion and hypothermic circulatory arrest in a chronic porcine model. J Cardiovasc Surg 1994;9:560–75.

26. Katz MG, Khazin V, Steinmetz A, et al. Distribution of cerebral flow using retrograde versus antegrade cerebral perfusion. Ann Thorac Surg 1999;67:1065–9.

27. Boeckxstaens CJ, Flameng WJ. Retrograde cerebral perfusion does not protect the brain in non-human primates. Ann Thorac Surg 1995;60:319–28.

28. Bonser RS, Wong CH, Harrington D, et al. Failure of retrograde cerebral perfusion to attenuate metabolic changes associated with hypothermic circulatory arrest. J Thorac Cardiovasc Surg 2002;123:943–50.

29. Safi HJ, Letsou GV, Iliopoulos DC, et al. Impact of retrograde cerebral perfusion on ascending aortic and arch aneurysm repair. Ann Thorac Surg 1997;63:1601–7.

30. Coselli JS. Retrograde cerebral perfusion is an effective means of neural support during deep hypothermic circulatory arrest. Ann Thorac Surg 1997;64:908–12.

31. Bavaria JE, Woo YJ, Hall RA, et al. Retrograde cerebral and distal aortic perfusion during ascending and thoracoabdominal aortic operations. Ann Thorac Surg 1995;60:345–53.

32. Usui A, Abe T, Murase M. Early clinical results of retrograde cerebral perfusion for aortic arch operations in Japan. Ann Thorac Surg 1996;62:94–103.

33. Okita Y, Takamoyo M, Ando S, et al. Mortality and cerebral outcome in patients who underwent aortic arch operations using deep hypothermic circulatory arrest with retrograde cerebral perfusion: no relation of early death, stroke, and delirium to the duration of circulatory arrest. J Thorac Cardiovasc Surg 1998;115:129–38.

34. Strauch JT, Lauten A, Spielvogel D, et al. Mild hypothermia protects the spinal cord from ischemic injury in a chronic porcine model. Eur J Cardiothorac Surg 2004;25:708–15.

35. Saritas A, Kervan U, Vural KM, et al. Visceral protection during moderately hypothermic selective antegrade cerebral perfusion through right brachial artery. Eur J Cardiothorac Surg 2009;37:669–76.

36. Guilmet D, Roux PM, Bachet J, et al. Nouvelle technique de protection cérébrale: chirurgie de la crosse aortique. Nouv Presse Med 1986;15:2191–5 [in French].

37. Bachet J, Guilmet D, Goudot B, et al. Cold cerebroplegia: a new technique of cerebral protection during operations on the transverse aortic arch. J Thorac Cardiovasc Surg 1991;102:85–94.

38. Kazui T, Inoue N, Yamada O, et al. Selective cerebral perfusion during operation for aneurysms of the aortic arch: a reassessment. Ann Thorac Surg 1992;53:109–14.

39. Bachet J, Guilmet D, Goudot B, et al. Antegrade cerebral perfusion with cold blood: a 13-year experience. Ann Thorac Surg 1999;67:1874–8.

40. Scorsin M, Menasché P, Nataf P, et al. Pressure adjusted antegrade brain perfusion for surgery of the aortic aneurysm. Eur J Cardiothorac Surg 2001;19:108–10.

41. Crawford ES, Saleh SA, Schuelsser JS, et al. Treatment of aneurysm of transverse aortic arch. J Thorac Cardiovasc Surg 1979;78:383–93.

42. DeBakey ME, Henly WS, Cooley DA, et al. Aneurysms of the aortic arch: factors influencing operative risk. Surg Clin North Am 1962;42:1543–54.

43. Swain JA, McDonald TJ, Griffith PK, et al. Low-flow hypothermic cardiopulmonary by pass protects the brain. J Thorac Cardiovasc Surg 1991;102:76–84.

44. Ye J, Yang J, Del Bigio MR, et al. Neuronal damage after hypothermic circulatory arrest and retrograde cerebral perfusion in the pig. Ann Thorac Surg 1996;61:1316–22.

45. Sakurada T, Kazui T, Tanaka H, et al. Comparative experimental study of cerebral protection during aortic arch reconstruction. Ann Thorac Surg 1996; 61:1348–54.

46. Filgueras CL, Winsborrow B, Ye J, et al. A P-magnetic resonance study of antegrade and retrograde cerebral perfusion during aortic arch surgery in pigs. J Thorac Cardiovasc Surg 1995;110:55–62.

47. Hagl C, Khaladj N, Peterss S, et al. Hypothermic circulatory arrest with and without cold selective antegrade cerebral perfusion: impact on neurological recovery and tissue metabolism in an acute porcine model. Eur J Cardiothorac Surg 2004;26: 73–80.

48. Kazui T, Yamashita K, Washiyama N, et al. Usefulness of antegrade selective cerebral perfusion during aortic arch operations. Ann Thorac Surg 2002;74:S1806–9.

49. Di Eusanio M, Schepens MA, Morshuis WJ, et al. Antegrade selective cerebral perfusion during operations on the thoracic aorta: factors influencing survival and neurologic outcome in 413 patients. J Thorac Cardiovasc Surg 2002;124:1080–6.

50. Di Eusanio M, Schepens MA, Morshuis WJ, et al. Brain protection using antegrade selective cerebral perfusion: a multicenter study. Ann Thorac Surg 2003;76:1181–8.

51. Numata S, Ogino H, Sasaki H, et al. Total arch replacement using antegrade selective cerebral perfusion with right axillary artery perfusion. Eur J Cardiothorac Surg 2003;23:771–5.

52. Pacini D, Leone A, Di Marco L, et al. Antegrade selective cerebral perfusion in thoracic aorta surgery: safety of moderate hypothermia. Eur J Cardiothorac Surg 2007;31:618–22.

53. Bakhtiary F, Dogan S, Zierer A, et al. Antegrade cerebral perfusion for acute type A aortic dissection in 120 consecutive patients. Ann Thorac Surg 2008; 85:465–9.

54. Harrington DK, Walker AS, Kaukuntla H, et al. Selective antegrade cerebral perfusion attenuates brain metabolic deficit in aortic arch surgery: a prospective randomized trial. Circulation 2004;110(11 Suppl 1):II231–6.

55. Sundt TM 3rd, Orszulak TA, Cook DJ, et al. Improving results of open arch replacement. Ann Thorac Surg 2008;86:787–96 [discussion: 787–96].

56. Strauch JT, Haldenwang PL, Müllem K, et al. Temperature dependence of cerebral blood flow for isolated regions of the brain during selective cerebral perfusion in pigs. Ann Thorac Surg 2009; 88:1506–13.

57. Khaladj N, Shrestha M, Meck S, et al. Hypothermic circulatory arrest with selective antegrade cerebral perfusion in ascending aortic and aortic arch surgery: a risk factor analysis for adverse outcome in 501 patients. J Thorac Cardiovasc Surg 2008; 135:908–14.

58. Strauch JT, Spielvogel D, Lauten A, et al. Optimal temperature for selective cerebral perfusion. J Thorac Cardiovasc Surg 2005;130:74–82.

59. Khaladj N, Peterss S, Oetjen P, et al. Hypothermic circulatory arrest with moderate, deep or profound hypothermic selective antegrade cerebral perfusion: which temperature provides best brain protection? Eur J Cardiothorac Surg 2006;30:492–8.

60. Touati GD, Marticho P, Farag M, et al. Totally normothermic aortic arch replacement without circulatory arrest. Eur J Cardiothorac Surg 2007; 32:263–8.

61. Küçüker SA, Ozatik MA, Saritaş A, et al. Arch repair with unilateral antegrade cerebral perfusion. Eur J Cardiothorac Surg 2005;27:638–43.

62. Ozatik MA, Küçüker SA, Tülüce H, et al. Neurocognitive functions after aortic arch repair with right brachial artery perfusion [review]. Ann Thorac Surg 2004;78:591–5.

63. Halkos ME, Kerendi F, Myung R, et al. Selective antegrade cerebral perfusion via right axillary artery cannulation reduces morbidity and mortality after proximal aortic surgery. J Thorac Cardiovasc Surg 2009;138:1081–9.

64. Ogino H, Sasaki H, Minatoya K, et al. Evolving arch surgery using integrated antegrade selective cerebral perfusion: impact of axillary artery perfusion. J Thorac Cardiovasc Surg 2008;136:641–8 [discussion: 948–9].

65. Immer FF, Moser B, Krähenbühl ES, et al. Arterial access through the right subclavian artery in surgery of the aortic arch improves neurologic outcome and mid-term quality of life. Ann Thorac Surg 2008;85:1614–8.

66. Olsson C, Thelin S. Antegrade cerebral perfusion with a simplified technique: unilateral versus bilateral perfusion. Ann Thorac Surg 2006;81:868–74.

67. Urbanski PP. Cannulation of the left common carotid artery for proximal aortic repair. J Thorac Cardiovasc Surg 2003;126:887–8.

68. Urbanski PP, Lenos A, Blume JC, et al. Does anatomical completeness of the circle of Willis correlate with sufficient cross-perfusion during unilateral cerebral perfusion? Eur J Cardiothorac Surg 2008; 33:402–8.

69. Griepp RB, Ergin MA, Galla JD, et al. Looking for the artery of Adamkiewicz: a quest to minimize paraplegia after operations for aneurysms of the descending thoracic and thoracoabdominal aorta. Thorac Cardiovasc Surg 1996;112:1202–13 [discussion: 1213–5].

70. Griepp RB, Griepp EB. Spinal cord perfusion and protection during descending thoracic and thoracoabdominal aortic surgery: the collateral network concept [review]. Ann Thorac Surg 2007; 83:S865–9 [discussion: S890–2].

71. Biglioli P, Roberto M, Cannata A, et al. Upper and lower spinal cord blood supply: the continuity of the anterior spinal artery and the relevance of the lumbar arteries. J Thorac Cardiovasc Surg 2004;127:1188–92.

72. Griepp RB. Cerebral protection during aortic surgery. J Thorac Cardiovasc Surg 2003;125:36–8.

Editorial Comment: What is the Best Method for Brain Protection in Surgery of the Aortic Arch?

John A. Elefteriades, MD

The conventional wisdom on the street (to mix metaphors) is that retrograde cerebral perfusion is useless, not providing any significant amount of blood flow or oxygen substrate to the brain. In his article in this issue of *Cardiology Clinics*, however, Dr Yuichi Ueda, a pioneer of this technique, in giving his particular interpretation of animal and clinical data, provides a more positive perspective.

In his article, Dr John A. Elefteriades shows that at his institution straight deep hypothermic circulatory arrest (DHCA) delivers excellent results. The simplicity is laudable. Although his group performs even total arch replacement with elephant trunk with straight DHCA, antegrade perfusion provides an extra safeguard in case of obstacles to completion of requisite anastomoses. In extremely long arrest time settings, straight DHCA may not suffice.

Antegrade perfusion provides safety and security at the expense of complexity and some potential for complications directly related to cannulas and perfusion. Antegrade perfusion is probably not required for straightforward hemiarch replacement, in elective cases or in acute type A aortic dissection.

Although all three techniques are used effectively by proponents, antegrade perfusion (discussed in the article by Dr Jean Bachet in this issue) probably is preferable at most institutions (**Fig. 1**).

Section of Cardiac Surgery, Department of Surgery, Yale University School of Medicine, Yale-New Haven Hospital, PO Box 208039, New Haven, CT 06520-8039, USA
E-mail address: john.elefteriades@yale.edu

Cardiol Clin 28 (2010) 403–404
doi:10.1016/j.ccl.2010.02.013
0733-8651/10/$ – see front matter © 2010 Elsevier Inc. All rights reserved.

Retrograde Perfusion (Ueda)	Straight DHCA (Elefteriades)	Antegrade Cerebral Perfusion (Bachet)
Ueda and Safi results are excellent	Retrograde perfusion probably does not deliver much blood to brain (at least in animal experiments)	Perfusion is good
Discouraging animal studies may not be representative of human setting	Antegrade perfusion has unique problems: • How fast to flow? • How many vessels to include? • Brain edema? • Non-uniform perfusion • Vessel trauma • Embolization	Antegrade perfusion provides essentially unlimited duration for arch repair
Effective route for retrograde flushing of debris	Results with straight DHCA equal or surpass those with other methods	Moderate hypothermia suffices, eliminating need for and limits of straight DHCA
Negative animal studies explained by inherent differences in venous circulation among species (due to bending of neck to graze in farm animals)	Most strokes are embolic, not related to inadequate flow or preservation	Axillary cannulation makes antegrade perfusion easy
	Bloodless, uncluttered field	
	Simplicity—surgery is the focus; perfusion techniques do not become the operation	

Fig. 1. Antegrade perfusion probably is preferable at most institutions.

Endovascular Therapy for Thoracic Aneurysm Diseases: PRO

Rossella Fattori, MD

KEYWORDS

• Thoracic aortic disease • Stent-graft treatment
• Endovascular therapy

Traditional treatment of patients with descending thoracic aortic aneurysms and dissections has long been open surgical graft replacement. Despite progressive advances in surgery and anesthesiology, conventional surgical repair is still associated with considerable morbidity and mortality, resulting in prolonged hospitalization and high costs. Endoluminal stent-graft (TEVAR) in patients with thoracic aortic disease emerged a decade ago as a revolutionary approach, stimulated by the need to avoid inherent surgical risks in elderly patients with other major medical conditions. The interest and clinical effect of this therapeutic innovation can be compared with the introduction of coronary angioplasty 30 years ago; furthermore, TEVAR focused the attention of radiologists, cardiologists, and vascular-cardiac surgeons and led to a progressive fusion of different experiences and cultures. Nevertheless, controversies regarding the long-term benefit and durability have stimulated extensive debate in the literature.

EARLY RESULTS

Early clinical experience with stent grafting of the thoracic aorta was hampered by primitive technology, based on rigid homemade devices requiring large delivery systems.

However, the Stanford pivotal clinical trial in 1994[1] reported a favorable 30-day mortality of 9% in a series of 103 patients at high risk for open surgery with different aortic diseases including atherosclerotic aneurysms, aortic dissection, penetrating ulcers, and posttraumatic lesions.

The introduction in 1996 of commercially manufactured endoprostheses allowed TEVAR to be used in clinical practice, contributing to technical growth and aortic disease knowledge in many centers.

Results of TEVAR for first-generation stent grafts are available from many single-center series and multicenter controlled registries, such as Talent Thoracic Retrospective (TTR) and EUROSTAR, or GORE-TAG, Zenith TX2,[2–5] which compared the results of TEVAR with an open surgical control cohort (**Table 1**). Perioperative mortality ranged from 1.5%[4] to 9.3%,[3] with a significant difference between emergency and elective cases; major complications included paraplegia (1.8%–4%), stroke (1.7%–4%), vascular injuries (4%–16%), and systemic problems (pulmonary, renal, cardiac) in approximately one-fourth of patients (see **Table 1**). Similar data are reported in a recent meta-analysis[6] that compared literature results of TEVAR with open surgery in 17 eligible series comprising 1109 patients (538 stents). Reduced mortality (5.4% in TEVAR vs 14% in the open surgical arm) and neurologic complications were reported for the stent arm, resulting in reduced length of hospital stay. Major reinterventions, considered a major limitation of TEVAR, were required in 29 stent patients (7%) and 30 surgical patients (8.4%).

Cardiovascular Radiology Unit-Cardiovascular Department (pad 21), University Hospital S. Orsola, Via Massarenti 9, 40128 Bologna, Italy
E-mail address: rossella.fattori@unibo.it

Cardiol Clin 28 (2010) 405–412
doi:10.1016/j.ccl.2010.01.011

Table 1
Results of major observational registries investigating first-generation commercial devices

Name of the Study, Year of Publication	No. of Patients	Emergency Procedures Included	Follow-up (Months)	Mortality at 30 Days (%)	Paraplegia (%)	Endoleak at 30 Days (%)	Device Alterations (no.)
EUROSTAR, 2004	443	Yes	12	9.2	2.4	7.2	NR
TTR, 2006	457	Yes	24	5	1.7	9.6	2
GORE-TAG, 2005	142	No	24	2	3	7	20
ZENITH, 2008	160	No	12	1.9	1.2	13	1

Even if early clinical results have generally been encouraging, concerns have emerged regarding the long-term efficacy and durability of TEVAR, as follow-up is still limited (from 2 to 5 years in the largest series).

Endoleak represents the main cause of procedural failure and has been reported with a variable incidence, either early after the procedure or during later follow-up. Type I (proximal) endoleak, causing reperfusion of the aneurysm sac or false lumen in aortic dissection, is strongly associated with risk of aortic rupture and needs immediate treatment. Conversely, type II endoleak (reperfusion of the aneurysm sac as a result of collateral circulation from the left subclavian or intercostal arteries) may resolve with spontaneous thrombosis of the inflow vessel. With technical improvements and growing experience, the incidence of endoleak is decreasing from 25% with the first homemade graft[1] to 3% to 10% with recent commercial devices.[2–7]

Similarly, the initial drawbacks of thoracic devices, such as large sheath size and rigidity, potential modular disconnection, uncertain fabric integrity, and graft porosity, have been progressively reduced as technical refinements have evolved.[7]

In clinical practice, any novel therapy is faced with a series of problems, such as imperfect materials, insufficient technical skill of the users, and uncertain confirmation of therapeutic competence. This aspect has been particularly remarkable for TEVAR, which has been approached by many different specialists,[8] sometimes without the necessary technical and clinical background. Nevertheless, the results of TEVAR can be considered satisfactory even at the beginning of the learning curve; therefore, it is reasonable to think that with technical refinements and growing experience, clinical results will further improve.

ASSESSMENT OF PROPER ANATOMY FOR STENT GRAFT: THE ROLE OF IMAGING

One of the major potential causes of TEVAR failure originates from unsuitable anatomic indication; vascular imaging is therefore crucial for patient selection, choice of endoprosthesis, and treatment planning. The major anatomic prerequisites to be considered include morphology of the aortic lesions, vascular access, and integrity of the aortic wall at the neck sites, crucial components in treatment planning. Degenerative atherosclerotic alterations, thrombus, and calcifications, as well as excessive aortic tortuosity in the landing zone may be causes of procedural failure.

Several excellent imaging techniques are currently available in pretreatment evaluation, during surgery, and in postprocedural follow-up. However, with recent technical advances of multidetector computed tomography (MDCT), which allows submillimetric spatial resolution and long field of view, computed tomography (CT) can be considered the method of choice for aortic evaluation before treatment.[9] High-resolution CT angiograms with 1-mm slice thickness are required. Software reconstructions as maximum intensity projection and volume-rendering images are essential for displaying complex three-dimensional anatomy at the aortic arch and supraortic or visceral abdominal vessels (**Fig. 1**). Angiography is rarely necessary in this preliminary evaluation; its role is limited to the endovascular procedure for fluoroscopic guidance and angiographic road maps. Transesophageal echocardiography (TEE) is also essential during TEVAR, allowing a real-time assessment of safe advancement and positioning of the stent graft and high-definition information regarding the aortic wall at the neck sites.[10] After stent-graft delivery, TEE with color Doppler can identify even minimal

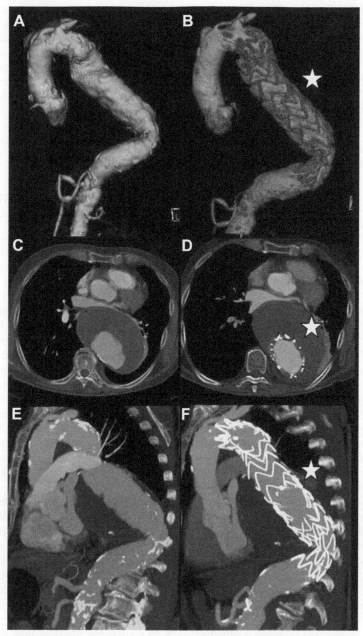

Fig. 1. MDCT volume-rendering (*A, B*), axial (*C, D*), and multiplanar reconstruction (*E, F*) images of a large TAA before (*A, C, E*) and after (*B, D, F*) endovascular therapy. The aneurysm sac is completely excluded from blood flow by the endograft (*star*).

flow inside the aneurysm sac (endoleak), or desired initial thrombosis (echo-contrast effect) outside the endograft, as an indicator of the efficacy of the procedure. In addition, periprocedural TEE avoids radiation and contrast medium, thus increasing procedural success. Magnetic resonance imaging (MRI) can also be used to assess vascular anatomy before stent-graft placement, even if calcifications are not visualized. The possibility of a functional analysis from MRI and rendering of anatomic details[11] may be useful in displaying flow dynamics in aortic dissection. During follow-up, as an alternative to MDCT, MRI can be used in young patients to avoid radiation, or in patients with renal insufficiency, which can be aggravated by repeated use of iodinated contrast medium.

APPROACHING THE AORTIC ARCH AND VISCERAL VESSELS: HYBRID PROCEDURES AND BRANCHED GRAFTS

Extension of the anatomic coverage of the proximal neck into the aortic arch is sometimes necessary to obtain better sealing. Left subclavian artery bypass or transposition can be performed with a supraclavicular surgical approach. This technique is minimally invasive and can protect from potential complications; specifically, occlusion of the left subclavian and left vertebral arteries without previous revascularization is associate with a higher risk of neurologic complications,[12] paraplegia,[13] and subclavian-vertebral steal syndrome.[14] Moreover, the risk of type II endoleak originating from the left subclavian artery may hamper aneurysm sealing. To further extend the proximal landing zone, extra-anatomic bypass of the carotid or innominate artery (total debranching) can be performed with sternotomy access. The results of combined open and endovascular strategies (hybrid procedures) are acceptable, with mortality and stroke rates of 0% to 20%, and 0% to 8%, respectively.[15] However, considering the efficacy and limited mortality of modern aortic arch surgery, endovascular therapy should be reserved for patients with a high risk from open surgery.

The combination of endovascular exclusion with visceral branch revascularization for the treatment of thoracoabdominal aortic aneurysms (TAA) involving the visceral aorta has also been attempted.[16,17] Although not specifically evaluated in any of the major clinical trials, adjunctive techniques are being increasingly used to expand the applicability of stent-graft technology to patients with more extensive aortic aneurysms and dissections. Visceral hybrid procedures offer an attractive alternative to open repair because potential benefits may be gained by the avoidance of thoracotomy and supraceliac cross-clamping. The key principle of this procedure is that retrograde revascularization of the visceral and/or renal arteries is effected via an abdominal approach; the abdominal aorta or common iliac or external iliac arteries can be used as the inflow sites for the visceral bypasses. However, there are some major concerns regarding long-term patency of visceral bypass and devastating complications associated with visceral graft occlusion have been reported, which suggests caution in wider proliferation of these complex operations. Endografts with branches represent a new alternative for treatment of TAA. This technology was first used in 2000 and continues to evolve. Multibranched stent grafts are modular devices with preattached limbs targeted for aortic side branches. These branches, which can be extended into the visceral and renal arteries using covered stents, allow a longer zone for hemostatic seal of the main aortic graft. Even if only small numbers of patients and short follow-up are available, this technical approach to expand endovascular treatment to TAA seems to be feasible, with limited mortality (<10%) and paraplegia rates.[18,19] With growing experience and the refinement of the devices, it is likely that endovascular repair will become a safe treatment option in selected patients with TAA.

CHANGING PARADIGMS IN THE MANAGEMENT OF ACUTE AORTIC DISEASE
Aortic Dissection

The emerging role of endovascular strategies for management of acute thoracic aortic pathologies has gained wide acceptance considering the unsatisfactory results of open repair. In acute type B dissection, medical treatment has long been the only treatment option for uncomplicated cases. Unfortunately, about 30% of acute type B dissections are complicated by peripheral vascular ischemia or hemodynamic instability at clinical presentation, with a subsequent high risk of spontaneous death; emergent open surgical repair of acute complicated dissection has a high mortality (25%–50%) only a few single-center series have reported more favorable results.[20–23] In such settings, TEVAR represents a less invasive alternative, promising encouraging results.[24,25] According to the results of the International Registry of Acute Aortic Dissections (IRAD) registry,[26] in 125 patients with acute type B dissection complicated by hemodynamic instability or malperfusion, TEVAR provided a better outcome, with 9.3% mortality in patients treated with stent graft and 33.9% mortality in patients submitted to open surgery. Malperfusion is 1 of the most important causes of morbidity and mortality in type B dissection and constitutes a challenge for medical and surgical treatment. Stent-graft occlusion of the entry site usually results in flow increase in the true lumen, restoring branch vessels patency. Therefore, direct resolution of malperfusion syndrome may be the first benefit of TEVAR in aortic dissection. Relief of visceral ischemia was observed in 16 of 17 patients in the IRAD population with malperfusion syndrome submitted to stent-graft placement only in 9 of 18 of those treated with percutaneous fenestration, and in just 4 of 14 patients treated with open surgery.[26] When malperfusion persists, a stent graft may be used in conjunction with other endovascular techniques, including branch vessel stenting, aortic stenting with bare or uncovered stents, and percutaneous wire slicing and balloon fenestration of the dissection septum.

Endovascular repair has been considered a milestone[27] in the history of management of type B dissection. The rationale for endovascular treatment of aortic dissection was originally based on evidence in the literature of a protective effect of false lumen thrombosis against false lumen expansion and risk of rupture. Closure of the entry tear of dissection may promote depressurization and shrinkage of the false lumen, with subsequent thrombosis, fibrous transformation, remodeling, and stabilization of the aorta (**Fig. 2**). Several series confirm the feasibility and a relative low rate of complications of TEVAR in acute type B dissection. However, long-term follow-up and outcome information to document a sustained benefit of endovascular repair are still lacking. Late aneurysmal degeneration of the thrombosed false lumen has been reported by Kato and colleagues,[28] and several case reports have highlighted the risk of retrograde extension of the dissection into the ascending aorta, potentially caused by stent-graft–induced intimal injury.[29] Even though extension of dissection is a known event in the natural course of type B dissection disease,[30] wire or sheath manipulation during the endovascular procedure could increase the risk of this dreadful complication. Continuous progress in stent-graft technology, improving morphology and flexibility, may lead to more suitable stent-graft configurations for aortic dissection. However, these unexpected

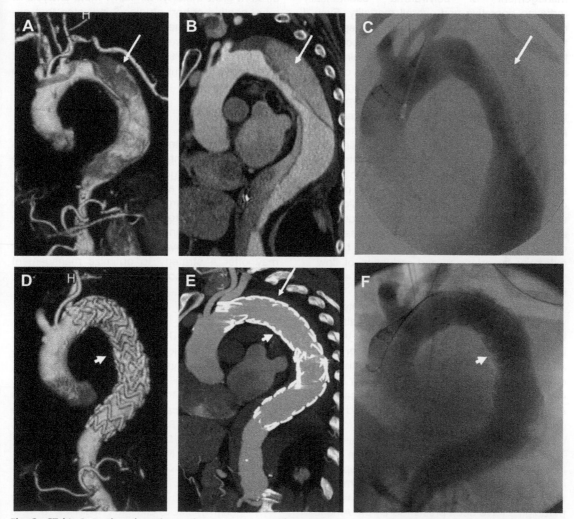

Fig. 2. CT (*A, B, D, E*) and angiography (*C, F*) images of an acute type B aortic dissection before (*A–C*) and after (*D–F*) endovascular treatment. The false lumen (*arrow* in *A–C*) is completely thrombosed and shrunken (*arrow* in *E*) after endovascular treatment, with complete expansion of the true lumen (*arrowhead* in *D–F*).

complications underline the particular fragility of the aortic wall and the need for careful selection criteria and rigorous follow-up.

Traumatic Aortic Injury

Traumatic aortic injury is not a rare pathologic entity, occurring in 10% to 30% of adults sustaining fatal blunt trauma[31]; it therefore represents 1 of the most common causes of death at the scene of vehicular accidents, accounting for 8000 victims per year in the United States. The more sophisticated prehospital care and the proliferation of rapid transport for patients have resulted in an increase in the number of patients treated. In the past few years, initial medical management and delayed surgery of the aortic traumatic injury represented an important advance in the difficult management of polytrauma, substantially reducing operative and overall mortality. Even if most patients with traumatic aortic injuries survive the initial impact and the first 6 hours become relatively stable, the risk of rupture may remain high for several days in approximately 5 to 10% of cases. On CT images,[32] unstable lesions at high risk of rupture involve the entire aortic circumference, usually present large periaortic hematoma and/or bilateral hemothorax, and, most important of all, show a discontinuity of the parietal profile, sometimes with contrast extravasation outside the adventitial wall. Usually, these imaging findings are associated with uncontrollable blood pressure, characterized by hypertensive crisis followed by severe hypotension. Sometimes the aortic tear, acting with a valve mechanism, may cause a pseudocoarctation syndrome, contributing to upper extremity hypertension and reduction of flow in the descending aorta with lower extremity ischemia.[33]

In these unstable polytrauma patients, endovascular techniques offer a suitable alternative to emergency open repair. Because of the lower invasiveness, there is no requirement for heparin and the blood loss is minimal, without the risk of destabilizing pulmonary, intracranial, or abdominal traumatic lesions. The risk of paraplegia seems to be low because of the limited longitudinal extension of a traumatic lesion, for which only 1 short segment of stent graft is necessary. Therefore, mortality and morbidity are notably less than in open surgery, as initially reported in case series and subsequently in comparative trials and meta-analyses.[34–38] New management paradigms have been presented by the American Association for the Surgery of Trauma. Comparing 2 observational multicentric studies,[39,40] covering a 10-year time interval, there was almost complete elimination of aortography and TEE, with increasing use of CT scans as the method of definitive diagnosis of traumatic injury. The percentage of patients who had CT scan diagnosis of the aortic injury increased from 34.8% to 93.3%. Moreover the time from admission to definitive repair increased significantly (16.5 ± 70.8 hours vs 54.6 ± 106.6 hours, $P<.001$); the method of definitive repair shifted from exclusively open techniques in 1997 to predominantly endovascular repairs in 2007. Most important, there were major outcome differences between the 2 studies: a significant reduction in the overall mortality during the second study period (from 31% in the first study 1997 to 13.0% in the second study), along with a significant reduction of procedure-related paraplegia (from 8.7% to 1.6%), as a result of the advent of stent-graft therapy. Similarly, meta-analysis of retrospective cohort studies[38] indicates that endovascular treatment of descending thoracic aortic trauma with respect to open repair provides lower mortality (2% vs 14%) and is associated with lower ischemic spinal cord complication rates (0% vs 7%).

SUMMARY

Although the long-term durability of stent grafts is still a concern, stent-graft treatment is already the best option in a large number of patients with descending thoracic aortic diseases who are poor candidates for surgical repair, or in an acute setting. With improved capability to recognize proper anatomy and select clinical candidates, the choice of endovascular stent-graft placement may offer a strategy to optimize management and improve prognosis.

REFERENCES

1. Dake MD, Miller DC, Semba CP, et al. Transluminal placement of endovascular stent-grafts for the treatment of descending thoracic aortic aneurysms. N Engl J Med 1994;331:1729–34.
2. Fattori R, Nienaber CA, Rousseau H, et al. Results of endovascular repair of the thoracic aorta with the Talent Thoracic Retrospective Registry. J Thorac Cardiovasc Surg 2006;132:332–9.
3. Leurs LJ, Bell R, Degrieck Y, et al. UK Thoracic Endograft Registry collaborators. Endovascular treatment of thoracic aortic diseases: combined experience from the EUROSTAR and United Kingdom Thoracic Endograft registries. J Vasc Surg 2004;40(4):670–9.
4. Makaroun MS, Dillavou ED, Kee ST, et al. Endovascular treatment of thoracic aortic aneurysms: results

of the phase II multicenter trial of the GORE TAG thoracic endoprosthesis. J Vasc Surg 2005;41(1): 1–9.

5. Matsumura JS, Cambria RP, Dake MD, et al. International controlled clinical trial of thoracic endovascular aneurysm repair with the Zenith TX2 endovascular graft: 1-year results. J Vasc Surg 2008;47:1094–8.

6. Walsh SR, Tang TY, Sadat U, et al. Endovascular stenting versus open surgery for thoracic aortic disease: systematic review and meta-analysis of perioperative results. J Vasc Surg 2008;47: 1094–8.

7. Thompson M, Ivaz S, Cheshire N, et al. Early results of endovascular treatment of the thoracic aorta using the valiant endograft. Cardiovasc Intervent Radiol 2007;30:1130–8.

8. Eggebrecht H, Pamler R, Zipfel B, et al. Thoracic aorta endografts: variations in practice among medical specialists. Catheter Cardiovasc Interv 2006;68(6):843–52.

9. Hoang JK, Martinez S, Hurwitz LM. MDCT angiography of thoracic aorta endovascular stent-grafts: pearls and pitfalls. AJR Am J Roentgenol 2009; 192(2):515–24.

10. Rocchi G, Lofiego C, Biagini E, et al. Transesophageal echocardiography-guided algorithm for stent-graft implantation in aortic dissection. J Vasc Surg 2004;40:880–5.

11. van Prehn J, van Herwaarden JA, Vincken KL, et al. Asymmetric aortic expansion of the aneurysm neck: analysis and visualization of shape changes with electrocardiogram-gated magnetic resonance imaging. J Vasc Surg 2009;49(6):1395–402.

12. Peterson BG, Eskandari MK, Gleason TG, et al. Utility of left subclavian artery revascularization in association with endoluminal repair of acute and chronic thoracic aortic pathology. J Vasc Surg 2006;43(3):433–9.

13. Buth J, Harris PL, Hobo R, et al. Neurologic complications associated with endovascular repair of thoracic aortic pathology: Incidence and risk factors. A study from the European Collaborators on Stent/Graft Techniques for Aortic Aneurysm Repair (EUROSTAR) registry. J Vasc Surg 2007; 46(6):1103–10.

14. Ferreira M, Monteiro M, Lanziotti L, et al. Deliberate subclavian artery occlusion during aortic endovascular repair: is it really that safe? Eur J Vasc Endovasc Surg 2007;33(6):664–7.

15. Schoder M, Lammer J, Czerny M. Endovascular aortic arch repair: hopes and certainties. Eur J Vasc Endovasc Surg 2009;38(3):255–61.

16. Chiesa R, Tshomba Y, Melissano G, et al. Is hybrid procedure the best treatment option for thoraco-abdominal aortic aneurysm? Eur J Vasc Endovasc Surg 2009;38(1):26–34.

17. Greenberg RK, Lytle B. Endovascular repair of thoracoabdominal aneurysms. Circulation 2008;117: 2288–96.

18. Verhoeven EL, Tielliu IF, Bos WT, et al. Present and future of branched stent grafts in thoraco-abdominal aortic aneurysm repair: a single-centre experience. Eur J Vasc Endovasc Surg 2009;38(2):155–61.

19. Greenberg RK, West K, Pfaff K, et al. Beyond the aortic bifurcation: branched endovascular grafts for thoracoabdominal and aortoiliac aneurysms. J Vasc Surg 2006;43:879–86.

20. Safi HJ, Miller CC 3rd, Reardon MJ, et al. Operations for acute and chronic dissection: recent outcomes in regard to neurological deficit and early death. Ann Thorac Surg 1998;66:401–11.

21. Marui A, Mochizuki T, Mitsui N, et al. Toward the best treatment of uncomplicated patients with type B acute aortic dissection: a consideration for sound surgical indication. Circulation 1999;100:II275–80.

22. Elefteriades JA, Hartleroad J, Gusberg RJ, et al. Long-term experience with descending aortic dissection: the complication-specific approach. Ann Thorac Surg 1992;53(1):11–20.

23. Schor JS, Yerlioglu E, Galla JD, et al. Selective management of acute type B aortic dissection: long-term follow-up. Ann Thorac Surg 1996;61: 1339–41.

24. Dake MD, Kato N, Mitchell RS, et al. Endovascular stent-graft placement for the treatment of acute aortic dissection. N Engl J Med 1999;340: 1546–52.

25. Nienaber CA, Fattori R, Lund G, et al. Nonsurgical reconstruction of thoracic aortic dissection by stent-graft placement. N Engl J Med 1999;340: 1539–45.

26. Fattori R, Tsai TT, Myrmel T, et al. Complicated acute type B dissection: is surgery still the best option?: a report from the International Registry of acute aortic dissection. JACC Cardiovasc Interv 2008;1: 395–402.

27. Vlahakes GJ. Catheter-based treatment of aortic dissection. N Engl J Med 1999;340(20):1585–6.

28. Kato N, Shimono T, Hirano T, et al. Midterm results of stent-graft repair of acute and chronic aortic dissection with descending tear: the complication-specific approach. J Thorac Cardiovasc Surg 2002;124:306–12.

29. Eggebrecht H, Thompson M, Rousseau H, et al. Retrograde ascending aortic dissection during or after thoracic aortic stent graft placement: insight from the European registry on endovascular aortic repair complications. Circulation 2009; 120:S276–81.

30. Winnerkvist A, Lockowandt U, Rasmussen E, et al. A prospective study of medically treated acute type B aortic dissection. Eur J Vasc Endovasc Surg 2006; 32(4):349–55.

31. Bertrand S, Cuny S, Petit P, et al. Traumatic rupture of thoracic aorta in real-world motor vehicle crashes. Traffic Inj Prev 2008;9:153–61.

32. Gavant ML. Helical CT grading of traumatic aortic injuries. Impact on clinical guidelines for medical and surgical management. Radiol Clin North Am 1999;37:553–74.

33. Malm JR, Deterling RH. Traumatic aneurysm of the thoracic aorta simulating coarctation. J Thorac Cardiovasc Surg 1960;40:271–8.

34. Rousseau H, Soula P, Perreault P, et al. Delayed treatment of traumatic rupture of the thoracic aorta with endoluminal covered stent. Circulation 1999;99:498–504.

35. Fattori R, Russo V, Lovato L, et al. Optimal management of traumatic aortic injury. Eur J Vasc Endovasc Surg 2009;37(1):8–14.

36. Doss M, Balzer J, Martens S, et al. Surgical versus endovascular treatment of acute thoracic aortic rupture: a single-center experience. Ann Thorac Surg 2003;76:1465–9.

37. Andrassy J, Weidenhagen R, Meimarakis G, et al. Stent versus open surgery for acute and chronic traumatic injury of the thoracic aorta: a single-center experience. J Trauma 2006;60:765–71.

38. Xenos ES, Abedi NN, Davenport DL, et al. Meta-analysis of endovascular vs open repair for traumatic descending thoracic aortic rupture. J Vasc Surg 2008;48:1343–51.

39. Demetriades D, Velmahos GC, Scalea TM, et al. Diagnosis and treatment of blunt thoracic aortic injuries: changing perspectives. J Trauma 2008;64: 1415–8.

40. Fabian TC, Richardson JD, Croce MA, et al. Prospective study of blunt aortic injury: multicenter trial of the American Association for the Surgery of Trauma. J Trauma 1997;42:374–80.

Endovascular Therapy for Thoracic Aneurysm Diseases: CON

John A. Elefteriades, MD

KEYWORDS

• Endovascular • Aorta • Endograft • Aneurysm

Federal Reserve Chairman Alan Greenspan 1996 coined the term "Irrational Exuberance" to describe the state of the US securities market, and, subsequently, Yale Economist Robert Shiller elaborated on this concept in his 2005 book of the same name.

It is important for heart specialists to regard the less-invasive modality of stent therapy for aneurysm disease with enthusiasm and, at the same time, with a grain of skepticism or at least realism. One needs to guard against an irrational exuberance in application of this modality. Multiple reasons for caution can be cited.

CONCEPTUAL ISSUES

(1) The fundamental rationale of endovascular therapy for degenerative aneurysms is questionable.[1] Specifically, one may question how a device inside the aorta, and not attached to the aorta, can prevent the enlargement of the aorta. Stents were designed originally to prevent atheroma from encroaching on the lumen of a vessel. In the case of aneurysm, stents do the opposite: prevent the outward expansion of the aorta. How can a graft placed inside an enlarging aorta and not attached to the aorta prevent the inexorable expansion of that aorta? One would think that any potential restraining device would need to be placed outside, not inside, the aorta. To control a herd of cattle, the analogy goes, the wooden pen has to go outside the cows; an internal endograft is like putting the pen inside the herd.

This concern is compounded by the fact that stents for aortic aneurysm exert a radially directed force, which would be anticipated to encourage outward enlargement of the aorta. The concern is that the inexorable expansion of the aorta will ultimately leave the endograft behind, ignoring it.

(2) Another conceptual issue concerns continued pressurization of the aneurysmal sac by intercostal or lumbar vessels. Such pressurization, which permits continued exposure of the weak aneurysm wall to arterial forces, essentially implies that the aneurysm has not been effectively treated.

(3) Yet another conceptual issue concerns the fact that the strength of the aorta resides in the adventitia, which is not incorporated in any way by the endograft. Any surgeon knows that stitches that do not "grab" the aorta will have no strength. So, how can an endograft restrain the aorta from inexorable expansion? The conceptual answer is elusive.

SHORT DURATION OF FOLLOW-UP OF AN INDOLENT DISEASE

Thoracic aortic aneurysm, although virulent and ultimately lethal, is an indolent disease. Several years are generally required from the time of diagnosis to the time of aneurysm-related death (in asymptomatic patients), especially with small to moderate-sized aneurysms (**Fig. 1**).[2] To have patients alive at 1 or 2 years (or even less, as in so many endograft reports) is not at all reassuring.

Section of Cardiac Surgery, Department of Surgery, Yale University School of Medicine, Yale-New Haven Hospital, PO Box 208039, New Haven, CT 06520-8039, USA
E-mail address: john.elefteriades@yale.edu

Cardiol Clin 28 (2010) 413–417
doi:10.1016/j.ccl.2010.01.016

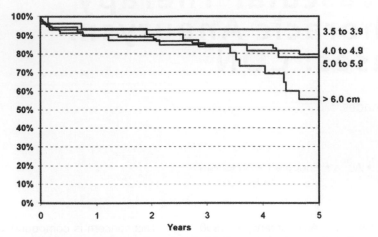

Fig. 1. Indolent nature of thoracic aortic aneurysm. Survival before operative repair is shown for different size classes. Note that the mortality risk expresses itself after years, even for large aneurysms. (*Reprinted from* Davies RR, Goldstein LJ, Coady MA, et al. Yearly rupture or dissection rates for thoracic aortic aneurysms: simple prediction based on size. Ann Thorac Surg 2002;73(1):25; with permission.)

Early effectiveness is meaningless, as most patients would be alive at 1, 2, or 3 years even without any therapy, as demonstrated in **Fig. 1**. This means that the mere presence of a small thoracic aneurysm is not a valid indication for endovascular therapy just because stent therapy is available.

DISCOURAGING MIDTERM FOLLOW-UP

In fact, the generally sparse stent data available to date that have matured to midterm or beyond are very discouraging in terms of the effectiveness of endovascular therapy for degenerative aneurysm.

At the recent International Aortic Symposium in Liege, Belgium,[3] where the latest midterm data

on abdominal aortic aneurysms (AAAs) were presented, the conclusion was frankly that endovascular therapy is not effective, in essence representing sham therapy (low risk, no benefit). This conclusion was based on data from 3 studies (representing the best scientific evidence available):

(1) The Endovascular Aneurysm Repair (EVAR) 2 trial. This trial compared EVAR with the use of no specific therapy (medical therapy). The key graph[4] presented in **Fig. 2** shows no benefit from stent grafting as compared with no therapy. (This was a trial for AAA). The all-cause mortality curves for EVAR and medical

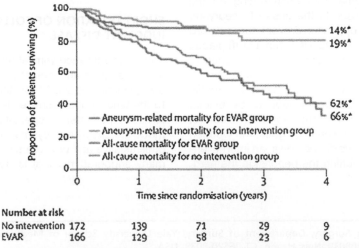

Fig. 2. Mortality curves in EVAR 2, showing no benefit from endovascular therapy of AAA. (*Reprinted from* EVAR trial participants. Endovascular aneurysm repair and outcome in patients unfit for open repair of abdominal aortic aneurysm (EVAR trial 2): randomized trial. Lancet 2005;365(9478):2189; with permission.)

therapy are superimposable, as are the curves for aneurysm-related mortality. There is simply no evidence of benefit.

(2) The Dutch Randomised Endovascular Aneurysm Management (DREAM) trial. The DREAM trial compared EVAR with traditional surgical therapy. The midterm follow-up in the DREAM trial found that at 2 years, the survival curves cross, and, from that point on, patients treated with a stent have poorer survival than surgically treated patients.[5] (This was a trial for AAA). That is, EVAR shows an early advantage because surgery has some mortality, but this advantage is lost because EVAR has no durable benefit. (The graph shows very significant results. It was presented at the International Aortic Symposium in Liege, Belgium, and will be published soon).

(3) The Investigation of Stent Grafts in Aortic Dissection (INSTEAD) trial. INSTEAD, conducted by Professor Neinaber in Germany, investigated stent therapy for patients who did well for more than 2 weeks after uncomplicated type B aortic dissection. It was hoped that tacking down the dissection flap would lead to a later benefit. Contrary to expectations, INSTEAD found severe early mortality and complications subsequent to stent therapy. There was no survival advantage over medical therapy alone. This study, showing negative results, were also presented in Belgium and has yet to be published.

The main concern indicated by these data is mortality. Patients die at least as commonly after endovascular therapy as after conventional surgery or even after no therapy at all. What about the patients who do survive endovascular therapy? Are there concerns in surviving patients?

Endoleak

In **Fig. 3** it can be noted that endoleak becomes increasingly common as duration of follow-up is extended.[6] It seems that nearly half the patients will experience diagnosed endoleak as follow-up becomes extended toward the 5-year point. In this context, the term endoleak is itself a euphemism for failure of treatment. It has been demonstrated that endoleak predicts the need for surgical conversion, rupture, and death and according to one European Collaborators Registry on Stent-Graft Techniques for Abdominal Aortic Aneurysm Repair (EUROSTAR) publication affected, respectively, 14%, 13%, and 27% of patients by 5 years after the procedure among patients presenting originally with large aneurysms.[7] These postendograft therapy statistics are of concern, as are the substantial rates of aneurysm-related death after endograft therapy when follow-up extends to 4 years, especially for large aneurysms.[8] This is shown vividly in **Fig. 4,**

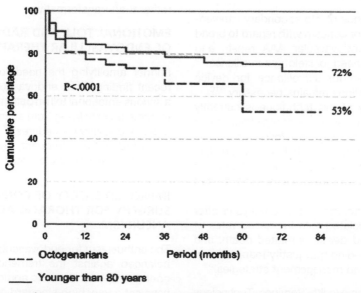

Fig. 3. Kaplan–Meier graph representing cumulative freedom from any endoleak in patients operated on for AAA with endovascular aneurysm repair. (*Reprinted from* Lange C, Leurs LJ, Buth J, et al. Endovascular repair of abdominal aortic aneurysm in octogenarians: an analysis based on EUROSTAR data. J Vasc Surg 2005;42:628; with permission.)

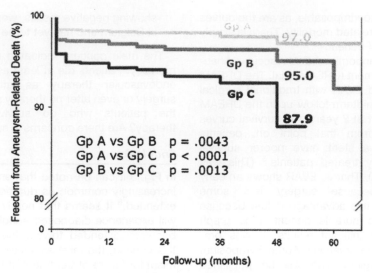

Fig. 4. Cumulative freedom from aneurysm-related death. Note low attrition of survival in first 3 years of follow-up and rapid attrition in fourth year. Groups represent increasing initial aneurysm size: group (Gp) A, 4.0 to 5.4 cm; Gp B, 5.5 to 6.4 cm; Gp C, 6.5 cm or larger. (*Reprinted from* Peppelenbosch N, Buth J, Harris PL, et al. Diameter of abdominal aortic aneurysm and outcome of endovascular aneurysm repair: does size matter? A report from EUROSTAR. J Vasc Surg 2004;39:291; with permission.)

which suggests that the aneurysm is indeed ignoring the endograft and merely expressing its natural tendency to rupture.

In recognition of these sobering statistics, several major EUROSTAR publications end with serious cautions about endograft therapy, calling attention to concerns about the long-term effectiveness and safety:

- "The high incidence of late secondary interventions is a cause for concern with regard to broad application of endovascular AAA repair, and emphasizes the need for lifelong surveillance."[9]
- "Continuing need for surveillance for device related complications remains necessary."[10]
- "...the durability of this technique is currently unknown, and continued use of registries should provide data from long-term follow-up... Only long duration studies can tell us whether this type of therapy really works—whether it prevents aneurysm growth and rupture and patient death."[11]
- "The midterm outcome of large aneurysms after EVAR was associated with increased rates of aneurysm related death, unrelated death, and rupture... This finding may justify reappraisal of currently accepted management strategies."[8]

The encyclopedic Health Services Technology Assessment Text of the Guide to Clinical Preventive Services, third edition, issued the following concluding statement on endografting: "Long-term

complications, including AAA rupture... may result in significant long-term morbidity and mortality."[12]

These extremely discouraging midterm data should raise a serious flag of caution regarding endovascular therapy, in the current state of the art, for degenerative aneurysms. Of course, endovascular technology will improve over time, but thus far, the improvements have been incremental rather than transformative.

EMOTIONAL TOLL AND RADIATION BURDEN OF ENDOVASCULAR THERAPY

Further amplifying the need for caution are the recent findings that endovascular therapy exerts a serious emotional toll on patients (who experience extreme anxiety living from scan to scan, in fear of need for ancillary procedures)[13] and that the radiation burden from frequent, repeated scans for surveillance of unreliable stents is of concern.[14–16]

IMPROVED SAFETY OF CONVENTIONAL SURGERY FOR THORACIC AORTIC ANEURYSM

The enthusiasm for endovascular therapy must be balanced against the tremendous advances in open therapy for thoracic aortic aneurysm, which have set a very high standard of safety and effectiveness. Elective open operations for ascending arch or descending aorta can now be accomplished with a mortality at or below 3%. It will be hard for endovascular therapies to exceed or even meet these surgical standards.

SUMMARY

There are many reasons, both conceptual and evidence based, to be concerned about the effectiveness, durability, and overall validity of endograft therapy for degenerative aneurysms. Stent therapy for degenerative aneurysms is burgeoning, but is it a case of "The Emperor's New Clothes"? The therapy is certainly propelled by profits to industry, hospitals, and practitioners.

This CON argument begs that endovascular therapies for degenerative aneurysms, while pursued enthusiastically, be subjected to careful scientific scrutiny. This CON argument also points out vividly that the available data are certainly of the highest concern regarding effectiveness in arresting the aneurysmal process, durability, and, especially, ability to forestall aneurysm rupture and death. At a very minimum, it is fairly argued, the decision to treat an aneurysm must be made with the same rigor for endovascular therapy as for open surgical therapy. One must balance the intense pressure from departments, hospitals, and industry to perform procedures and use devices with a full understanding of the disease of thoracic aortic aneurysm and a respect for the patient.

If a proponent of endovascular therapy argues forcefully for this modality (and against traditional surgery), one need only ask the proponent for tangible, scientific evidence of midterm effectiveness and patient benefit from stent treatment of aneurysm disease. Such evidence is sorely lacking.

REFERENCES

1. Elefteriades JA, Percy A. Endovascular stenting for descending aneurysms: wave of the future or the emperor's new clothes? J Thorac Cardiovasc Surg 2007;133(2):285–8.
2. Coady MA, Rizzo JA, Hammond GL, et al. What is the appropriate size criterion for resection of thoracic aortic aneurysms? J Thorac Cardiovasc Surg 1997;113:476–91.
3. International meeting on aortic aneurysms: new insights into an old problem. Palais des Congres, Liege (Belgium), September19–20, 2008.
4. EVAR trial participants. Endovascular aneurysm repair and outcome in patients unfit for open repair of abdominal aortic aneurysm (EVAR trial 2): randomized trial. Lancet 2005;365(9478):2187–92.

5. Blankensteijn J. Late results of endovascular aneurysm repair versus open aneurysm repair. International meeting on aortic aneurysms: new insights into an old problem. Palais des Congres, Liege (Belgium), September 19–20, 2008.
6. Lange C, Leurs LJ, Buth J, et al. Endovascular repair of abdominal aortic aneurysm in octogenarians: an analysis based on EUROSTAR data. J Vasc Surg 2005;42:624–30.
7. Waasderp EJ, de Vries JP, Hobo R, et al. Aneurysm diameter and proximal aortic neck diameter influence clinical outcome of endovascular abdominal aortic repair: a 4-year EUROSTAR experience. Ann Vasc Surg 2005;19:757–9.
8. Peppelenbosch N, Buth J, Harris PL, et al. Diameter of abdominal aortic aneurysm and outcome of endovascular aneurysm repair: does size matter? A report from EUROSTAR. J Vasc Surg 2004;39:288–97.
9. Laheij RJ, Buth J, Harris PL, et al. Need for secondary interventions after endovascular repair of abdominal aortic aneurysm. Intermediate-term follow-up results of a European collaborative registry (EUROSTAR). Br J Surg 2000;87:1666–73.
10. Hobo R, Buth J, The EUROSTAR Investigators. Secondary interventions following endovascular abdominal aortic aneurysm repair using current endografts. A EUROSTAR report. J Vasc Surg 2006;43: 896–902.
11. Leurs LJ, Bell R, Degrieck Y, et al. Endovascular treatment of thoracic aortic diseases: combined experience from the EUROSTAR and United Kingdom Thoracic Endograft registries. J Vasc Surg 2004;40:670–80.
12. Health Services/Technology Assessment Text (HSTAT). Guide to clinical preventative services, 3rd ed. Evidence syntheses, formerly systematic evidence reviews. National Library of Medicine and NCBI. Available at: http://hstat.nlm.nih.gov. Accessed September 24, 2006.
13. Aliabri B, Al Wahaibi K, Abner D, et al. Patient-reported quality of life after abdominal aortic aneurysm surgery: a prospective comparison of endovascular and open repair. J Vasc Surg 2006; 44:1182–7.
14. Kalef_Ezra JA, Karavasilis S, Ziogas D, et al. Radiation burden of patients undergoing endovascular abdominal aortic aneurysm repair. J Vasc Surg 2009;49(2):283–7 Epub.
15. Achneck HE, Rizzo JA, Tranquilli M, et al. Safety of thoracic surgery in the present era. Ann Thorac Surg 2007;84(4):1180–5.
16. Clagett GP. EVAR, TEVAR, FEVAR, too far? Perspect Vasc Surg Endovasc Ther 2008;20(2):115–9.

Editorial Comment: Endovascular Therapy for Thoracic Aneurysm Diseases

John A. Elefteriades, MD

Despite the steamrolling of endovascular therapy in clinical practice, the mid-term results are extremely discouraging, and the theoretic concerns are legion (**Table 1**). In overall assessment, it is fair to say that the ultimate fate of this therapy, without transformative improvements, remains guarded (**Fig. 1**).

Table 1
Endovascular therapy for degenerative aneurysms of the thoracic aorta

Pro: In Favor of Endovascular Therapy (Rossella Fatori)*	Con: Against Endovascular Therapy (John A. Elefteriades)*
Periprocedural "success" rates are high	Fundamental theoretic concerns include the following: • Any restraining device would need to go outside, not inside, the aorta • Intercostal arteries remain patent, pressurizing the aneurysm • Even the so-called neck of the aneurysm, where the landing zones are placed, dilate over time, leading to endograft failure
Devices improve progressively	Mid-term results are abysmal, with high incidence of endoleak and aneurysm-related death
Radiographic imaging, on which endovascular therapy is predicated, improves progressively	EVAR-II, DREAM, and EUROSTAR all showed that in mid-term follow-up, survival of endografted patients fell below that of medically or surgically treated patients
State-of-the art devices and techniques are described in this article	
Valid role in complicated type B acute aortic dissection	
Valid role in acute aortic transaction	
Acknowledges long-term effectiveness is a concern	

Abbreviations: DREAM, Dutch Randomized Endovascular Aneurysm Management; EUROSTAR, European Collaborators on Stent Graft Techniques for Abdominal Aortic Aneurysm and Dissection Repair; EVAR-II, Endovascular Aneurysm Repair-II.
  * See the article elsewhere in this issue of *Cardiology Clinics.*

Section of Cardiac Surgery, Department of Surgery, Yale University School of Medicine, Yale-New Haven Hospital, PO Box 208039, New Haven, CT 06520-8039, USA
E-mail address: john.elefteriades@yale.edu

Cardiol Clin 28 (2010) 419–420
doi:10.1016/j.ccl.2010.02.011

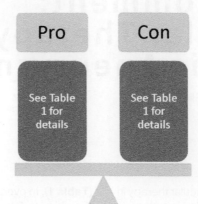

Fig. 1. The ultimate fate of this therapy remains guarded.

Index

Note: Page numbers of article titles are in **boldface** type.

A

ACE inhibitor. See *Angiotensin-converting enzyme (ACE) inhibitors.*

α-Actin, smooth muscle–specific isoforms of, mutations in genes for, 194–195

Acute aortic disease, management of, changing paradigms in, 408–410

Acute aortic dissection
"anti-pulse" therapy for, history of, 255–257
medical therapy for, pro, 259
type A
cerebral malperfusion, 318
extended arch resection in
con, **343–347**
described, 343–344
higher mortality, 345
inherently lethal condition, 346
necessity of tear resection, 345–346
no evidence of decreased incidence of late distal aneurysms, 345
no evidence of survival benefit, 345
reoperation rate factors, 346
editorial comment, 349–350
pro, **335–342**
described, 335
diagnostics, 335–337
surgical strategy, 337–341
initial presentation of, 317–318
surgical intervention for
con, **325–331**
age-related issues, 326
delayed presentation, 326
permament nonoperative management, 327–330
prior aortic valve replacement, 327
stroke issues, 325–326
editorial comment, 333–334
pro, **317–323**
age-related issues, 319
cerebral monitoring, 318–319
described, 317
indications, 319–320
previous cardiac surgery, 320–321
stroke issues, 319
type B, medical therapy for, pro, 258–259

Acute aortic syndrome
causes of, 231–232
incidence of, clinicians' role in reducing, 234–235

Age, as factor for surgical intervention for type A acute aortic dissection, 319, 326

Anesthesia/anesthetics, during TC-MEP monitoring, 362–363

Aneurysm(s)
aortic, thoracic, genetic testing in, pro, 193–194
formation of, 261–262
pathogenesis of, 273–274
routine screening for, in young athletes
con, **229–236.** See also *Young athletes, routine screening for aneurysm, con.*
editorial comment, 237–238
pro, **223–228**

Aneurysm parity, 265–266

Angiotensin receptor blockers (ARBs), for thoracic aortic aneurysm, 281–283

Angiotensin-converting enzyme (ACE) inhibitors, for thoracic aortic aneurysm, 280–283

Antegrade selective perfusion
in brain protection during aortic arch surgery, 392–394
core temperature in, 392–393
perfusate temperature in, 393
with cold blood, 393–394

"Anti-pulse" therapy, for acute aortic dissection, history of, 255–257

Aorta
ascending, pathology of, 290–291
normal size, described, 233–234

Aortic aneurysm(s), thoracic, genetic testing in, pro, 193–194

Aortic aneurysm disease, genetic testing in
con, **199–204**
editorial comment, 205–206
pro, **191–197**
described, 191
familial thoracic aortic aneurysms and dissections, 193–194
Loeys-Dietz syndrome, 192–193
Marfan syndrome, 192–193
mutations in genes for smooth muscle–specific isoforms of α-actin and ß-myosin, 194–195

Aortic arch surgery, brain protection during
antegrade selective perfusion in, 392–394
current techniques, 390–392
DHCA in, 390–391
editorial comment, 403–404
Kazui technique, 392
retrograde cerebral perfusion in, **371–379**

Cardiol Clin 28 (2010) 421–425
doi:10.1016/S0733-8651(10)00057-3

Moving?

Make sure your subscription moves with you!

To notify us of your new address, find your Clinics Account Number (located on your mailing label above your name), and contact customer service at:

Email: journalscustomerservice-usa@elsevier.com

800-654-2452 (subscribers in the U.S. & Canada)
314-447-8871 (subscribers outside of the U.S. & Canada)

Fax number: 314-447-8029

Elsevier Health Sciences Division
Subscription Customer Service
3251 Riverport Lane
Maryland Heights, MO 63043

To ensure uninterrupted delivery of your subscription, please notify us at least 4 weeks in advance of move.

Printed and bound by CPI Group (UK) Ltd, Croydon, CR0 4YY

03/10/2024

01040360-0010